Neurology and Neurobiology

EDITORS

Victoria Chan-Palay
University Hospital, Zurich

Sanford L. Palay
The Harvard Medical School

ADVISORY BOARD

Albert J. Aguayo
McGill University

Günter Baumgartner
University Hospital, Zurich

Masao Ito
Tokyo University

Tong H. Joh
Cornell University Medical
College, New York

Bruce McEwen
Rockefeller University

William D. Willis, Jr.
The University of Texas,
Galveston

NEUROTROPHIC ACTIVITY OF GABA DURING DEVELOPMENT

NEUROTROPHIC ACTIVITY OF GABA DURING DEVELOPMENT

Based Primarily on the Proceedings of a Symposium Entitled
Neurotrophic Activity of GABA at the International Society of
Developmental Neuroscience Meeting Held in Mexico City
July 8–12, 1986

Editors

Dianna A. Redburn

Department of Neurobiology and Anatomy
University of Texas Medical School
Houston, Texas

Arne Schousboe

Department of Biochemistry
Panum Institute
University of Copenhagen
Copenhagen, Denmark

ALAN R. LISS, INC., NEW YORK

Address all Inquiries to the Publisher
Alan R. Liss, Inc., 41 East 11th Street, New York, NY 10003

Library of Congress Cataloging-in-Publication Data

Neurotrophic activity of GABA during development.

(Neurology and neurobiology ; v. 32)
Based on a symposium held in Mexico City in
July 1986.
Includes bibliographies and index.
1. GABA—Physiological effect—Congresses.
2. Developmental neurology—Congresses. I. Redburn,
Dianna A. II. Schousboe, Arne. III. Series.
[DNLM: 1. GABA—physiology—congresses. 2. Nerve
Growth Factors—physiology—congresses.
W1 NE337B v.32 / WL 104 N49455 1986]
QP563.G32N48   1987   612'.8   87-3024
ISBN 0-8451-2734-9

Contents

Contributors

Jens Abraham, Department of Biochemistry A, Panum Institute, University of Copenhagen, DK-2200 Copenhagen, Denmark **[109]**

Vladimir J. Balcar, Department of Pharmacology, University of Sydney, Sydney, N.S.W. 2006, Australia **[57]**

Bo Belhage, Department of Biochemistry A, Panum Institute, University of Copenhagen, DK-2200 Copenhagen, Denmark **[139]**

Jørgen Drejer, Department of Biochemistry A, Panum Institute, University of Copenhagen, DK-2200 Copenhagen, Denmark; present address: Research Division, A/S Ferrosan, DK-2860 Soeborg, Denmark **[139]**

Gert H. Hansen, Department of Biochemistry A, Panum Institute, University of Copenhagen, DK-2200 Copenhagen, Denmark **[109]**

Graham A.R. Johnston, Department of Pharmacology, University of Sydney, Sydney, N.S.W. 2006, Australia **[57]**

Ferenc Joo, Laboratory of Molecular Neurobiology, Institute of Biophysics, Biological Research Center, Szeged, Hungary **[221]**

Peter Kasa, Central Research Laboratory, University Medical School, Szeged, Hungary **[221]**

M. Elizabeth Keith, Department of Neurobiology and Anatomy, University of Texas Medical School, Houston, TX 77025 **[79]**

Abel Lajtha, Center for Neurochemistry, Division of the N.S. Kline Institute for Psychiatric Research, Wards Island, NY 10035 **[1]**

Paul Madtes, Jr., Departments of Biology and Chemistry, Point Loma Nazarene College, San Diego, CA 92106 **[161]**

Eddi Meier, Department of Biochemistry A, Panum Institute, University of Copenhagen, DK-2200 Copenhagen, Denmark; present address: Department of Pharmacology, H. Lundbeck and Co., DK-2500 Valby, Denmark **[109,139]**

A. Michler-Stuke, Department of Anatomy, Developmental Neurobiology Unit, University of Göttingen, D-3400 Göttingen, Federal Republic of Germany **[253]**

Dianna A. Redburn, Department of Neurobiology and Anatomy, University of Texas Medical School, Houston, TX 77025 **[xi, 79]**

Arne Schousboe, Department of Biochemistry A, Panum Institute, University of Copenhagen, DK-2200 Copenhagen, Denmark **[xi, 109,139]**

The numbers in brackets are the opening page numbers of the contributors' articles.

Nikolaus Seiler, Merrell Dow Research Institute, Strasbourg Center, 67084 Strasbourg-Cedex, France **[1]**

P.E. Spoerri, Department of Neurosurgery, University of Göttingen, D-3400 Göttingen, Federal Republic of Germany **[189]**

Joachim R. Wolff, Department of Anatomy, Developmental Neurobiology Unit, University of Göttingen, D-3400 Göttingen, Federal Republic of Germany **[221, 253]**

Preface

This volume has been written primarily by participants in a symposium at the International Society of Developmental Neuroscience, held in Mexico, July 1986, entitled Neurotrophic Activity of GABA. The symposium and the book represent the first time to our knowledge that this particular topic has been recognized and that workers in the field have been brought together specifically to exchange data and ideas about the role of GABA in development. Recognizing the newness of the field, some of us had misgivings about whether or not the attempt to produce this volume was premature. However, these misgivings were quickly dispelled as each of us became aware of the breadth and depth of the available data that emerged at the meeting and in the course of the reviewing the literature for these chapters. Of course, as in any new field, there are many questions as yet unanswered. Many of the studies to date have concentrated on demonstrating the phenomenon and establishing where and when GABA expresses trophic actions. The more mechanistic questions are just beginning to be addressed. One of our goals for this book has been to establish a starting point for the field–to define the problem and provide a foundation for further studies. Another one of our goals for this book has already been accomplished. It has already provided a means for increasing communication among those actively working in the field and from this, alone, should come some advancements in our common study of the trophic actions of GABA. As a final goal, it is our hope to establish recognition for GABA among the rapidly expanding number of classical neurotransmitters which are currently recognized not only for information processing in the adult, but for developmental information processing as well.

The editors wish to thank the authors not only for their contributions, but also for their support, enthusiasm, and willingness to respect deadlines, enabling us to provide a volume that is not only valuable but timely. Since the authors cover three continents, very early morning or late night phone calls were often the rule rather than the exception, and telephone lines were not always cooperative. The good-natured attitude of all the contributors is most gratefully appreciated.

We are very grateful to Alan R. Liss, Inc. for its interest in our endeavor, for its financial support, for its willingness to try a new approach to the "camera-ready format", and for providing a very pleasant and efficient contact person, Mr. Glen Campbell.

Very special recognition goes to two people who played key roles in making this project possible. Ms. Cheryl Mitchell made time in her busy research schedule to assume major responsibilities in proofreading, formating and assembling the chapters. Her patience with colleagues working on this book and her attention to detail have contributed significantly to whatever success this book may enjoy. Ms. Diana Parker assumed the difficult task of typing the entire volume on a word processor and following through on multiple rounds of drafts and corrections. She accomplished this with incredible speed and accuracy; at the same time, fitting it in with her other considerable workload. Without her special talents, this format simply would not have been possible.

Dianna A. Redburn
Arne Schousboe

Neurotrophic Activity of GABA During Development, pages 1–56
© **1987 Alan R. Liss, Inc.**

FUNCTIONS OF GABA IN THE VERTEBRATE ORGANISM

Nikolaus Seiler and Abel Lajtha[1]

Merrell Dow Research Institute, Strasbourg Center, 16, rue d'Ankara, 67084 STRASBOURG-CEDEX, France

THE METABOLIC ORIGIN OF GABA

GABA (4-aminobutyric acid) is ubiquitous in the living world. It has been found in bacteria, plants, and a great variety of animal species (Meister, 1965). Low concentrations of GABA can be found in all vertebrate tissues and blood (Seiler and Wiechmann, 1969; Tanaka, 1985). It is, therefore, not surprising that GABA is formed along more than one metabolic route.

Formation

Probably the most general GABA-forming pathway is the oxidative deamination of putrescine (1,4-diaminobutane) to 4-aminobutyraldehyde and its subsequent oxidation to GABA or pyrrolidin-2-one, the lactam of GABA (Seiler, 1980). In spite of observations which seemed to suggest specific functions during early development of retina and brain (De Mello et al., 1976; Sobue and Nakajima, 1979), it has not been possible up to now to assign any role to this reaction, other than the elimination of exogenous or excessive endogenous putrescine. Even in early stages of brain development, decarboxylation of glutamate seems the only reaction that forms functionally important GABA (Seiler and Sarhan, 1983).

---

[1]   Center for Neurochemistry, Division of the N.S. Kline Institute for Psychiatric Research, Wards Island, New York 10035

Decarboxylation of L-glutamate by GAD (L-glutamate-1-carboxyylase, E.C. 4.1.1.15), which turned out to be the key reaction of GABA formation in the CNS, was first described by Roberts and Frankel (1950). GAD, a pyridoxalphosphate-dependent enzyme, forms GABA within the nerve endings by an anaerobic reaction and is considered the marker for GABAergic neurons (Wu, 1983). However, in spite of the fact that more than 35 years have passed since its identification, there is still no agreement about the key regulatory function of this enzyme, which controls GABA synthesis in the vertebrate nervous system (Tunnicliff and Ngo, 1986). Feedback regulation of GAD activity by brain GABA concentrations is probably the most important mechanism, but others may contribute as well. Pyridoxalphosphate deficiency caused by inadequate nutrition may initiate seizures because of decreased GAD activity; it is also a frequent result of convulsant drugs which act as pyridoxal scavengers (Tapia, 1983).

Considerable GABA formation from L-glutamate can be demonstrated with a number of tissue preparations, including brain and liver, by an aerobic, NAD^+-dependent multistep reaction (Seiler and Wagner, 1976). It is, however, not known whether this reaction is important in vivo.

There is little doubt about the metabolic origin of the neurotransmitter pool of GABA. However, the pathway along which glutamate is made available in GABAergic (and glutamatergic) neurons is a matter of debate. Glucose, glutamine, and ornithine are currently being discussed (Shank and Campbell, 1983). Most arguments are in favor of glutamine, which appears to be preferentially formed in astrocytes, the cell type with the highest glutamine synthase activity (Norenberg, 1979). It can be transported by three different amino acid carriers into nerve endings (Shank et al., 1982). The preferential formation of glutamate from glutamine is suggested by the fact that the phosphate-dependent form of glutaminase is prevalent in nerve endings (Kvamme, 1983).

Radioactive ornithine is transformed within the brain into GABA along the glutamate pathway, and evidence that vertebrate brain contains the entire enzymatic and transport machinery for the utilization of L-ornithine as precursor of glutamate and GABA, has been demonstrated

(Seiler, 1980). The potential role of ornithine as precursor of neurotransmitter glutamate is, therefore, currently being examined. Metabolism of ornithine leads to two molecules of glutamate. One is derived from transfer of an amino group to 2-oxoglutarate, and the second from subsequent oxidation of glutamic acid semialdehyde. This pathway seems, therefore, attractive and also fits the hypothesis according to which 2-oxyglutarate is the actual precursor of glutamate (Shank and Campbell, 1983).

Distribution

GABA is a major constituent of the brain; its levels are not as high as those of taurine, glutamate, aspartate, or glutamine, but are above most other amino acids. The values reported in the literature, in units of μmol/g wet weight in adult brain, are 1.8-2.5 in mouse and rat, 1.5 in rabbit, 1.9-2.0 in guinea pig, 0.9-1.4 in cat, 0.8-3.3 in dog, and 0.9-1.4 in monkey (Himwich and Agrawal, 1969; Perry, 1982). Developmental changes seem to be species dependent; a significant increase during development was found in mouse and dog brain, while no such change was noted in rabbit, guinea pig, or cat brain (Himwich and Agrawal, 1969). It is not homogeneously distributed in the brain; analyses of gross areas show levels to be about twice as high in the midbrain as in the hindbrain or cerebellum (Himrich and Agrawal, 1969). A recent report (Elekes et al., 1969) measured GABA and glycine levels in 44 microdissected rat brain areas. GABA was highest in the medial preoptic and anterior hypothalamic nuclei (184 nmol/mg protein), lowest in pontine nuclei (21 nmol/mg protein), but in most other areas values varied between 70 and 100 nmol/mg, indicating a fairly even distribution except in a few areas. Glycine distribution was somewhat more homogeneous than that of GABA in these assays. These distributions are similar to those found in previous reports (Fahn and Cote, 1968; Okada et al., 1971; Perry et al., 1971; Van der Heyden et al., 1979; Frankfurt et al., 1984) and indicated a low level in most white matter areas, and high levels in the substantia nigra and hypothalamus. In human autopsied brain, GABA levels as μmol/g wet weight, varied from 1.4 and 1.7 in the inferior olivary nucleus and frontal and cerebellar cortex to 6.1 and 7.2 in the substantia nigra and the globus pallidus, respectively (Perry, 1982). High levels of GABA were also found in synaptosomes (Wood and Kurylo, 1984). They showed similar regional heterogeneity, with the synaptosomal level in the cerebellum 25 percent of that in the mesencephalon. The authors suggest that this regional heterogeneity does not indicate great differences in the level of GABA in different cells, but rather, heterogeneity in the distribution of the cells containing GABA. The regional distributions of GABA in a number of species has been measured in several laboratories, but little is known of regional alterations of GABA levels. Immobilization-induced stress caused increases in striatum and hypothalamus but not in other regions (Yoneda et al., 1983), pain-induced stress caused increases in cortex but not in basal ganglia, thalamus, or hypothalamus (Sherman and Gebhart, 1974), and insulin-induced stress decreased levels in the hypothalamus (Butterworth et al., 1982).

An important consideration in GABA level determinations is the possible changes in GABA post mortem, since glutamate levels and GAD activity are high in brain. Elekes et al. (1986) report 3 to 5-fold higher GABA levels in brains of decapitated animals as compared to those killed by microwave irradiaton, and many other laboratories indicate a significant and rapid post-mortem increase of GABA (Lajtha and Toth, 1974; Perry et al., 1981; Perry, 1982), although Van der Heyden et al. (1978, 1979) indicated that microwave irradiation may decrease existing GABA levels. Since GABA formation may itself show regional heterogeneity, not necessarily parallel with GABA levels, the post-mortem changes may not be proportional in each brain area. In some studies regional distribution was different in frozen as compared to microwave-treated brain (Tappaz et al., 1977).

From this analysis, it is clear that GABA is present at fairly high levels throughout the brain, and its distribution is heterogeneous. It is likely that the regional heterogeneity of distribution also represents regional heterogeneity in functional activity and heterogeneity of GABA pools. When inhibitors of GABA synthesis or of GABA catabolism are administered the changes observed are fairly similar in all areas and synaptosomal changes are parallel with those of the rest of the brain. Such observations indicate that the various pools rapidly equilibrate under most conditions. The fact that the synaptosomal pool of glutamate + glutamine +

aspartate + GABA is fairly constant under a number of conditions suggests that metabolic conversions play an active role in the regulation of GABA pools. Clearly, synaptosomal changes are functionally the most important, but are at present less well known. The high levels of this neurotransmitter in nerve endings are puzzling and suggest that there are also heterogeneous pools in this structure. This is indicated by observations such as that aminooxyacetic acid increased a different synaptosomal GABA pool from the one increased by valproic acid (Loscher and Vetter, 1985).

Release from nerve endings

Depolarization of brain slices or synaptosomes by high K^+ concentrations leads to release of GABA. This release is Ca^{2+} dependent. Using push-pull cannulae for the determination of GABA release from deep nuclei (substantia nigra, striatum) or cups for the determination of GABA release from superficial structures, the Ca^{2+}-dependence of GABA release could be confirmed in vivo after electrical stimulation or depolarization with K^+ (Tapia, 1983). The spontaneous release of GABA from the posterior hypothalamus could also be shown (Dietl, Philippu, 1980), however, in order to detect spontaneous release from the sensorimotor and visual cortices it was necessary to prevent GABA degradation; i.e., only after administrations of vinyl GABA (vigabatrin) a specific inactivator of GABA-T (4-aminobutyrate:2-oxoglutarate aminotransferase, E.C. 2.6.1.19) was GABA detectable in the superfusate (Abdul-Ghani et al., 1980).

Spontaneous release of GABA from the substantia nigra and striatum was decreased by 50-60% after superfusion with 3-mercaptopropionic acid (Van der Heyden et al., 1979, 1980) an inhibitor of GAD (Wu, 1976), suggesting that the amount of releasable GABA is directly dependent of the activity of GAD.

GABA release is similar in many aspects to the release of other neurotransmitters, but there is no evidence that the released GABA is stored in vesicles within the nerve endings. The comparison of the specific radioactivities of precursors and GABA in subcellular fractions indicated that the cytoplasm is the most probable source of the GABA that is released by depolarization (DeBelleroche,

Bradford, 1977).

Transport systems and removal from the synaptic cleft

Several transport systems for amino acids are present in brain tissue (Sershen and Lajtha, 1979). In their properties, (a) that a system transports a number of structurally related amino acids, and (b) that some amino acids may have affinity to more than one transport system, these systems in the brain are similar or identical to the systems present in other tissues (Christensen, 1975). The transport systems are not uniformly distributed. A number of systems present in brain cells are absent from brain capillaries (Oldendorf and Szabo, 1976; Sershen and Lajtha, 1976); that is, they do not play a role in blood brain barrier transport. GABA is not transported through the blood-brain-barrier and therefore it is usually not taken up by the brain. However, when plasma levels are greatly elevated an increase in brain can be found (Toth and Lajtha, 1981).

Although the cerebral GABA transport system has been shown to be fairly specific for GABA, it is not clear whether it exists in several modified forms or whether several different GABA systems exist, and it is not well investigated whether such systems are present outside the nervous system. In respect to the heterogeneity of the GABA transport systems the questions that have not been finally settled are the differences in development, in cell types, in subcellular elements, and in affinity.

The systems that are studied may not always be comparable: tissue slices are a complex system, and may represent multiple uptake systems (glial, synaptosomal, etc.), while cultured cells although a more heterogeneous system may represent a system that was altered in culture. For example, retinal cells, which in culture accumulate only GABA, are shown to accumulate glycine or serotonin additionally when the intact cells are studied (Osborne and Beaton, 1985). The need for caution in deducing in vivo activity from in vitro values is shown by the finding of an increase of uptake of amino acids, among them GABA, when hand-sliced tissue is further cut by chopping. Our interpretation was that transport capacity that is latent in vivo is activated by tissue damage (Bracco et al., 1982). Developmental changes may also add complexity, as the high-affinity GABA transport component may disappear from some cells during development, depending on species and maturation patterns, with glial transport decreasing with maturation (Levi, 1972; Schousboe, 1979).

Differences between glial and neuronal GABA uptake were found some time ago (Schon and Kelly, 1975; Roberts, 1980) and it was proposed that model compounds (β-alanine and diaminobutyric acid) may be cell-type specific. More recent work suggests that the inhibition of GABA uptake by β-alanine and taurine in either astrocyte or neuron culture is not competitive, and therefore they are not transported by the GABA carrier in either cell type (Larsson et al., 1986); on the other hand the structural requirements of substrate for the neuronal GABA carrier were found to differ from those in astrocytes (Schousboe, 1979). Differences are also indicated by such findings as that homocysteine inhibits high-affinity GABA uptake in astrocytes but not in neuronal or in synaptosomal preparations (Allen et al., 1986). There may be species differences in astrocytic GABA transport: β-alanine and taurine are competitive inhibitors of GABA uptake in rat astrocyte cultures, indicating transport of both species by the GABA system (Holopainen and Kontro, 1986), but are noncompetitive inhibitors in mouse astrocytes, thus representing a different system (Larsson et al., 1986). In cortical synaptosomes GABA and taurine represent separate systems (Debler and Lajtha, 1987). We found a single high-affinity system for GABA in synaptosomes (Debler and Lajtha, 1987); others report three synaptosomal uptake systems based on affinity (Sidhu and Wood, 1986).

A number of laboratories measuring the kinetic constants of GABA uptake reported high- and low-affinity components (Martin, 1976; Lahdesmaki et al., 1981; Larsson et al., 1983; Tapia, 1983; Yunger et al., 1983); in general the K_M of high-affinity and of low-affinity transport was in the micromolar range, but within each range several values were found. In cerebral astrocytes K_M for GABA was 13-40 μM, in cortical neurons 5-11 μM (Larsson et al., 1986; Yu and Hertz, 1982; Schousboe, 1979). In general high-affinity K_M values varied from 0.5 to 100 μM, with most in the 10-40 μM range, and the low-affinity K_M was over 400 μM (Tapia, 1983). V_{max}

values seemed to depend on the age of the brain and on the age of the culture, showing both increases and decreases with age (Schousboe, 1979; Tapia, 1983).

The mechanisms of GABA uptake into nerve endings are not fully established. That high-affinity uptake of GABA into synaptosomes in vitro is normally a 1:1 exchange between extra and intrasynaptosomal GABA. This casts doubts about the physiological role of GABA uptake into presynaptic terminals. To find a way out of this dilemma Levi and Raiteri (Levi et al., 1978; Levi, Raiteri, 1978) proposed, on the basis of homoexchange experiments with superfused synaptosomes in which Na^+ and Ca^{2+}-fluxes were modified, that GABA transport in nerve ending is modulated both by extracellular-GABA concentrations and by the magnitude of changes of Na^+ and Ca^{2+}-fluxes during the depolarization-repolarization cycle. Under resting conditions homoexchange prevails. However, after depolarization the enhanced inward fluxes of Na^+ and Ca^{2+} favor enhancement of efflux over influx, which increases GABA concentration in the synaptic cleft. The inverse cation fluxes during repolarization of the nerve terminal invert the stoichiometry of efflux/influx; at high extrasynaptic GABA concentrations low-affinity uptake of GABA may also come into play.

Na^+/GABA coupling of transport is also known for glial cells: in most systems the coupling ratio is 2 or higher (Larsson et al., 1983), although the high-affinity net uptake into cultured astrocytes has a 1:1 ratio (Hertz et al., 1978). This astrocytic uptake is K^+-independent.

GABA uptake into synaptic plasma vesicles was found to be Cl^--dependent with a $Na^+:Cl^-:GABA$ ratio of 2-3:1:1 (Radian and Kanner, 1983), while the presynaptic GABA uptake showed a $Na^+:K^+:GABA$ stoichiometry of 3:1:1 (Cupello and Hyden, 1986).

The numerous mechanistic studies did not clarify the relative importance of glial and neuronal uptake of GABA from the synaptic cleft under physiological conditions. GABA uptake inhibitors (Schousboe, 1979; Krogsgaard-Larsen, 1980) were not very efficient tools in this regard either, although a transient increase of GABA concentration in nerve endings in vivo was noticed (Wood et al., 1980a). From biochemical, pharmacological, and electrophysiological findings Cupello and Hyden (1986) came to the conclusion that presynaptic uptake could not function to inactivate GABA, but that uptake by the postsynaptic neuron (Deiter's neuron) could have such a function.

Specific inactivators of GABA-T, the enzyme responsible for the major route of GABA degradation, produce up to ten-fold increases of brain GABA concentrations. GABA accumulates under these conditions both in nerve endings and in non-synaptosomal compartments, i.e., in glial cells (Sarhan, Seiler, 1979; Wood et al., 1980b). GABA-T is present in both neurons and glia, but prevails in the latter (Sellstrom et al., 1975) and is also present in most tissues including liver and kidney (Tews et al., 1980). From the metabolic and pharmacologic effects of inactivators of GABA-T and of inhibitors of GAD it was suggested (Seiler, Sarhan, 1980) that normal functioning of the brain GABA system depends on a continuous flux of GABA from the nerve ending, the site of its production, into the synaptic cleft, and from the synaptic cleft into the glial cell. Re-uptake into presynaptic endings is assumed to play a minor role normally. The flux is supported by the uptake and rapid transamination of GABA within the glial cells, whereby GABA is shunted into the citrate cycle. At the same time, one molecule of glutamate is formed from 2-oxoglutarate for each molecule of GABA that is degraded. This glutamate can be amidated and the resulting glutamine transported into the nerve endings, where it may serve as GABA precursor (Hertz, Schousboe, 1980).

Ca^{2+}-independent release of GABA from glial cells has been repeatedly observed (Tapia, 1983), but there is evidence that it plays no physiologic role (Bowery et al., 1979; Adams, Brown, 1979). However, GABA may well be released from glial cells by depolarization, if GABA concentrations are elevated, for example, because of inactivation of GABA-T. In this situation, GABA uptake into glial cells is presumably impaired, and owing to increased GABA concentrations within the synaptic cleft, GABA re-uptake into the presynaptic terminals is favored. Enhanced GABA concentrations in the nerve endings will diminish the activity of GAD by feed-back inhibition and the rate of the GABA-flux will be reduced. Due to its release from glial cells, GABA is able to interact with receptors rather distant from the site of its production, with which it cannot interact under physiologic conditions. The fact that chromodacryorrhea and chromorhinorrhea were observed in rats with elevated brain GABA levels (Schechter, Tranier, 1978) indicates that GABA interacts under unphysiological conditions not only with GABA receptors, but presumably also with acetylcholine receptors.

THE PRINCIPLES OF INHIBITION AND DISINHIBITION

GABA receptors are general constituents of neuronal membranes and exist independently, whether or not the neuron is innervated by GABAergic synapses. In contrast, glial cells seem not to have GABA receptors.

Pharmacologically two major groups of GABA receptors can be distinguished (Johnston, 1986; Enna, Karbon, 1986).

Isoguvacine is an agonist, and bicuculline is the typical antagonist of the $GABA_A$ receptors. They are found both presynaptically (axo-axonic receptors) and postsynaptically (axo-somatic and axo-dendritic receptors) and as was mentioned, there is evidence for non-synaptic bicuculline-binding receptors. A further subdivision of $GABA_A$ receptors is possible according to their relative sensitivity to GABA agonists (Krogsgaard-Larsen et al., 1986).

$GABA_B$ receptors are insensitive to bicuculline, but they bind the lipophilic GABA analogue baclofen (3-(4-chlorophenyl)4-aminobutyric acid), which depresses neuronal firing (Bowery et al., 1981; Curtis, 1978a). There is evidence that other bicuculline-insensitive GABA receptors exist in addition to $GABA_B$ receptors.

The ionic events following the interaction of GABA with the bicuculline sensitive receptor are remarkably similar in invertebrates and vertebrates (Krnjevic, 1976; Takeuchi, 1976).

The amount of GABA released from the lobster neuromuscular junction has been estimated to be in the order of 5 to 20×10^{-17} moles per impulse per muscle fiber (Takeuchi, 1976). This amount of GABA is considered to be sufficient to produce an increase in the

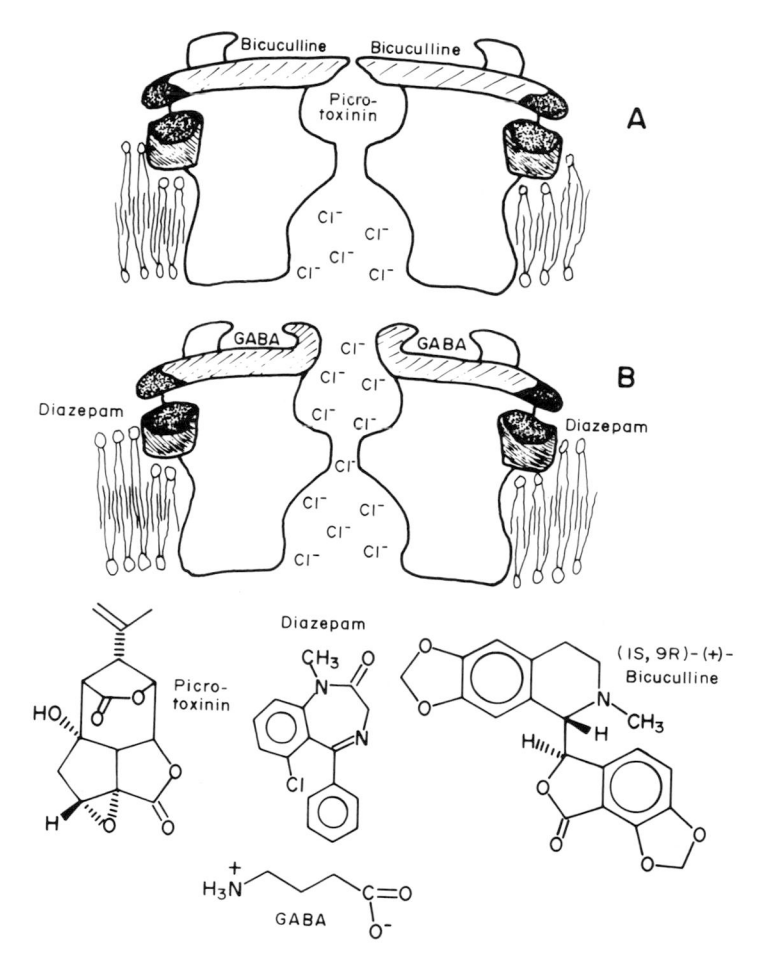

Fig. 1. Legend on next page

Cl⁻-conductance of the nerve terminal membrane, and thus an inhibitory effect.

The inhibitory action of GABA is, in contrast with that of glycine, or the excitatory action of glutamate, of slow onset and of remarkably long duration of action (> 100 msec) (Krnjevic, 1976).

From very numerous biochemical, pharmacological, and electrophysiological studies it appears that the bicuculline-sensitive $GABA_A$ receptor is a complex unit. A Cl⁻-ionophore is controlled by the GABA receptor, which interacts at the same time with a binding site of benzodiazepines. Barbiturates and related depressant agents and picrotoxin and related excitatory compounds bind to the Cl⁻-ionophore. GABA, benzodiazepine, and picrotoxinin (barbiturate) receptors, show reciprocal Cl⁻-dependent allosteric interactions, even in a partially purified protein complex, thus demonstrating the existence of the three receptor Cl⁻-channel complex, which mediates the postsynaptic effects of GABA (Braestrup et al., 1983; Ticku et al. 1983; Krogsgaard-Larsen et al., 1986; Fischer and Olsen, 1986; Stephenson and Barnard, 1986). In Fig. 1, a model of the GABA receptor is demonstrated. It illustrates the interaction of its units and the sites where drugs are assumed to exert their effects. The physiological role of the benzodiazepine binding receptor is not known. The detection of

---

Figure 1. GABA/benzodiaepine/chloride receptor.

A. Closed Cl⁻-channel
B. Open Cl⁻-channel (GABA bound to the receptor).

Two molecules of GABA seem to be required per receptor in order to open the Cl⁻-channel. The site of bicuculline binding indicates its function as GABA antagonist; the site of picrotoxinin binding, its role as channel blocker. The benzodiazepine binding sites are arranged such that they are able not to open the Cl⁻-channel, but to enhance the ability of GABA to carry out this event. Benzodiazepine antagonists would make the transition from closed to open channel conformation unfavorable. (According to Tallman, 1986).

low-molecular-weight endogenous ligands (Mohler et al., 1979) and of two peptides, which bind specifically to benzodiazepine recognition sites (Costa and Guidotti, 1985), may assist in elucidating functions of these highly interesting drug binding sites.

In contrast with the GABA$_A$ system, which produces a reduction in spike amplitudes by opening Cl$^-$-conductance, activation of GABA$_B$ receptors by GABA or baclofen markedly reduces the duration of Ca^{2+}-spikes (Dunlap and Fischbach, 1981); i.e., GABA reduces the availability of extracellular Ca^{2+} at intraneuronal sites.

There is evidence for excitatory effects of GABA in ganglion cells (Obata, 1979), but the effects of GABA on neurons are in general hyperpolarization and inhibition (Krnjevic, 1976), as is the case with most neurotransmitters (glycine, dopamine, norepinephrine, serotonin, enkephalins, etc.) (McGeer et al., 1978). Excitatory effects are mainly mediated by glutamate (Cotman et al., 1981; Fagg and Foster, 1983) and in many instances by acetylcholine (at nicotinic and muscarinic receptors) although acetylcholine also mediates inhibitory effects via muscarinic receptors (McGeer et al., 1978).

The excitatory synapses outnumber the inhibitory ones in the CNS; nevertheless it appears that excitatory effects are produced not only directly by activation of excitatory synapses, but also via inhibitory neuronal networks. Noting the ubiquitous occurrence of GABAergic neurons in the vertebrate CNS, E. Roberts has suggested disinhibition of pacesetter neurons, whose activity is under the control of tonically active inhibitory command neurons, as an organizing principle. Disinhibition can be best understood by following the description of Roberts (1976) of the following simple model:

In a linear series of three neurons A, B, and C and a muscle fiber, neuron A controls through the interneuron B the activity of the motor neuron C. If C is left alone, it could discharge spontaneously at a high rate, causing the muscle fiber to contract. If the interneuron B is tonically active, and if B is liberating the inhibitory transmitter at such a rate that the membrane potential of the motor neuron C is decreased to a level below firing level, the muscle fiber will not contract. If neuron A is inhibitory, an increase in its rate of discharge will decrease the firing rate of B, and thus decrease the inhibitory effect on C, and C will fire. This in turn will cause contraction of the muscle fiber.

If the muscle fiber in the above model is substituted by an entire genetically preprogrammed neuronal circuit, the pacesetter for the firing of the preprogrammed circuit is then neuron C, with the tonically active interneuron B of the preceding model taking over the role of the command neuron for the circuit, while the inhibitory neuron A is acting on B as disinhibitory neuron, coming from a circuit higher in the control hierarchy, or from one preceding it in a temporal sequence.

Of course we have to assume multiple excitatory and inhibitory inputs to both the pacesetter and command action. The model requires that decreases or cessation of the inhibitory signal from the command neuron would be a necessary, but not always sufficient, condition for the firing of the pacesetter neuron. Excitatory input may be required for the depolarization of the pacesetter neuron to the firing level, even when the tonic inhibitory influence of A has been removed.

GABAERGIC NEURONAL SYSTEMS IN THE CNS

Autoradiographic localization of labelled GABA, although somewhat problematic because of the uptake of GABA into both nervous and glial cells (Ottersen and Storm-Mathisen, 1984a); localization of GABA and GAD in single cells by micromethods (Okada and Shimada, 1976), and more recently by immunohistochemical methods (Ottersen and Storm-Mathisen, 1984b; Mugnaini and Oertel, 1985; Somogyi et al., 1985); and quantitative receptor autoradiography (Boast et al., 1986) in conjunction with surgical or chemical lesions of afferent pathways were the most important methods for the establishment of GABAergic pathways in the CNS and retina. Among these methods the immunohistochemical localization of GAD proved most successful. It was initiated by the purification of GAD (Wu, 1976) and subsequent production of antibodies against this enzyme. It allowed the localization of GAD both at light microscopic (Saito, 1976) and electron microscopic (Wood et al., 1976) levels and led to the establishment of the most extensive atlas of GABAergic neurons and terminals (Mugnaini, Oertel, 1985). A very useful compilation of GABA-mediated inhibitions was published by Curtis (1978b).

In most areas of the brain postsynaptic inhibition predominates and is mediated by axo-dendritic and axo-somatic terminals. In the spinal cord GAD-immunoreactive terminals are found presynaptic to primary afferents and represent presumably the morphological correlate for presynaptic inhibition; they may modulate the release of transmitters from individual presynaptic terminals in the serial synapses. An example for lateral inhibition can be found in the retina (amacrine cells) (Vaughan et al., 1981) where GABA is known to inhibit the firing of ganglion cells (Straschell and Perwein, 1969).

If the intensity of staining of GAD were proportional to the extent of GABA synthesis and release, the following structures could be among the most active GABAergic elements in rat brain (Mugnaini and Oertel, 1985): peridendritic boutons in the deep fibrocellular layer of the pallidum ventrale, the boutons in the neuropil of the nucleus interpeduncularis, in the nucleus habenulae lateralis, in the nucleus ventralis corporis trapezoidei, in the β-subnucleus of the oliva inferior, and in the substantia gelatinosa of the nucleus tractus spinalis n. trigemini.

As has been discussed above, disinhibition occurs when an inhibitory neuron innervates a second inhibitory neuron. Immunocytochemical localization of GAD has revealed numerous examples of direct interactions between GABAergic neurons all over the brain, suggesting that disinhibition is indeed a major principle of information processing in the vertebrate CNS, even if we disregard the existence of glycinergic interneurons which may interact with GABAergic neurons (Pycock et al., 1981).

Depending on the GABAergic cell types that are interacting, one may distinguish between the following cases:

    (a) Interaction between local circuit neurons that belong either to the same cell class or to

different cell classes.
Example: Olfactory bulb (Ribak et al., 1977).

(b)   Interaction between local circuit neurons and projection neurons.
Example: In the cerebellar cortex basket cell axon terminals synapses on Purkinje cell bodies and their initial axon segment (Oertel et al., 1981).

(c)   Interaction between different types of projection neurons.
Example: Striatal GABAergic projection neurons terminate monosynaptically on pallidal GABAergic projection neurons (Oertel et al., 1984).

The neocortex contains GABAergic interneurons, and it receives GAD-positive projections from the posterior hypothalamus (Vincent et al., 1982).

The majority of GAD-positive cells in the striatum are projection neurons with extensive collaterals in the striatum, but GABAergic interneurons are also present (Oertel and Mugnaini, 1984).

The colliculus superior receives at least one GABAergic projection from the substantia nigra (pars reticulata) and possesses numerous GABAergic interneurons (Chevalier et al., 1981; Houser et al., 1983).

In the thalamus, three different GABAergic systems have been found: an input from pallidal areas (Penny and Young, 1981; Kutlas-Ilinsky, 1985), from the nucleus reticularis thalami to the thalamic relay nuclei (Frigyesi, 1972), and GABAergic interneurons (Kultas-Ilinsky, 1985).

The number of GABAergic interneurons in the thalamus increases very markedly from rodents to primates, suggesting a change in the role of intrinsic inhibitory control with brain evolution (Penny et al., 1983, 1984).

GABA and CNS Disorders

Disease states are, in analogy to artificial lesions in experimental animals, a potential source of insight into physiological functions of GABAergic systems in the human brain. Moreover, one may hope to obtain from the knowledge of the pathophysiology of diseases, bases for new therapies.

From the ubiquitous inhibitory action of GABAergic neurons upon a multitude of neuronal circuits, one might expect the involvement of GABA in a great variety of behavioral patterns and a more or less direct role in various CNS dysfunctions. It is, therefore, not surprising that at an early stage of research a defect of the GABA system was suggested as a basis of schizophrenia (Roberts, 1972).

Information about specific functions of GABAergic systems in distinct behavioral patterns is, however, rather scarce, and dysfunctions of GABAergic neurons as the major basis of CNS diseases are not known. But there is considerable evidence in a number of diseases for a role of GABA.

Brain GABA and aging

From detailed determinations of GAD activity in post-mortem human brains, McGeer and McGeer (1978) came to the conclusion that there is a significant decline of GAD activity with age, with a steeper decline of activity at young age. The areas showing greatest loss in GAD were thalamic areas, followed by cortical and rhinencephalic areas, whereas the basal ganglia showed less decline of GAD activity with age. In contrast, choline acetyltransferase and tyrosine hydroxylase activities showed the sharpest decline in the caudate, putamen, and nucleus accumbens.

GABA determinations (Perry, 1982) are basically in agreement with the enzyme determinations and support the idea that in normal aging there is a major loss of GABAergic neuronal activity in the thalamic areas.

Movement disorders

There is a wealth of anatomical, biochemical, and pharmacological information on the role of GABA as a major transmitter of the extrapyramidal system and thus the control of certain movements (Walaas and Fonnum, 1978; Cattabeni et al., 1978; Fuxe et al., 1978; Feger, 1981; Kitai, 1981; Ribak, 1981; Yoshida, 1981; Bartholini et al., 1981; Bernardi et al., 1981; DiChiara et al., 1981; Korf et al., 1981; Waszczak et al., 1981; Scheel-Kruger, 1984). Briefly, the extrapyramidal system consists of two major sections, the basal ganglia and the cerebellum. The striatum is the integrating unit for the basal ganglia, the cerebellar cortex for the cerebellum. These structures receive diverse excitatory inputs from the cortex, thalamus, and substantia nigra.

GABAergic neurons play a paramount role in both integrating systems, as local circuit and as projection neurons. Through the projection neurons, information is transmitted to discrete nuclei (substantia nigra, globus pallidus), and from the Purkinje cells to deep cerebellar nuclei. These project out of the system the motor information that has evolved in the integrating units. Through their thalamic projections the basal ganglia and the cerebellum influence cortical and motor functions, and they can directly influence motor activity at a spinal level through the bulbo-mesencephalic branch. Physiological, pathological, or drug-induced changes at any of these sites potentially influence extrapyramidal motor function.

Most information on GABAergic neurons in motor behavior concerns the striato-nigral GABA neurons, for the following reasons:

Highest GABA concentrations are found in the subtantia nigra and in the nucleus accumbens (Fahn and Cote, 1968; Balcom et al., 1975). The substantia nigra contains the cell bodies of nigro-neostriatal dopamine neurons; the nucleus accumbens has a dense network of dopamine nerve terminals which belong to the mesolimbic dopamine neurons. Hence, interrelations between these systems are noticed early and the role of striato-nigral GABA neurons in the regulation of muscle tone and coordination behavior by nigro-striatal dopamine pathways was extensively studied (Marshall and Ungerstedt, 1977; DiChiara et al., 1981; Kilpatrick, 1981; Reavill et al., 1981; Scheel-Kruger, 1984). The stereotypic behavior of intrareticularly administered GABA agonists (muscimol, THIP), which mimic the behavioral syndrome produced by dopamine receptor stimulation, and the circling produced by unilateral injections of GABA agonists (including GABA-T inhibitors) or antagonists (bicuculline, picrotoxinin) into the substantia nigra appeared to be most useful for exploring which of the various nigral output pathways support such influences on behavior.

Losses of GABAergic neurons in Huntington's chorea was assumed, based on abnormally low GABA levels in the caudate, putamen, globus pallidus, substantia nigra, and occipital cortex (Perry et al., 1973) and a severe decrease of GAD activity in the extrapyramidal nuclei, while tyrosine hydroxylase activity did not change. Choline acetyltransferase activity was specifically reduced in the caudate and was lower in the putamen. GABA receptors were either normal or decreased, and the number of muscarinic receptors was markedly decreased (McGeer and McGeer, 1978).

There were numerous attempts to substitute for the lack of GABA function by administration of direct and indirect GABA agonist (Marsden and Sheehy, 1981), without convincing results, however. The reason for this is most probably not only the difficulty in the use of GABA agonists, which owing to the ubiquitous occurrence of GABA receptors, tend to have numerous side effects. It appears that in Huntington's chorea a general loss of neurons in the caudate and putamen, and to a lower extent in the globus pallidus, occurs, which resembles the morphological and biochemical picture that is obtained by intrastriatal injections of kainic acid, an analogue of glutamic acid. This analogy led to the assumption that the destruction of the neurons in the neostriatum that occurs is due to the overactivity of the excitatory (glutamatergic) cortico-striatal tract (Coyle et al., 1978).

Significantly lowered GABA concentrations in lumbar CSF indicated GABA deficits not only in patients with Huntington's disease, but also in those with Parkinson's disease, adult onset dystonia, and drug-induced tardive dyskinesia (Chase, Tamminga, 1978). Treatment with GABA agonists was disappointing (Marsden, Sheehy, 1981; Bartholini, 1985) except in the case of tardive dyskinesia, where a certain alleviation of the syndrome was observed after muscimol administration, or after elevation of brain GABA levels by inhibition of GABA-T (Thaker et al., 1983). This is not too surprising: Parkinson's syndrome is an example of an extrapyramidal disease, in which the general enhancement of GABAergic

consistent with impaired GABAergic function within the mesolimbic system (Stevens et al., 1974). However, biochemical findings concerning GABA content in CSF and the nucleus accumbens of the thalamus and GAD activity in certain brain regions were conflicting, and did not contribute definitive evidence for or against the GABA deficit hypothesis of schizophrenia. Furthermore, treatment of schizophrenic patients with GABA agonists showed no therapeutic action against the symptoms of the disease, but were, on the contrary, capable of producing acute psychoses (Meldrum, 1982; Bartholini, 1985).

A few years ago alterations in the timing of the circadian system were postulated to play a key role in the pathogenesis of bipolar affective disorders (Wehr et al., 1983). The identification of the circadian pacemaker in the hypothalamus (Rusak, Zucker, 1979) prompted Borsook et al. (1986) to review the potential implications of GABAergic transmission in the circadian time keeping and to formulate strategies for treatment of patients with manic-depressive illness and certain sleep disorders with GABA mimetics. On the basis of the influence of clinically effective antimanic drugs on GABA turnover, Bernasconi (1982) previously formulated a GABA hypothesis of affective illness, and Lloyd et al. (1983) reported preliminary clinical data on a GABA mimetic in depression, which resembled the reduction of symptoms by imipramine. It is premature to draw conclusions, but exciting new developments may arise from more detailed studies of GABAergic control functions in circadian events.

Epilepsy

Impairment of GABAergic transmission in experimental animals, by inhibition of GAD or reduction of brain pyridoxal phosphate levels, by blockade of postsynaptic bicuculline sensitive receptors, or by a block of GABA-mediated changes of Cl^- conductance, invariably leads to generalized convulsive seizures. On the other hand, GABA and GABA agonists have anticonvulsant properties in a number of experimental seizures. In view of these facts a central role of GABA in the pathophysiology of a variety of types can be assumed although they do not provide direct evidence for an involvement of GABA in seizure disorders (Meldrum, 1975; Snead, 1983; Roberts, 1986a).

Epilepsy is a heterogeneous group of disorders. For simplification we are separating it into two categories: focal epilepsy and generalized types.

Focal epilepsy. Neurons belonging to an acute epileptic focus show paroxysmal depolarization shifts. These seem to be responsible for the appearance of electroencephalographic interictal spikes, upon which epileptic activity is built.

More and more evidence has accumulated suggesting that impairment of GABA transmission is a major pathogenetic factor in focal epilepsy. In experimental foci a decreased number of synaptic boutons containing GAD (Ribak et al., 1979) and decreased GABA concentrations, and reduced GABA binding sites (Bakay and Harris, 1981) were observed. In human epileptic foci reduced GAD activity and reduced numbers of GABA receptors were reported (Lloyd et al., 1985).

Primary generalized epilepsy of petit mal type. The major pathophysiological difference between focal and primary generalized epilepsy is the absence of paroxysmal depolarization shifts; therefore it is not possible to distinguish between normal and "epileptic" neurons (Pollen, 1964). In contrast to generalized convulsive and partial seizures, augmentation of GABAergic neurotransmission in models of generalized absence seizures (which resemble petit mal seizures) appears to exacerbate the symptoms (Snead, 1983). For example, GABA-T inhibitors potentiate pentylenetetrazol-induced spike-wave seizures (Myslobodsky et al., 1979), and muscimol may even induce absence-like seizure activity (Pedley et al., 1979). These findings can be taken as arguments against a GABA-deficit hypothesis of primary, generalized seizures. Clinical results with vigabatrin, a specific irreversible inhibitor of GABA-T are, however, evidence against this notion. This compound is known to elevate brain GABA levels in patients (as determined from elevated GABA concentration in the CSF) (Grove et al., 1981). Its anticonvulsant actions are believed to be due to the preferential elevation of GABA within the nerve endings (Sarhan and Seiler, 1979; Seiler and Sarhan, 1980). Patients with complex partial seizures or primary or secondary generalized seizures who were refractory to conventional anticonvulsant therapy showed striking reductions of seizure frequencies (Schechter et al., 1984; Loiseau et al., 1986). Results with progabide, a compound considered a pro-drug of GABA (Bartholini et al., 1985) and the effective treatment of epilepsies with sodium valproate (Chapman et al., 1982) may also be quoted in this connection, although there is some controversy about the mode of action of these compounds. Administration of sodium valproate causes a significant increase of GABA levels in various parts of the brain of experimental animals (Mandel et al., 1981). The fact that the GABA accumulates exclusively within the nerve endings (Sarhan, Seiler, 1979) is strong evidence in favor of an indirect GABA-agonist action. However, a number of other mechanisms have also been postulated, among which action through glutamate antagonisms seems most interesting (Chapman et al., 1982; 1983).

Quite obviously GABA does not play an equally important role in the pathogenetic mechanism of all seizure disorders, as has been established for focal epilepsy. It is not surprising that a considerable number of neurotransmitters and their respective neuronal networks are currently discussed in connection with epilepsy (Snead, 1983).

On the role of the substantia nigra in the propagation of seizures. Hayashi (1953) was the first to present evidence that the efferent pathways of epileptic seizures following cortical stimulation can be interrupted by lesions of the rostral midbrain, including the substantia nigra. The notion of a mediating role of the substantia nigra in the spread and generalization of cortical epileptiform activity was developed further by Gale and Iadarola (1980). There is now a great deal of evidence that prevention of nigral outflow by selective lesions (Garant and Gale, 1983) or enhancement of nigral GABAergic activity by direct or indirect GABA-agonists (Kaniff et al., 1981; Le Gal La Salle et al., 1983; McNamara et al., 1984; Gale, 1985; Turski et al., 1986) causes a decreased sensitivity to a variety of chemically or electrically induced seizures, without precluding the animal's ability to exhibit motor components of a seizure. By local injections of vigabatrin, the aforementioned selective inactivator of GABA-T, the importance of presynaptically accumulating GABA for the anticonvulsant activity was evidenced (Gale, 1985). Since not only GABA agonists, but also glutamate agonists and antagonists (N-methyl-D-aspartic acid; 2-amino-7-phosphonoheptanoic acid) modulate the threshold against seizures in a model of temporal lobe epilepsy (Cavalheiro et al., 1985), it appears that mediation of seizures by the substantia nigra is due to an imbalance of excitatory and inhibitory inputs.

GABA AND ENDOCRINE FUNCTION

In the course of the last decade evidence has accumulated suggesting the involvement of GABA in the regulation of adenohypophyseal, hypothalamic, thyroid, and pancreatic hormones (DeFeudis, 1984a). A great deal of this evidence is of pharmacological nature. Therefore, it is not always possible to decide whether the observed effects of GABA are of primary physiological importance, are ancillary, or are merely pharmacological curiosities.

A relatively simplistic description of potential GABA functions in the regulation of hormones is given throughout this review whenever complex behavioral patterns are described that necessarily cannot be the result of one major regulatory influence. We have to keep in mind the complexity of the neurotransmitter interrelationships in the subcortical areas that ultimately regulate the activity of the hypothalamic nuclei (Leonard, 1984) and, therefore, help to regulate pituitary adrenal function.

Hypothalamic neurons of the arcuate nucleus and other nuclei of the median eminence secrete specific releasing hormones: corticotropin-releasing hormone (CRH), gonado-tropin-releasing hormone (Gn-RH), thyrotropin-releasing hormone (TRH), growth hormone-releasing hormone (GH-RH), melanocyte-stimulating hormone (MSH-RH) and release-inhibiting hormones: prolactin release-inhibiting hormone (PRL-RIH), growth hormone release-inhibiting hormone (GH-RIH, somatostatin), melanocyte-stimulating hormone release-inhibiting hormone (MSH-RIH) into the hypophyseal portal system. These factors are then transported to cells of the adenohypophysis, where they enhance or inhibit the release of the appropriate hormones (Schally et al., 1973). Isolation of GABA from pig hypothalami and demonstration of its capacity to inhibit prolactin (PRL) release from the adenohypophysis (Schally et al., 1977) indicated a role of GABA as a release-inhibiting hormone and induced a great interest in the regulation of PRL by this neurotransmitter, in spite of the fact that it is less potent than dopamine (Enjalbert et al., 1979). Disturbed PRL-regulation is a frequent clinical problem. Since the adenohypophysis contains, not GAD, but GABA binding sites (Grandison and Guidotti, 1979; Racagni et al., 1982) one has to assume that GABA formed in the median eminence arrives at the anterior pituitary glandular cells via the portal system.

GABA has a dual effect on PRL release. Injection of GABA into the third ventricle increases plasma prolactin levels. The current explanation is that the stimulation of PRL-release by GABA occurs at CNS sites. It might involve inhibition of the tubero-infundibular dopaminergic system and action on the serotonin system (Casanueva et al., 1981), whereas PRL-release inhibition is a direct effect of GABA on the glandular cells.

High concentrations of GABA in various parts of the hypothalamus (Okada et al., 1971) and the distribution of markers of GABAergic neurons within the hypothalamus and the pituitary are consistent with a general involvement of GABAergic regulation, not only of PRL but of the entire hypothalamo-hypo- physeal axis (Tappaz et al., 1982). Thus it is not surprising that pharmacologic manipulations of the hypothalamic GABA neurons produce alterations in the secretion of adenocorticotrophic hormone (ACTH) (Makara and Stark, 1974; Jones et al., 1984), growth hormone (GH) (Vijayan and McCann, 1978; Racagni et al., 1982), luteinizing hormone (LH) (Ondo, 1974), thyroid stimulating hormone (TSH) (Vijayan, McCann, 1978), and melanocyte-stimulating hormone (MSH) (Hadley et al., 1977).

As in the case of PRL, exogenous GABA has dual actions on GH release. It has been suggested (Fiok et al., 1981) that intraventricularly administered GABA influences the periventricularly localized GH-RIH neuronal elements, but not the GH-RH in the more distant ventromedial nuclei. Thus intraventricularly administered GABA agonists might release GH by inhibiting the release of GH-LRH. A general increase of brain GABA levels as obtained after inhibition of GABA-T was, however, associated with a decrease of GH plasma levels, which is most probably due to inhibition of GH-LH release. These examples may be sufficient to demonstrate that the effects of GABA on neuroendocrine regulation are dependent on local changes of GABA. It has to be clarified in the future where and how local changes of GABAergic activity within the hypothalamic nuclei occur under physiological and pathological conditions to such an extent as to affect adenohypophyseal hormones.

Release of vasopressin from the neurohypophysis is controlled by many factors, among which GABA may also play a role. Evidence for this was based on the occurrence of GABA binding sites on the peptidergic axons of the hypothalamo-neurohypophyseal tract (Mathison, Dreifus, 1980), a decrease of GABA content and GABA uptake in the pituitary of water-deprived rats (Hamberger et al., 1979), and attenuation of vasopressin release in response to carotid occlusion after application of GABA or glycine to a release at the transition between medulla and spinal cord (Feldberg, Rocha e Silva, 1981).

Considering the prominent role of hypothalamic structures in the control of body temperature, it may be appropriate to mention here that direct (muscimol) and indirect (vigabatrin) GABA agonists produce hypothermia. The evidence for a physiologic function of GABA in central thermoregulation is, however, only circumstantial (DeFeudis, 1984b).

The observation that injection of GABA into the marginal ear vein of rabbits produces hypotension and first depresses and then stimulates respiration, is more than 30 years old (Takahashi et al., 1955). Later, these early observations were confirmed and considerably extended (for reviews see DeFeudis, 1981; 1984c; Roberts, Krause, 1982).

It was shown, among other things, that the hypotensive effect of intracerebroventricularly injected GABA and of GABA agonists is antagonized in a variety of species by bicuculline (Antonaccio et al., 1978a, b; Bousquet et al., 1985). Inhibition of GABA formation by 3-mercaptopropionic acid produced an elevation of blood pressure or heart rate if it was given intraperitoneally (Fan et al., 1985). While inhibition of GABA-T antagonized the effect of 3-mercaptopropionic acid, global increase of brain GABA levels by GABA-T inhibitors produced no significant changes in the cardiovascular or respiratory system in one laboratory (Palfreyman et al.,

1981); in another, sustained hypotension and bradycardia were observed with a series of these compounds in rats, cats, and dogs (Loscher, 1982). The latter results are, however, in disagreement with clinical experience with vigabatrin (Hammond and Wilder, 1985). On the other hand oral doses of GABA have been reported to produce a remarkable lowering of blood pressure in hospitalized patients with essential hypertension, while the blood pressure of normotensive individuals was not affected (Shibata et al., 1960). These results suggest that not just a single GABAergic mechanism is involved in the regulation of cardiovascular effects and further work indicates that this is indeed the case. Microinjections of nanogram quantities of bicuculline into the nucleus ambiguus of the brain suggested that the parasympathetic cardio-inhibitory effects which arise from this structure are modulated by GABA. These cholinergic neurons in the nucleus ambiguus are assumed to be tonically inhibited by GABA which is released from terminals projecting to them either from other sectors or from intrinsic neurons (DiMicco et al., 1979). There is also convincing evidence for tonically active GABAergic inhibition of central sympathetic outflow from the forebrain (Williford et al., 1980).

Maximal respiratory depressant effects were elicited by GABA and muscimol if applied on Schlaefke's area of the ventral surface of the medulla. Bicuculline administration antagonized these effects. The respiratory stimulation by bicuculline in Schlaefke's area indicates that this brain region contains tonically active GABAergic neurons (at least under the conditions of the experiments) (Yamada et al., 1982). One may conclude that neurons originating in the nucleus tractus solitarius synapse on GABAergic interneurons in Schlaefke's area. These interneurons control neurons of the same region that project to both the phrenic motor nucleus and the preganglionic sympathetic neurons in the intermediolateral cell column of the spinal cord (DeFeudis, 1984c) and thus control respiration.

GABAERGIC ANALGESIA

Short exposure of experimental animals to hot-plate stimulus caused an increase of GABA levels in certain brain areas; restraint stress, however, had no effect

(Sherman and Gebhart, 1974). When a number of GABA-manipulating drugs were administered, alterations in morphine analgesia and morphine dependence were found (Ho et al., 1976) and morpine administration produced elevation of GABA levels in thalamic nuclei (Yoneda et al., 1977) and the dorsal horn in the spinal cord (Kuriyama and Yoneda, 1978), suggesting that an enhanced GABAergic inhibitory input by these interneurons may account in part for the action of morphine. From numerous reports it is now apparent that nearly all direct and indirect GABA agonists have (moderate) analgesic effects and they enhance opiate-induced analgesia (Sivam, Ho, 1985). However, the GABAergic analgesia is not opiate-like; it is not affected by naloxone. The development of new analgesics on the basis of GABAergic compounds has not been possible owing to the global conflicting effects of GABA mimetics in the CNS.

Disregarding the above mentioned interactions of GABAergic neurons with endogenous opiate systems, feeding and drinking behavior is the most important example of GABA-endorphin interrelations. However, we are far from understanding the underlying mechanisms (Cooper, 1983).

GABA IN PERIPHERAL TISSUES

The detection of GABA in virtually all tissues (Seiler, Wiechmann, 1969; Erdo et al., 1982) and especially in the reported high concentrations of GABA in the islets of Langerhans of the pancreas (Okada et al., 1976) and in female reproductive organs (Erdo et al., 1982), together with the high GAD activities in these tissues (Okada et al., 1976; Erdo, Laszlo, 1984), have attracted considerable interest after a long period during which GABA was considered to be a CNS compound exclusively.

GAD activity, GABA uptake and release upon stimulation, GABA binding sites, and even functional responses to GABA have been observed now in a number of tissues: blood vessels, adrenals, pancreas, gut, kidney, ovary, oviduct, urinary bladder, and stomach, indicating that GABA might have physiological functions in these organs.

GABAergic mechanisms in smooth muscles

A relatively clear picture of a neurotransmitter role of GABA is presently available for the myenteric plexus (Jessen, 1981; Jessen et al., 1983; Tanaka, 1985). The contractility of various segments of the gut can be modulated via GABA$_A$ receptors by local administration of GABA. These receptors are located on postganglionic cholinergic neurons in the myenteric plexus. GABA$_B$ receptors mediate relaxation through inhibition of post-ganglionic cholinergic nerves; thus GABA has a dual effect on the gut, which is further evidenced by the facilitatory and inhibitory effects of GABA on acetylcholine release from the guinea pig ileum (Tanaka, 1985). Interactions of GABA with serotonergic neurons of the gut are also known.

The machinery necessary for GABAergic transmission is present in the gall bladder, and GABA may act on parasympathetic ganglia of the urinary bladder as well (Tanaka, 1985).

The spontaneous motility in the longitudinal and circular muscle preparations of rabbit oviducts from virgin rabbits was stimulated by GABA and baclofen, indicating the involvement of GABA$_B$ receptors in this tissue. These observations and those concerning the active uptake of [^{3}H]GABA into slices of rat ovary (Erdo, 1984) suggest the innervation of the female reproductive organs by GABAergic neurons. The functional role of these GABAergic neurons has yet to be established.

In addition to the central mechanisms that regulate the cardiovascular system, circulating GABA may elicit direct effects. GABA receptors are located in blood vessels and in cardiac tissue (DeFeudis, 1981; Roberts and Krause, 1982; Tanaka, 1985). In vitro experiments revealed relaxation by GABA and GABA agonists in strips of basilar and middle cerebral arteries, but not the aorta, mesenteric artery, or portal vein (Anwar and Mason, 1982); these effects are mediated by GABA$_A$ receptors. In contrast, the release of noradrenaline and the corresponding contraction caused by electrical stimulation in isolated vas deferens is mediated by GABA$_B$ receptors which are located on adrenergic nerve terminals, whereas in the pulmonary artery GABA inhibits the contractile response and the release of norepinephrine via bicuculline-insensitive receptors (Bowery et al., 1981;

Starke and Weitzell, 1980).

It remains a task for the future to determine to what extent GABAergic mechanisms are involved in the physiologic control of smooth muscle functions.

Pancreas, thyroid, adrenals

From studies of pancreatic islet cells (Taniguchi et al., 1979), it appears that GABA is localized in the B cells. In the perfused rat pancreas GABA and muscimol inhibited glucose-mediated somatostatin release, in the dog pancreas GABA increased the release of somatostatin at 10-100 µM, and insulin secretion was inhibited by 1 µM GABA. The latter effect was bicuculline insensitive. In clinical studies GABA and baclofen, but not muscimol, increased plasma levels of insulin and glucagon (Tanaka, 1985). These results clearly indicate involvement of GABAergic mechanisms in the regulation of pancreatic endocrine function, although the mechanisms seem to differ, and may be of different importance in different species.

Autoradiographic studies have revealed high-affinity uptake sites in the follicle cells of the thyroid gland. The properties of the GABA uptake system change with the functional status of the gland (Gebauer and Haas, 1980).

A direct role of GABA in the regulation of adrenal medullary function is indicated by the fact that GABA releases catecholamines from perfused bovine adrenal gland. GABA antagonists (picro- toxinin) inhibit catecholamine release (Yamanaka et al., 1983). Recently it was reported that both cholinergic and GABAergic mechanisms are important in the regulation of dopamine-β-hydroxylase activity in rat adrenal glands (Lima and Sourkes, 1986).

In view of the rather general occurrence of GABA receptors in peripheral tissues, it is surprising that treatment of patients with inhibitors of GABA-T, such as vigabatrin (Loiseau et al., 1986), a compound that is known to elevate circulating GABA and has GABA antagonistic properties (Robin et al., 1979) or progabide, a GABA agonist (Bartholini et al., 1985), did not provide evidence for significant peripheral effects of these compounds.

EFFECT ON METABOLISM

The possibility that GABA can affect protein metabolism was raised by the finding of stimulation by GABA and glycine of amino acid incorporation in a ribosomal system from immature brain (Campbell et al., 1966; Tewari and Baxter, 1969). Stimulation of incorporation was also found in other systems such as slices from brain (Snodgrass, 1973) and mitochondria (Goertz, 1979). In these studies GABA had no effect on similar preparations from liver, and its effect was different from that of dopamine, which was reported to inhibit amino acid incorporation in such systems (Tapia and Sandoval, 1977). It is difficult to reach conclusions from the above reports, partially because the effect seems to be dependent on experimental circumstances and is not always reproducible, and partially because it is not possible to predict from in vivo observations what the in vitro effects would be. In vivo experiments that indicated the influence of GABA on proteins used GAD inhibitors that reduced brain GABA levels and also reduced leucine incorporation into brain protein (Tapia and Sandoval, 1974). In another set of experiments both inhibitors of GABA synthesis (lowering its level) and inhibitors of GABA catabolism (increasing its level) stimulated amino acid incorporation into proteins (Lapinjoki et al., 1980). The authors concluded that there is no clear connection between GABA and protein synthesis. When GABA, taurine, or glycine levels in the brain were increased by administration of large doses, brain protein synthesis in vivo was unaffected (Toth and Lajtha, 1984).

It is attractive to think that neurotransmitter-regulated alterations of protein synthesis participate in synaptic function, but at the present time there is no convincing proof that GABA plays such a role. On the other hand, GABA-induced changes in polyamine levels are likely to influence protein synthesis.

GABA AND DEVELOPMENT

As exemplified in the rat visual cortex (Wolff et al., 1984) at least four phases can be distinguished in the development of GABAergic neurons:

(1)   During mitosis, migration, and positioning none of the biochemical properties of GABAergic nerve cells (GAD, GABA uptake) are expressed.

(2)   After the cells have arrived at their permanent positions, dendrites are formed and small amounts of GAD and uptake of [^{3}H]GABA become detectable.

(3)   Non-pyramidal aspinous neurons start to develop axons and form increasing numbers of varicosities and potential presynaptic terminals at the end of the first postnatal week. Varicosities and potential presynaptic terminals contain GAD and accumulate GABA. Ca^{2+}-dependent GABA release can be observed at this stage.

(4)   Formation of synapses completes differentiation. About 75 percent of the GABAergic synapses in the visual cortex of the rat are formed between the 2nd and 8th post- natal week, i.e., after the eyes have opened.

These data reveal that there is a period during which GABA is formed, and can be replaced, and taken up by the neurons before synapses are formed. The question arises whether the GABA that exists in the CNS at very early stages of development has a function in the development of the GABAergic system.

The capacity of GABA to affect cell differentiation in general has been demonstrated by showing that GABA induces metamorphosis in planktonic abalone larvae (Morse et al., 1979). Exposure of the superior cervical ganglion of freely moving rats to nanomolar amounts of GABA demonstrated the formation of numerous densities along the extrasynaptic membranes, which resembled the postsynaptic densities of Gray's type 1 synapses (Wolff, 1981). Subsequently Meier et al. (1983) found a requirement of GABA in the culture medium for the development of low-affinity GABA binding sites in cultured granule cells, binding sites which are normally present in cerebellar membranes. These and other workers (Madtes, Redburn, 1983) have thus revealed a new aspect of the functional significance of GABA, apart from its role as inhibitory neurotransmitter.

CONCLUSIONS

About 40 years have passed since the first observation of elevated GABA concentration in tumor tissue (Roberts, 1986b) to the firm establishment of GABA as the major inhibitory neurotransmitter in the CNS (Roberts, 1986c). High concentrations of GABA are not restricted to brain as has been believed for decades, but can be found in pancreas and female reproductive organs as well, and more evidence is accumulating in favor of a transmitter role of GABA in different peripheral tissues, among which the gut is of special importance.

At least two different receptor types are transmitting GABA-linked message from the presynaptic terminals to postsynaptic neurons. Compounds suitable for the specific modulation of the activity of these receptors and of other functional or metabolic units that are involved in GABAergic neurotransmission (e.g. glial and neuronal uptake systems, GABA forming and metabolizing enzymes) became an important target of research, because insights into functions of specific GABAergic neurons can be expected from their selective activation or inactivation.

New immunohistochemical methods allowed the subcellular localization of GABA and GAD, and the demonstration of the very numerous contacts of GABAergic nerve endings with a great variety of neurons in all brain areas. These methods are also a basis for the establishment of GABAergic pathways. The numerous direct contacts that have been identified between GABAergic neurons, i.e., between two inhibitory nerve cells, are morphological evidence in favor of the notion that disinhibition is a major principle of information processing in the CNS.

There is no doubt that GABAergic neurons together with aminergic and other neuronal networks are involved in the control of various motor functions and of complex behaviors. As evidenced from the facilitation of GABAergic neurotransmission by the anxiolytic benzodiazepines, and the existence of a benzodiazepine binding site that is an integral part of the GABA receptor complex, affective behavior is under the control of GABAergic neurons. A prominent role of GABA in aggressive behavior has been demonstrated.

Central and peripheral effects of GABA on the

cardiovascular, respiratory, and nociceptive systems, and the involvement of GABA in the control of a multitude of endocrine functions underline the universal role of GABA in physiology. Specific losses of GABAergic neurons in Huntington's chorea and a GABA deficit in epileptic foci are examples of its pathogenetic role in movement disorders. Substitution of GABA deficits by GABA agonists, and especially elevation of brain GABA levels by inactivation of its major catabolic pathway has been a successful therapeutic measure in certain epilepsies. However, this approach was less effective in other movement disorders, presumably due to the fact that enhancement of GABAergic function all over the brain may produce conflicting effects.

Development of the GABA area is still progressing in many directions. Recent work, for example, indicates a role of GABA in the sexual differentiation of the brain (Flugge et al., 1986b). Much can be hoped from more sophisticated studies of diseases (Roberts, 1986b), and the role of GABA in the modulation of endocrine function is rapidly developing (Racagni, Donoso, 1986). Even GABA derived from gastrointestinal bacteria may under certain conditions play a major pathogenetic role (Jones et al., 1984). Drug-induced alterations or psychological and physical dependencies, as are involved in the abuse of alcohol (Kulonen, 1983), may be better understood on the basis of functional roles of GABA and their aberrations.

The present development of GABA as a trophic factor seems to close the circle, suggesting that GABA not only may be important in nervous system function, but, as was indicated by its elevated concentration in tumors, may have more general functions as a cell constituent.

REFERENCES

Abdul-Ghani AS, Coutinho-Netto J, Bradford HF (1980). The action of γ-vinyl-GABA and γ-acetylenic GABA on the resting and stimulated release of GABA in vivo. Brain Res 191: 471–481.

Adams PR, Brown DA (1979). Electrical responses of presumed sympathetic neuroglial cells to K^+ ions and to preganglionic nerve stimulation. J Physiol (Lond) 293: 95–101.

Allen IC, Schousboe A, Griffiths R (1986). Effects of

L-homocysteine and derivatives on the high-affinity uptake of taurine and GABA into synaptosomes and cultured neurons and astrocytes. Neurochem Res 11: 1487–1496.

Antonaccio MJ, Kerwin L, Taylor DG (1978a). Effect of central GABA receptor antagonism and antagonism on evoked diencephalic cardiovascular responses. Neuropharmacology 17: 597–603.

Antonaccio MJ, Kerwin K, Taylor DG (1978b). Reductions in blood pressure, heart rate and renal sympathetic nerve discharges in cats after central administration of muscimol, a GABA agonist. Neuropharmacology 17: 783–791.

Anwar N, Mason BR (1982). Two actions of γ-aminobutyric acid on responses of the isolated basilar artery from the rabbit. Br J Pharmacol 75: 177–181.

Bakay RAE, Harris AB (1981). Neurotransmitter, receptor and biochemical changes in monkey cortical epileptic foci. Brain Res 206: 387–404.

Balcom GJ, Lenox RH, Meyerhoff JL (1975). Regional γ-aminobutyric acid levels in rat brain determined after micro wave fixation. J Neurochem 245: 609–613.

Bartholini G (1975). GABA receptor agonists: pharmacological spectrum and therapeutic actions. Medicinal Res Rev 5: 55–75.

Bartholini G, Scatton B, Worms P, Zivkovic B, Lloyd KG (1981). Interactions between GABA, dopamine, acetylcholine, and glutamate-containing neurons in the extrapyramidal and limbic system. In DiChiara G, Gessa GL (eds): "GABA and the Basal Ganglia" New York: Raven Press, pp 119–128.

Bartholini G, Bossi L, Lloyd KG, Morselli PL (1985). Epilepsy and GABA Receptor Agonists. Basic and Therapeutic Research. New York, Raven Press.

Bernardi G, Marciani MG, Stanzione P, Cherubini E, Mercuri N (1981). Evidence in favor of GABA as an inhibitory transmitter in the rat striatum. In DiChiari G, Gessa GL (eds): GABA and the Basal Ganglia" New York: Raven Press, pp 69–77.

Bernasconi R (1982). The GABA hypothesis of affective illness: Influence of clinically effective antimanic drugs on GABA turnover. In Emrich IHM, Aldenhof JB, Lux HD (eds): "Basic Mechanisms in the Action of Lithium" Amsterdam: Excerpta Medica, pp 183–192.

Boast CA, Snowhill EW, Altar CA (eds) (1986). "Quantitative Receptor Autoradiography" New York: Alan R Liss.

Borsook D, Richardson GS, Moore-Ede MC, Brennan MJW

(1986). GABA and circadian timekeeping: implications for manic-depression and sleep disorders. Med. Hypotheses 19: 185–197.

Bousquet P, Feldman J, Schwartz J (1985). GABA et regulation centrale de la fonction cardiovasculaire. J. Pharmacol. (Paris) 16, suppl II: 29–50.

Bowery NG, Brown DA, Marsh S (1979). γ-Aminobutyric acid efflux from sympathetic glial cells: Effect of "depolarizing" agents. J Physiol (Lond) 293: 75–101.

Bowery NG, Doble A, Hill DR, Hudson AL, Shaw SS, Turnbull MJ, Warrington R (1981). Bicuculline-insensitive GABA receptors on peripheral autonomic nerve terminals. Eur J Pharmacol 71: 53–70.

Bracco F, Gennaro J Jr, Lajtha A (1982). Relationship of morphologic damage and amino acid uptake in incubated slices of brain. Exp Neurol 76: 606–622.

Braestrup C, Nielsen M, Honore T (1983). Benzodiazepine receptor ligands with positive and negative efficacy. In Mandel P, DeFeudis FV (eds): "CNS Receptors: From Molecular Pharmacology to Behavior" New York: Raven Press, pp 237–245.

Butterworth RF, Merkel AD, Landrewille F (1982). Regional amino acid distribution in relation to function in insulin hyperglycaemia. J Neurochem 38: 1483–1489.

Campbell MD, Mahler HR, Moore WJ, Tewari S (1966). Protein synthesis systems from rat brain. Biochemistry 5: 1174–1184.

Casanueva F, Apuid J, Locatelli V, Martinez-Campos A, Cirati C, Racagni G, Cocchi D, Muller E (1981). Mechanisms subserving the stimulatory and inhibitory components of γ-Aminobutyric acid-ergic control of prolactin secretion in the rat. Endocrinology 109: 567–575.

Cattabeni F, Bugatti A, Gropetti A, Maggi A, Parenti M, Racagni G (1978). GABA and dopamine: their mutual regulation in the nigro-striatal system. In Krogsgaard-Larsen P, Scheel-Kruger J, Kofod H (eds): "GABA-Neurotransmitters. Pharmacochemical, Biochemical and Pharmacological Aspects" Copenhagen: Munksgaard, pp 107–117.

Cavalheiro EA, Meldrum BS, Turski L (1985). Effect of intranigral 2-amino-7-phosphonoheptanoate and N-methyl-D-aspartate on seizures produced by pilocarpine in rats. Br J Pharmacol 85: 367P.

Chapman A, Keane PE, Meldrum BS, Simiand J, Vernieres JC (1982). Mechanisms of anticonvulsant action of valproate. Progr Neurobiol 19: 315–359.

Chapman AG, Meldrum BS, Mendes E (1983): Acute anticonvulsant activity of structural analogues of valproic acid and changes in brain GABA and aspartate content. Life Sci 32: 2023–2031.

Chase TN, Tamminga CA (1978). GABA system participation in human motor, cognitive and endocrine function. In Krogsgaard-Larsen P, Scheel-Kruger J, Kofod H (eds): "GABA-Neurotransmitters. Pharmacochemical, Biochemical and Pharmacological Aspects" Copenhagen: Munksgaard, pp 283–294.

Chevalier G, Deniau JM, Thierry AM, Feger J (1981). The nigrostriatal pathway. An electrophysiological reinvestigation in the rat. Brain Res 213: 253–263.

Christensen HN (1975). Biological Transport, 2nd edition, W.A. Benjamin, Inc., Reading, Massachusetts.

Cooper SJ (1983). GABA and endorphin mechanism in relation to the effect of benzodiazepines on feeding and drinking. Progr Neuropsychopharmacol Biol Psychiatr 7: 495–503.

Costa E, Guidotti A (1985). Endogenous ligands for benzodiazepine recognition sites. Biochem. Pharmacol. 34: 3399–3403.

Costa E, Guidotti A, Mao CC (1975). Evidence for the involvement of GABA in the action of benzodiazepine: studies on rat cerebellum. In Costa E, Greengard P (eds): "Mechanisms of Action of Benzodiazepines" New York, Raven Press, pp 113–120.

Cotman CW, Foster A, Lanthorn T (1981). An overview of glutamate as a neurotransmitter. In DiChiara G, Gessa GL (eds): "Glutamate as a Neurotransmitter" New York, Raven Press, pp 1–27.

Coyle JT, McGeer EG, McGeer PL, Schwartz R (1978). Neostriatal injections: a model for Huntington's chorea. In McGeer EG, Olney JW, McGeer PL (eds): "Kainic Acid as a Tool in Neurobiology" New York, Raven Press, pp 139–160.

Cupello A, Hyden H (1986). γ-Aminobutyric acid (GABA) removal from the synaptic cleft: A postsynaptic event? Cell Mol Neurobiol 6: 1–16.

Curtis DR (1978a). Pre- and non-synaptic activities of GABA and related amino acids in the mammalian nervous system. In Fonnum F (ed): "Amino Acids as Chemical Transmitters" New York: Plenum Press, pp 55–86.

Curtis DR (1978b). GABAergic transmission in the mammalian central nervous system. In Krogsgaard-Larsen

P, Scheel-Kruger J, Kofod H (eds): "GABA-Neurotransmitters. Pharmacochemical, Biochemical and Pharmacological Aspects" Copenhagen, Munksgaard, pp 17-27.

De Belleroche JS, Bradford HF (1977). On the site of origin of transmitter amino acids released by depolarization of nerve terminals in vitro. J Neurochem 29: 335-343.

Debler EA, Lajtha A (1987). High-affinity transport of GABA, glycine, taurine, L-aspartic acid, and L-glutamic acid in synaptosomal (P_2) tissue: A kinetic and substrate specificity analysis. J Neurochem in press.

DeFeudis FV (1981). GABA and Neuro-cardiovascular mechanisms. Neurochem Int 3: 113-122.

DeFeudis FV (1984a). GABA and endocrine regulation. - Relation to neurologic-psychiatric disorders. Neurochem Int 6: 1-26.

DeFeudis FV (1984b). Involvement of GABA and other inhibitory amino acids in thermoregulation. Gen Pharmacol 15: 445-447.

DeFeudis FV (1984c). GABA and respiratory function. Gen Pharmacol 15: 441-444.

De Mello FG, Bachrach U, Nirenberg M (1976). Ornithine and glutamic acid decarboxylase activities in the developing chick retina. J Neurochem 27: 847-851.

DiChiara G, Porceddu ML, Imperato A, Morelli M (1981). Role of GABA neurons in the expression of striatal motor neurons. In DiChiara G, Gessa GL (eds): "GABA and the Basal Ganglia" New York, Raven Press, pp 129-163.

Dietl H, Philippu A (1979). In vivo release of endogenous GABA in the cat hypothamalus. Naunyn-Schmiedeberg's Arch Pharmacol 308: 143-147.

DiMicco JA, Gale K, Hamilton B, Gillis RA (1979). GABA receptor control of parasympathetic outflow to the heart: characterization and brain-stem localization. Science 204: 1106-1109.

Dunlap K, Fischbach GD (1981). Neurotransmitters decrease the calcium conductance activated by depolarization of embryonic chick sensory neurones. J Physiol (Lond) 317: 519-535.

Elekes I, Patthy A, Lang T, Palkovits M (1986). Concentrations of GABA and glycine in discrete brain nuclei. Neuropharmacology 25: 703-709.

Enjalbert A, Ruberg M, Arancibia S, Fiore L, Priam M, Kordon C (1979). Independent inhibition of prolactin secretion by dopamine and gamma-aminobutyric acid in vitro. Endocrinology 105: 823-826.

Enna SJ (1984). Role of γ-Aminobutyric acid in anxiety. Psychopathology 17 (suppl 1): 15–24.

Enna SJ, Karbon EW (1986). GABA receptors: an overview. In Olsen RW, Venter JC (eds): "Benzodiazepine/GABA Receptors and Chloride Channels: Structural and Functional Properties" New York: Alan R Liss, pp 41–56.

Erdo SL (1984). High affinity, sodium dependent γ-aminobutyric acid uptake by slices of rat ovary. J Neurochem 40: 582–584.

Erdo SL, Laszlo A (1984). High specific gamma-amino-butyric acid binding to membranes of the human ovary. J Neurochem 42: 1464–1467.

Erdo Sl, Rosdy B, Szporny L (1982). Higher GABA concentrations in fallopian tube than in brain of the rat. J Neurochem 38: 1174–1176.

Fagg GE, Foster AC (1983). Amino acid neurotransmitters and their pathways in the mammalian central nervous system. Neuroscience 9: 701–719.

Fahn S, Cote LJ (1968). Regional distribution of γ-Aminobutyric acid (GABA) in brain of the rhesus monkey. J Neurochem 15: 209–213.

Fan SG, Zhou JP, Xu H, Han JS (1985). The effect of intracerebroventricular 3-mercaptopropionic acid on blood pressure and heart rate in the rat. Brain Res 337: 184–187.

Feger J (1981). Electrophysiological studies of GABAergic neurons in the basal ganglia: Nigro-collicular, nigro-thalamic, and pallidosubthalamic neurons. In DiChiara G, Gessa GL (eds): "GABA and the Basal Ganglia" New York: Raven Press pp 53–68.

Feldberg W, Rocha e Silva M Jr (1981). Inhibition of vasopressin release to carotid occlusion by γ-aminobutyric acid and glycine. Br J Pharmacol 72: 17–24.

Fiok J, Acs Z, Stark E (1981). Possible inhibitory influence of gamma-aminobutyric acid on growth hormone secretion in the rat. J Endocrinol 91: 391–397.

Fischer JB, Olsen RW (1986). Biochemical aspects of GABA/benzodiazepine receptor function. In Olsen RW, Venter JC (eds): "Benzodiazepine/GABA Receptors and Chloride Channels: Structural and Functional Properties" New York: Alan R Liss, pp 241–259.

Flugge G, Wuttke W, Fuchs E (1986). Postnatal development of transmitter systems: sexual differentiation of the GABAergic system and effects of muscimol. Int J Devl Neurosci 4: 319–326.

Frankfurt M, Fuchs E, Wuttke W (1984). Sex differences in γ-aminobutyric acid and glutamate concentrations in discrete rat brain nuclei. Neurosci Lett 50: 245-250.

Frigyesi TL (1972). Intracellular recordings from neurons in the dorsolateral thalamic reticular nucleus during capsular, basal ganglia and midline thalamic stimulation. Brain Res 48: 157-172.

Fuxe K, Andersson K, Ogren S-O, Perez de la Mora M, Schwarcz R, Hokfelt T, Eneroth P, Gustafsson J-A, Skett P (1978). GABA neurons and their interaction with monoamine neurons. An anatomical, pharmacological and functional analysis. In Krogsgaard-Larsen P, Scheel-Kruger J, Kofod H (eds): "GABA Neurotransmitters. Pharmacochemical, Bio- chemical and Pharmacological Aspect" Copenhagen, Munksgaard, pp 74-94.

Gale K (1985). Mechanisms of seizure control mediated by γ-aminobutyric acid: role of the substantia nigra. Fed Proc 44: 2414-2424.

Gale K, Iadarola (MJ (1980). GABAergic denervation of rat substantia nigra: functional and pharmacological properties. Brain Res 183: 217-223.

Garant DS, Gale K (1983). Lesions of substantia nigra protect against experimentally induced seizures. Brain Res 273: 156-161.

Gebauer H, Haas K (1980). γ-Aminobutyric acid transport in thyroids of triiodothyronine and propylthiouracil-treated rats. Hoppe-Seyler's Z. Physiol Chem 361: 1284.

Goertz B (1979). Effect of γ-Aminobutyric acid on cell-free protein synthesizing systems from mouse brain. Exp Brain Res 34: 365-372.

Grandison L, Guidotti A (1979). Gamma-aminobutyric acid receptor function in rat anterior pituitary: evidence for control of prolactin release. Endocrinology 105: 754-759.

Grove J, Schechter PJ, Tell G, Koch-Weser J, Sjoerdsma A, Warter JM, Marescaux C, Rumbach L (1981). Increased gamma-aminobutyric acid (GABA), homocarnosine and beta-alanine in cerebrospinal fluid of patients treated with gamma-vinylGABA (4-aminohex-5-enoic acid). Life Sci 28: 2431-2439.

Hadley ME, Davis MD, Morgan CM (1977). Cellular control of melanocyte stimulating hormone secretion. Front Horm Res 4: 94-104.

Haefely W, Kulcsar A, Mohler H, Pieri L, Polc P, Schaffner R (1975). Possible involvement of GABA in the central action of benzodiazepines. In Costa E,

Greengard P (eds): "Mechanisms of Action of Benzodiazepines" New York: Raven Press, pp 131-151.

Hamberger A, Norstrom N, Sandberg M, Svanberg V (1979). In vitro GABA transport in the neurohypophysis from rat with hereditary diabetes insipidus and after osmotic stimulation. Brain Res 174: 341-344.

Hammond EJ, Wilder BJ (1985). Gamma-vinylGABA: a new antiepileptic drug. Clin Neuropharmacol 8: 1-12.

Hayashi T (1953). The efferent pathway of epileptic seizures for the face following cortical stimulation differs from that for limbs. Jap J Pharmacol 4: 306-321.

Heath RG (1955). Studies in schizophrenia. Harvard Univ. Press, Cambridge, Mass.

Hertz L, Schousboe A (1980). Interactions between neurons and astrocytes in the turnover of gamma amino butyric-acid and glutamate. Brain Res Bull 5 (Suppl 2): 389-395.

Hertz L, Wu PH, Schousboe A (1978). Evidence for net uptake of GABA into mouse astrocytes in primary cultures – its sodium dependence and potassium independence. Neurochem Res 3: 313-323.

Himwich WA, Agrawal HC (1969). Amino acids: In Lajtha A (ed): "Handbook of Neurochemistry" New York: Plenum Press, vol 1, pp 33-52.

Ho IK, Loh HH, Way EL (1976). Pharmacological manipulation of gamma-aminobutyric acid (GABA) in morphine analgesia, tolerance and physical dependence. Life Sci 18: 1111-1123.

Holopainen I, Kontro P (1986): High-affinity uptake of taurine and β-alanine in primary cultures of rat astrocytes. Neurochem Res 11: 207-215.

Houser CR, Lee M, Vaughn JE (1983). Immunocytochemical localization of glutamic acid decarboxylase in normal and deafferented superior colliculus: evidence for reorganization of γ-aminobutyric acid synapses. J Neurosci 3: 2030-2042.

Jessen KR (1981). GABA and the enteric nervous system. A neurotransmitter function. Mol Cell Biochem 38: 69-76.

Jessen KR, Hills JM, Dennison ME, Mirski R (1983). Gamma-aminobutyrate as an autonomic neurotransmitter: release and uptake of [^{3}H]gamma-aminobutyrate in guinea pig large intestine and cultured enteric neurons using physiological methods and electron microscopic autoradiography. Neuroscience 10: 1427-1442.

Johnston GAR (1986). Multiplicity of GABA receptors. In Olsen RW, Venter JC (ed): "Benzodiazepine/GABA Receptors and Chloride Channels. Structural and Functional

Properties" New York: Alan R Liss, pp 57-71.

Jones MT, Gillham B, Altaher ARH, Nicholson SA, Campbell EA, Watts SM, Thody A (1984a). Clinical and experimental studies on the role of GABA in the regulation of ACTH secretion: a review. Psychoneuroendocrinology 9: 107-123.

Jones EA, Schafer DR, Ferenci P, Pappas SC (1984b). The GABA hypothesis of the pathogenesis of hepatic encephalopathy: current status. Yale J Biol Med 57: 301-316.

Kaniff TE, Chuman CM, Neafsey EJ (1983). Substantia nigra single unit activity during penicillin-induced focal cortical epileptiform discharge in the rat. Brain Res Bull 11:11-13.

Kilpatrick IC, Starr MS, James TA, Mac Leod NK (1981). Evidence for the involvement of nigrothalamic GABA neurons in circling behavior in the rat. In DiChiara T, Gessa GL (eds): "GABA and the Basal Ganglia" New York: Raven Press, pp 205-224.

Kitai ST (1981). Anatomy and physiology of the neostriatum. In DiChiara G, Gessa GL (eds): "GABA and the Basal Ganglia" New York: Raven Press, pp 1-21.

Korf J, Van der Heyden JAM, Venema K, Postema F (1981). Distribution and release of GABA in the basal ganglia. In DiChiara G, Gessa GL (eds): "GABA and the Basal Ganglia" New York: Raven Press, pp 105-117.

Krnjevic K (1976). Inhibitory action of GABA and GABA-mimetics on vertebrate neurons. In Roberts E, Chase TN, Tower DB (eds): "GABA in Nervous System Function" New York: Raven Press, pp 269-281.

Krogsgaard-Larsen P (1980). Inhibitors of the GABA uptake systems. Mol. Cell. Biochem. 31: 105-121.

Krogsgaard-Larsen P, Nielsen L, Falch E (1986). The active site of GABA receptors. In Olsen RW, Venter JC (eds): "Benzodiazepine/GABA Receptors and Chloride Channels: Structural and Functional Properties" New York: Alan R Liss, pp 73-95.

Kulonen E (1983). Ethanol and GABA. Med. Biol. 61: 147-167.

Kultas-Ilinsky K, Ribak CE, Peterson GM, Oertel WH (1985). A description of the GABAergic neurons and axon terminals in the motor nuclei of the cat thalamus. J Neurosci. 5: 1346-1369.

Kuriyama K, Ito Y (1983): Some characteristics of solubilized and partially purified cerebral GABA and benzodiazepine receptors. In Mandel P, DeFeudis FV (eds): "CNS Receptors: From Molecular Pharmacology to Behavior" New York: Raven Press, pp 59–70.

Kuriyama K, Yoneda Y (1978). Morphine-induced alterations of γ-aminobutyric acid and taurine contents and L-glutamate decarboxylase activity in rat spinal cord and thalamus: possible correlates with analgesic action of morphine. Brain Res 148: 163–169.

Kvamme E (1983). Deaminases and amidases. In Lajtha A (ed): "Handbook of Neurochemistry" New York: Plenum Press, vol. 4, pp 85–110.

Lahdesmaki P, Pesonen I, Kumpulainen E (1981). The terms of "high affinity" and "high capacity" as conceptions in the interaction of amino acids with synaptic membranes. In DeFeudis FV, Mandel P (eds): "Amino Acid Neurotransmitters". New York: Raven Press, pp 429–435.

Lajtha A, Toth J (1974). Postmortem changes in the cerebral free amino acid pool. Brain Res 76: 546–551.

Lapinjoki SP, Pajunen AEI, Hietala OA, Piha RS (1980). The effect of changes in GABA metabolism on the activities of L-ornithine in decarboxylase mouse brain. Acta Univ Oul A97 Biochem 29: 31–38.

Larsson OM, Drejer J, Hertz L, Schousboe A (1983). Ion dependency of uptake and release of GABA and (RS)-nipecotic acid studied in cultured mouse brain cortex neurons. J. Neurosci. Res. 9: 291–302.

Larsson OM, Griffiths R, Allen IC, Schousboe A (1986). Mutual inhibition kinetic analysis of γ-aminobutyric acid, taurine and β-alanine high-affinity transport into neurons and astrocytes: Evidence for similarity between the taurine and β-alanine carriers in both cell types. J Neurochem 47: 426–432.

Le Gal La Salle G, Kaijima M, Feldblum S (1983). Abortive amygdaloic kindled seizures following microinjection of γ-vinylGABA in the vicinity of substantia nigra in rats. Neurosci Lett 36: 69–74.

Leonard BE (1984). GABA and endocrine regulation. Critique Neurochem Int 6: 17–22.

Levi G (1972). Transport systems for GABA and other amino acids in incubated chick brain tissue during development. Arch Biochem Biophys 151: 8–21.

Levi G, Raiteri M (1978). Modulation of γ-aminobutyric acid transport in nerve endings: Role of extracellular γ-aminobutyric acid and of cationic fluxes. Proc Natl Acad Sci 75: 2981–2985.

Levi G, Banay-Schwartz M, Raiteri M (1978). Uptake,

exchange and release of GABA in isolated nerve endings. In Fonnum F (ed): "Amino Acids as Chemical Transmitters" New York: Plenum Press, pp 326–350.

Lima L, Sourkes TL (1986). Cholinergic and GABAergic regulation of dopamine beta-hydroxylase activity in the adrenal gland of the rat. J Pharmacol Exp Therap 237: 265–270.

Lloyd KG, Morselli PL, Depoortere H, Fournier V, Zivkovic B, Scatton B, Broekkamp C, Worms P, Bartholini G (1983). The potential use of GABA agonists in psychiatric disorders: Evidence from studies with Progabide in animal models and clinical trials. Pharmacol Biochem Behav 18: 957–966.

Lloyd KD, Bossi L, Morselli PL, Rougier M, Loiseau P, Munari C (1985). Biochemical evidence for dysfunction of GABA neurons in human epilepsy. In Bartholini G, Bossi L, Lloyd KG, Morselli PL (eds): "Epilepsy and GABA Receptor Agonists. Basic and Therapeutic Research" New York: Raven Press, pp 43–51.

Loscher W (1982). Cardiovascular effects of GABA, GABA-aminotransferase inhibitors and valproic acid following systemic administration in rats, cats and dogs: pharmacological approach to localize the site of action. Arch Int Pharmacodyn Ther 259: 32–58.

Loscher W, Vetter M (1985). In vivo effects of aminooxyacetic acid and valproic acid on nerve terminal (synaptosomal) GABA levels in discrete brain areas of the rat. Biochem Pharmacol 34: 1747–1756.

Loiseau P, Hardenberg JP, Pestre M, Guyot M, Schechter PJ, Tell G (1986). Double blind, placebo-controlled study of vigabatrin (gamma-vinylGABA) in drug resistant epilepsy. Epilepsia 27: 115–120.

Madtes PC, Redburn DA (1983). GABA as a trophic factor during development. Life Sci 33: 979–984.

Makara GB, Stark E (1974). Effect of gamma-aminobutyric acid (GABA) and GABA antagonist drugs on ACTH release. Neuroendocrinology 16: 178–190.

Mandel P, Ciesielski L, Maitre M, Simler S, Kempf E, Mack G (1981). Inhibitory amino acids, aggressiveness and convulsions. In DeFeudis FV, Mandel P (eds): "Amino Acid Neurotransmitters" New York: Raven Press, pp 1–9.

Mandel P, Kempf E, Simler S, Puglisi S, Ciesielski L, Mack G (1983). Comparison of the effects of GABA-mimetic agents on two types of aggressive behavior. In Mandel P, DeFeudis FV (eds): "CNS Receptors: From Molecular Pharmacology to Behavior" New York: Raven Press, pp

149–161.

Marsden CD (1978). GABA in relation to extrapyramidal diseases, with particular relevance to animal models. In Krogsgaard-Larsen P, Scheel-Kruger J, Kofod H (eds): "GABA-Neurotransmitters. Pharmacochemical, Biochemical and Pharmacological Aspects" Copenhagen, Munksgaard, pp 295–307.

Marsden CD, Sheehy MP (1981). GABA and movement disorders. In DiChiara G, Gessa GL (eds): "GABA and the Basal Ganglia" New York: Raven Press, pp 225–234.

Marshall JF, Ungerstedt U (1977). Striatal efferent fibers play a role in maintaining rotational behavior in the rat. Science 198: 62–64.

Martin DL (1976): Carrier-mediated transport and removal of GABA from synaptic regions. In Roberts E, Chase TN, Tower DB (eds): "GABA in Nervous System Function" New York: Raven Press, pp 347–386.

Mathison RD, Dreifuss JJ (1980). Structure-activity relationship of a neurohypophyseal GABA receptor. Brain Res 187: 476–480.

McGeer EG, McGeer PL (1978). GABA-containing neurons in schizophrenia, Huntington's chorea and normal aging. In Krogsgaard-Larsen P, Scheel-Kruger J, Kofod H (eds): "GABA-Neurotransmitters. Pharmacochemical, Biochemical and Pharmacological Aspects: Copenhagen: Munksgaard, pp 340–356.

McGeer PL, Eccles C, McGeer EG (1978). Molecular Neurobiology of the Mammalian Brain. New York, London: Plenum Press.

McNamara JO, Galloway MT, Rigsbee LC, Shin C (1984). Evidence implicating substantia nigra in regulation of kindled seizure threshold. J Neurosci 4: 2410–2417.

Meier E, Drejer J, Schousboe A (1983). Trophic action of GABA on the development of physiologically active GABA receptors. In Mandel P, DeFeudis FV (eds): "CNS Receptors from Molecular Pharmacology to Behavior" New York: Raven Press, pp 47–58.

Meister A (1965). "Biochemistry of the Amino Acids" New York, London: Academic Press, vol 1, p 90.

Meldrum BS (1975). Epilepsy and gamma-aminobutyric acid-mediated inhibition. Int Rev Neurobiol 17: 1–36.

Meldrum BS (1982). GABA and acute psychoses. Psychol Med 12: 1–5.

Mohler H, Polc P, Cumin R, Pieri L, Kettler R (1979). Nicotinamide is a brain constituent with benzodiazepine-like actions. Nature (Lond) 278: 563–565.

Morse DE, Hooker, Duncan H, Jensen L (1979). γ-Aminobutyric acid, a neurotransmitter, induces planktonic abalone larvae to settle and begin metamorphosis. Science 204: 407-410.

Mugnaini E, Oertel WH (1985). An atlas of the distribution of GABAergic neurons and terminals in the rat CNS as revealed by GAD immunohistochemistry. In Bjorklund A, Hokfelt T (eds): "Handbook of Chemical Neuroanatomy" Amsterdam, New York, Oxford: Elsevier, vol 4, p 436-622.

Myslobodsky MS, Ackermann RF, Engel J (1979). Effects of gamma-acetylenic GABA and GABA on metrazol-activated, and kindled seizures. Pharmacol Biochem Behav 11: 265-271.

Nestoros JN (1984). GABAergic mechanisms of anxiety: An overview and a new neurophysiological model. Can J Psychiatry 29: 520-529.

Norenberg MD (1979). Distribution of glutamine synthetase in the rat central nervous system. J Histochem Cytochem 27: 756-762.

Obata K (1976): Excitatory effects of GABA. In Roberts E, Chase TN, Tower DB (eds): "GABA in Nervous System Function" New York: Raven Press, pp 283-286.

Oertel WH, Mugnaini E (1984). Immunocytochemical studies of GABAergic neurons in rat basal ganglia and their relations to other neuronal systems. Neurosci Lett 47: 233-238.

Oertel WH, Schmechel DE, Mugnaini E, Tappaz ML, Kopin IJ (1981). Immunocytochemical localization of glutamate decarboxylase in rat cerebellum with a new antiserum. Neuroscience 6: 2715-2735.

Oertel WH, Nitsch C, Mugnaini E (1984). The immunocytochemical demonstration of the GABAergic neurons in rat globus pallidus and nucleus entopeduncularis and their GABAergic innervation. Adv Neurol 40: 91-98.

Okada Y, Shimada C (1976). Intrahippocampal distribution of GABA and GAD activity in the guinea pig: microassay method for the determination of GAD activity. In Roberts E, Chase TN, Tower DB (eds): "GABA in Nervous System Function" New York, London: Raven Press, pp 223-228.

Okada Y, Nitsch-Hassler C, Kim JS, Bak IJ, Hassler R (1971). Role of γ-Aminobutyric acid (GABA) in the extrapyramidal motor system. I. Regional distribution of GABA in rabbit, guinea pig and baboon CNS. Exp.

Brain Res 13: 514–518.

Okada T, Taniguchi H, Shimada C (1976). High concentration of GABA and high glutamate decarboxylase activity in rat pancreatic islets and human insulinoma. Science 194: 620–622.

Oldendorf WH, Szabo J (1976). Amino acid assignment to one of three blood–brain barrier amino acid carriers. Am J Physiol 230: 94–98.

Ondo JG (1974). Gamma–aminobutyric acid effects on pituitary gonadotropin secretion. Science 186: 738–739.

Osborne NN, Beaton DW (1985). Selectivity of uptake of tritiated glycine, GABA, aspartate and serotonin by rabbit retinal cells in culture. Biogenic Amines 3: 169–179.

Ottersen OP, Storm–Mathisen J (1984a). Neurons containing or accumulating transmitter amino acids. In Bjorklund A, Hokfelt T, Kuhar MJ (eds): "Handbook of Chemical Neuroanatomy" Amsterdam, New York, Oxford: Elsevier, vol 3, part II, pp 141–246.

Ottersen OP, Storm–Mathisen J (1984b). Glutamate and GABA containing neurons in the mouse and rat brain, as demonstrated with a new immunocytochemical technique. J Comp Neurol 229: 374–392.

Palfreyman MG, Schechter PJ, Buckett WR, Tell GP, Koch–Weser J (1981). The pharmacology of GABA–transaminase inhibitors. Biochem Pharmacol 30: 817–824.

Pedley TA, Horton RW, Meldrum BS (1979). Electroencephalographic and behavioral effects of a GABA agonist (muscimol) on photosensitive epilepsy in the baboon, Papio papio. Epilepsia 20: 409–416.

Penney JB Jr, Young AB (1981). GABA as the pallido–thalamic neurotransmitter: implications for basal ganglia function. Brain Res 207: 195–199.

Penny GR, Fitzpatrick D, Schmechel DE, Diamond TT (1983). Glutamic acid decarboxylase immunoreactive neurons and horseradish peroxidase–labelled projection neurons in the ventral posterior nucleus of the cat and Galago senegalensis. J Neurosci 3: 1868–1887.

Penny GR, Conley M, Diamond IT, Schmechel DE (1984). The distribution of glutamic acid decarboxylase immunoreactivity in the diencephalon of the opossum and rabbit. J Comp Neurol 228: 38–57.

Perry TL (1982). Cerebral amino acid pools. In Lajtha A (ed): "Handbook of Neurochemistry" New York, London: Plenum Press, vol 1, pp 151–180.

Perry TL, Berry K, Hansen S, Diamond S, Mok C (1971).

Regional distribution of amino acids in human brain obtained at autopsy. J Neurochem 18: 513–519.

Perry TL, Hansen S, Kloster M (1973). Huntington's chorea, deficiency of γ-aminobutyric acid in brain. New Engl J Med 288: 337–342.

Perry TL, Hansen S, Gandham S (1981). Post mortem changes of amino acid compounds in human and rat brain. J Neurochem 36: 406–412.

Pollen DA (1964). Intracellular studies of cortical neurons during thalamic induced wave and spike. Electroenceph Clin Neurophysiol 17: 398–404.

Pycock CJ, Dawbarn D, Kerwin RW (1981). Roles of GABA and glycine in the substantia nigra. In DeFeudis FV, Mandel P (eds): "Amino Acid Neurotransmitters" New York: Raven Press, pp 77–87.

Racagni G, Donoso AO (eds) (1986). "GABA and Endocrine Function" New York: Raven Press.

Racagni G, Apud JA, Cocchi D, Locatelli V, Muller EE (1982). GABAergic control of anterior pituitary hormone secretion. Life Sci 31: 823–838.

Radian R, Kanner BI (1983). Stoichiometry of sodium and chloride-coupled gamma-aminobutyric acid transport by synaptic plasma membrane vesicles isolated from rat brain. Biochemistry 22: 1236–1241.

Reavill C, Leigh N, Jenner P, Marsden CD (1981). Critical role of mid-brain reticular formation in the expression of dopamine-mediated circling behavior. In DiChiara G, Gessa GL (eds): "GABA and the Basal Ganglia" New York, Raven Press, pp 187–204.

Ribak CE (1981). The GABAergic neurons of the extrapyramidal system as revealed by immunocytochemistry. In DiChiara G, Gessa GL (eds): "GABA and the Basal Ganglia" New York: Raven Press, pp 23–36.

Ribak CE, Vaughn JE, Saito K, Barber R, Roberts E (1977). Glutamate decarboxylase localization in neurons of the olfactory bulb. Brain Res 126: 1–18.

Ribak CE, Harris AB, Vaughn JE, Roberts E (1979). Inhibitory, GABAergic nerve terminals decrease at sites of focal epilepsy. Science 205: 211–240.

Roberts E (1972). An hypothesis suggesting that there is a defect in the GABA system in schizophrenia. Neurosci Res Program Bull 10: 468–481.

Roberts E (1976). Disinhibition as an organizing principle in the nervous system. The role of the GABA system. Application to neurologic and psychiatric disorders. In Roberts E, Chase TN, Tower DB (eds):

"GABA in Nervous System Function" New York: Raven Press, pp 515–539.

Roberts E (1986a). Failure of GABAergic inhibition: a key to local and global seizures. Adv Neurol 44: 319–341.

Roberts E (1986b). Metabolism and nerve system disease: a challenge for our times. Part I. Metabolic Brain Disease 1: 3–23.

Roberts E (1986c). GABA: the road to neurotransmitter status. In Olsen RW, Venter JC (eds): "Benzodiazepine/GABA Receptors and Chloride Channels. Structural and Functional Properties" New York: Alan R Liss, pp 1–39.

Roberts E, Frankel S (1950). γ-Aminobutyric acid in brain. Its formation from glutamic acid. J Biol Chem 187: 55–63.

Roberts E, Krause DN (1982). γ-Aminobutyric acid system in cardiovascular and cerebrovascular function. Isr J Med Sci 18: 75–81.

Roberts PJ (1980). Transport and binding of gamma aminobutyric-acid and related amino-acids by peripheral glial cells of dorsal root ganglia. Brain Res Bull 5 (Suppl 2): 83–88.

Robin MM, Palfreyman MG, Schechter PJ (1979). Dyskinetic effects of intrastriatally injected GABA-transaminase inhibitors. Life Sci 25: 1103–1110.

Rusak B, Zucker I (1979). Neural regulation of circadian rhythms. Physiol Rev 59: 449–526.

Saito K (1976). Immunochemical studies of GAD and GABA-T. In Roberts E, Chase TN, Tower DB (eds): "GABA in Nervous System Function" New York, London: Raven Press, pp 103–111.

Sanger DJ (1985). GABA and the behavioral effects of anxiolytic drugs. Life Sci. 36: 1503–1513.

Sarhan S, Seiler N (1979). Metabolic inhibitors and subcellular distribution of GABA. J Neurosci Res 4: 399–421.

Schally AV, Arimura A, Kastin AJ (1973). Hypothalamic regulatory hormones. Science 179: 341–350.

Schally AV, Redding TW, Arimura A, Dupont A, Linthianu GL (1977). Isolation of γ-Aminobutyric acid from pig hypothalami and demonstration of its prolactin release-inhibiting (PIF) activity in vivo and in vitro. Endocrinology 100: 681–691.

Schechter PJ, Tranier J (1978). The pharmacology of enzyme-activated inhibitors of GABA-transaminase. In

Seiler N, Jung MJ, Koch-Weser J (eds): "Enzyme-Activated Irreversible Inhibitors:" Amsterdam, New York, Oxford: Elsevier/North-Holland Biomedical Press, pp 149-162.

Schechter PJ, Hanke NFJ, Grove J, Huebert N, Sjoerdsma A (1984). Biochemical and clinical effects of γ-vinylGABA in patients with epilepsy. Neurology 34: 182-186.

Scheel-Kruger K (1984). GABA in striatonigral and striatopallidal systems as moderator and mediator of striatal functions. Adv Neurol 40: 85-90.

Schmidt RF, Vogel ME, Zimmermann M (1967). Die Wirkung von Diazepam auf die presynaptische Hemmung und andere Ruckenmarksreflexe. Naunyn-Schmiedeberg's Arch Pharmacol 258: 69-82.

Schon F, Kelly JS (1975). Selective uptake of [^{3}H]-β-alanine by glia: association with the glial uptake system for GABA. Brain Res 86: 243-257.

Schousboe A (1979). Effects of GABA analogues on the high affinity uptake of GABA in astrocytes in primary culture. In Mandel P, DeFeudis FV (eds): "GABA-Biochemistry and CNS Functions" New York: Plenum Press, pp 219-237.

Seiler N (1980). On the role of GABA in vertebrate polyamine metabolism. Physiol Chem Phys 12: 411-429.

Seiler N, Sarhan S (1980). Drugs affecting GABA. In Battistin L, Hashim G, Lajtha A (eds): "Neurochemistry and Clinical Neurology" New York: Alan R Liss, pp 425-439.

Seiler N, Sarhan S (1983). Metabolic routes of GABA formation in chick embryo brain. Neurochem Int 5: 625-633.

Seiler N, Wagner G (1976). NAD$^+$-dependent formation of γ-aminobutyrate (GABA) from glutamate. Neurochem Res 1: 113-131.

Seiler N, Wiechmann M (1969). Zum Vorkommen der γ-aminobuttersaure und der γ-amino-β-hydroxybutter-saure in tierischem Gewebe. Hoppe-Seyler's Z Physiol Chem 350: 1493-1500.

Sellstrom A, Sjoberg LB, Hamberger A (1975). Neuronal and glial systems for γ-Aminobutyric acid metabolism. J Neurochem 25: 393-398.

Sershen H, Lajtha A (1976). Capillary transport of amino acids in the developing brain. Exp Neurol 53: 465-474.

Sershen H, Lajtha A (1979). Inhibition pattern by analogs indicates the presence of ten or more transport

dietary gamma amino butyric-acid and protein on growth, food intake, and gamma-aminobutyric acid metabolism in the rat. Brain Res Bull 5 Suppl 2: 245-251.

Thaker GK, Hare TA, Tamminga CA (1983). GABA system: clinical research and treatment of tardive dyskinesia. Mod. Probl. Pharmacopsychiat. 21: 155-167.

Ticku MK, Burch TP, Thyagarajan R, Ramanjaneyulu R (1983). Barbiturate interactions with benzodiazepine-GABA-receptor-ionophore complex. In Mandel P, DeFeudis FV (eds): :"CNS Receptors: From Molecular Pharmacology to Behavior" New York: Raven Press, pp 81-91.

Toth E, Lajtha A (1981). Elevation of cerebral levels of nonessential amino acids in vivo by administration of large doses of GABA. Neurochem Res 6: 1303-1320.

Toth E, Lajtha A (1984). Brain protein synthesis rates are not sensitive to elevated GABA, taurine, or glycine. Neurochem Res 9: 173-179.

Tunnicliff G, Ngo TT (1986). Regulation of γ-Aminobutyric acid synthesis in the vertebrate nervous system. Neurochem Int 8: 287-297.

Turski L, Cavalheiro ZA, Schwarcz M, Turski WA, DeMoraes Mello LEA, Bortolotto ZA, Klockgether T, Sontag KH (1986). Susceptibility to seizures produced by pilocarpine in rats after microinjection of isoniacid or γ-vinylGABA into the substantia nigra. Brain Res 370: 294-309.

Van der Heyden JAM, Korf J (1978). Regional levels of GABA in the brain: rapid semiautomated assay and prevention of post mortem increase by 3-mercaptopropionic acid. J Neurochem 31: 197-203.

Van der Heyden JAM, Kloet ER de, Korf J, Versteeg DHG (1979). GABA content of discrete brain nuclei and spinal cord of the rat. J Neurochem 33: 857-861.

Van der Heyden JAM, Venema K, Korf J (1979). In vivo release of endogenous GABA from rat substantia nigra measured by a novel method. J Neurochem 32: 469-476.

Van der Heyden JAM, Venema K, Korf J (1980). In vivo release of endogenous γ-Aminobutyric acid from rat striatum: Effects of muscimol, oxotremorine and morphine. J Neurochem 34: 1648-1653.

Vaughn JE, Famiglietti EV Jr, Barber RP, Saito K, Roberts E, Ribak CE (1981). GABAergic amacrine cells in rat retina: immunocytochemical identification and synaptic connectivity. J Comp Neurol 197: 113-128.

Vincent SR, Hokfelt T, Wu J-Y (1982). GABA neuron systems in hypothalamus and pituitary gland: immunohistochemical demonstration using antibodies against glutamate decarboxylase. Neuroendocrinology 34: 117-125.

Vijayan E, McCann SM (1978). Effects of intraventricular injection of gamma-aminobutyric acid (GABA) on plasma growth hormone and thyrotropin in conscious ovariectomized rats. Endocrinology 103: 1888-1893.

Walaas I, Fonnum F (1978). The distribution of putative monoamine, GABA, acetylcholine and glutamate fibers in the mesolimbic system. In Krogsgaard-Larsen P, Scheel-Kruger J, Kofod H (eds): "GABA-Neurotransmitters: Pharmacochemical, Biochemical and Pharmacological Aspects" Copenhagen: Munksgaard, pp 60-73.

Waszczak BL, Bergstrom DA, Walters JR (1981). Single unit responses of substantia nigra and globus pallidus neurons to GABA agonist and antagonist drugs. In DiChiara G, Gessa GL (eds): "GABA and the Basal Ganglia" New York: Raven Press, pp 79-94.

Wehr TA, Sack D, Rosenthal N, Duncan W, Grillin JC (1983). Circadian rhythm disturbances in manic-depressive illness. Fed Proc 42: 2809-2814.

Williford DJ, DiMicco JA, Gillis RA (1980). Evidence for the presence of a tonically active forebrain GABA system influencing central sympathetic outflow in the cat. Neuropharmacology 19: 245-250.

Wolff JR (1981). Evidence for a dual role of GABA as a synaptic transmitter and promoter of synaptogenesis. In DeFeudis FV, Mandel P (eds): "Amino Acid Neurotransmitters" New York: Raven Press, pp 459-465.

Wolff JR, Balcar VJ, Zetzsche T, Bottcher H, Schmechel DE, Chronwall BM (1984). Development of GABAergic system in rat visual cortex. In Lauder JM, Nelson PG (eds): "Gene Expression and Cell-Cell Interactions in the Developing Nervous System" New York: Plenum Press, pp 215-239.

Wood JD, Kurylo E (1984). Amino acid content of nerve endings (synaptosomes) in different regions in brain: Effects of Gabaculine and isonicotinic acid hydrazide. J. Neurochem. 42: 420-425.

Wood JD, Schousboe A, Krogsgaard-Larsen P (1980a). In vivo changes in the GABA content of nerve endings (synaptosomes) induced by inhibitors of GABA uptake. Neuropharmacology 19: 1149-1152.

Wood JD, Russell MP, Kurylo E (1980b). The γ-amino-butyrate content of nerve endings (synaptosomes) in mice after intramuscular injection of γ-amino-butyrate-elevating agents: a possible role in anticonvulsant activity. J. Neurochem. 35: 125-130.

Wood JG, McLaughlin BJ, Vaughn JE (1979). Immunocyto-chemical localization of GAD in electron microscopic preparations of rodent CNS. In Roberts E, Chase TN, Tower DB (eds): "GABA in Central Nervous System Function" New York, London: Raven Press, pp 133-148.

Wu J-Y (1976). Purification, characterization and kinetic studies of GAD and GABA-T from mouse brain. In Roberts E, Chase TN, Tower DB (eds): "GABA in Nervous System Function" New York, Raven Press, pp 7-55.

Wu J-Y (1983). Decarboxylases: Brain glutamate decarboxylase as a model. In Lajtha A (ed): "Handbook of Neurochemistry" New York, London: Plenum Press, vol 4, pp 111-131.

Yamada KA, Norman WP, Hamosh P, Gillis RA (1982). Medullary ventral surface GABA receptors affect respiratory and cardiovascular function. Brain Res 248: 71-78.

Yamanaka K, Yamada S, Okada T, Hayashi E (1982): Effect of picrotoxin on adrenal catecholamine secretion. Jap J Pharmacol 33: 1049-1055.

Yoneda Y, Kuriyama K, Kurihara E (1977). Morphine alters distribution of GABA in thalamus. Brain Res 124: 373-378.

Yoneda Y, Kanmori K, Ida S, Kuryiama K (1983). Stress-induced alterations in metabolism of γ-aminobutyric acid in rat brain. J Neurochem 40: 350-356.

Yoshida M (1981). The GABAergic systems and the role of basal ganglia in motor control. In Dichiara G, Gessa GL (eds): "GABA and the Basal Ganglia" New York: Raven Press, pp 37-52.

Yu ACH, Hertz L (1982). Uptake of glutamate, GABA, and glutamine into a predominantly GABAergic and a predominantly glutamatergic nerve cell population in culture. J Neurosci Res 7: 23-35.

Yunger LM, Moonsammy GI, Rush JA (1983). Kinetic analysis of the accumulation of gamma-aminobutyric acid by particulate fractions of rat brain: Comparison of the effects of nipecotic acid and cis-3-aminocylohexane-1-carboxylic acid. Neurochem Res 8: 757-769.

Neurotrophic Activity of GABA During Development, pages 57–77
© **1987 Alan R. Liss, Inc.**

ONTOGENY OF GABAERGIC SYSTEMS IN THE BRAIN

Vladimir J. Balcar and Graham A.R. Johnston

Department of Pharmacology
University of Sydney,
N.S.W. 2006 AUSTRALIA

INTRODUCTION

The possibility that some of the neuroactive compounds may act as trophic factors during the development or regeneration of synaptic connections, has been discussed for some time (Kasematsu and Pettigrew, 1976; Jacobsen, 1978). However, the idea that the central synaptic transmitters, in particular those of inhibitory character, can have trophic effects, is of a more recent date. For example, Wolff (1981) attempted to explain some of the unusual properties of the most common central inhibitory synaptic transmitter, γ-aminobutyric acid (GABA), by proposing an additional role for it in the nervous tissue – that of a trophic factor.

This suggestion was supported by a study showing that externally applied GABA could produce distinct morphological changes in the superior cervical ganglion (SCG) (Wolff et al., 1978), a finding which has since been supported by physiological techniques and which may have major implications for the understanding of the mechanisms by which synaptogenesis in SCG is directed (Dames et al., 1985).

The central nervous system is much more complex than the sympathetic ganglia and, therefore, the first data, indicating that GABA could have trophic effects on central neurons, were obtained using simplified experimental models. Thus Spoerri and Wolff, (1981) reported GABA-elicited formation of postsynaptic-like densities in cultured neuroblastoma and other workers demonstrated increased growth of dendrites (Hansen et al., 1984), changes in the characteristics of GABA receptors (Meier et al., 1983; 1984) and altered expression of a neuron-specific protein (Meier and Jorgensen, 1986) in primary cultures of cerebellar granule cells exposed to exogeneous GABA.

However, similar studies using central nervous tissue in which GABA concentrations were artificially manipulated in vivo, have also been carried out (Madtes and Redburn, 1983; Sykes et al., 1984; Beart et al., 1985; Sykes and Horton, 1986).

In the present article we shall summarize the data on the ontogenetic development of neurochemical functions associated with GABAergic systems, examining a possibility that some of these functions may be involved in trophic effects of GABA rather than in synaptic transmission.

ONTOGENY OF GABAERGIC NEURONS AND SYNAPTIC CONTACTS

Immunohistochemical studies based on the assumption that the structures labelled by antibodies to GAD, the enzyme that catalyses GABA synthesis from L-glutamate, represent GABAergic neurons and corresponding synaptic terminals, have indicated that GABAergic neurons in the CNS are usually integrated into local inhibitory circuits and, with a few exceptions, do not form long projecting pathways (Ribak, 1978). The most typical GABAergic neurons in rat cerebral cortex are the small sparsely spinous (or aspinous) stellate cells but, in general, the anatomical type and physiological function of GABAergic neurons vary from one part of brain to another and, also from species to species.

The small neurons which form the local inhibitory circuits were thought to originate, migrate and differentiate later in the ontogenetic development than the larger cells (Jacobsen, 1978). This view was based mainly on anatomical and morphological studies using [^{3}H]thymidine labelling for the determination of the date at which the neurons had undergone the last mitotic division. However, when other criteria, such as expression of transmitter-related functions, were applied, different, more complex pattern began to emerge.

For example, in the rat cerebral cortex, it is accepted that all presumptive GABAergic neurons originate, migrate and settle by the time of birth (Wolff et al., 1984b). This precedes the period of the most intense formation of synapses by about two weeks (Aghajanian and Bloom, 1967). However, a large proportion of axodendritic inhibitory synaptic contacts formed during the period of rapid synaptogenesis, later disappear (Blue and Parnavelas, 1983), while the number of GABAergic axo-somatic synapses increases by about 50% after the postnatal day 20 (P20) (Bahr and Wolff, 1985). This raises some interesting questions, for instance − what is the functional state of the presumptive GABAergic neurons during their time between the migration/positioning and the formation of GABAergic synapses? Are the neurochemical characteristics of GABAergic neurons? expressed before their synapses are formed and, if so, does GABA have any specific role during this time which happens to coincide with the period of most rapid differentiation of cortical neurons? The results of morphological studies to date do not provide simple answers. Thus, the majority of GABAergic neurons probably migrate and settle during the whole period of cortical neurogenesis (Johnston and Coyle, 1980) and, accordingly, cells accumulating [^{3}H]GABA have been detected as early as on embryonic day 16 (E 16) (Chronwall and Wolff, 1980). The matter is made more complex by the fact that many small nonpyramidal cells (the majority of which are GABAergic in the adult cortex; Emson and Hunt, 1981) may not follow the characteristic temporo-spatial mode of migration described for the larger cortical cells ("inside-out layering", Berry and Rogers, 1965) and seem to travel to all cortical layers in a diffuse manner (Rickmann et al., 1977; Wolff et al., 1984b; but see also Miller, 1986b). Many presumptive GABAergic neurons seem to undergo massive morphological transformation during the first two to three weeks post partum, especially in terms of the dendritic arborization, but this is not necessarily paralleled by formation of synapses (Miller, 1986a).

Careful examination of GABA neurochemistry, including quantitative studies of GABA-related neurochemical markers, during the early postnatal development, may help to clarify some of the questions.

NEUROCHEMISTRY OF THE GABAERGIC INHIBITORY SYSTEM IN CNS

In the CNS, GABA is produced by an enzyme-catalyzed, pyridoxal phosphate-dependent 1-decarboxylation of L-glutamate (Roberts and Frankel, 1951) and, possibly, by other synthetic pathways of quantitatively minor importance (Seiler, 1981). The enzyme, glutamate-decarboxylase (EC 4.1.1.15, L-glutamate-1-carboxylyase, GAD) is thought to be localized in neuronal structures such as nerve endings (Fonnum, 1968).

Electrically- and K^+-stimulated release of [^{3}H]GABA from brain slices is Ca^{2+}-dependent and, based mainly on this criterion, it has been suggested that it represents the synaptic release of GABA (Srinivasan et al., 1969). In fact, K^+-stimulated, Ca^{2+}-dependent release of [^{3}H]GABA from preparations enriched in isolated nerve endings has been demonstrated (Levy et al., 1973), although stimulated Ca^{2+}-dependent release of GABA from other, non-synaptic (Jaffe and Cuello, 1981) or even non-neuronal structures (Roberts, 1974; Minchin and Iversen, 1975; Johnston, 1977), cannot be ruled out.

Following synaptic release, GABA interacts in a structurally highly specific manner, with the postsynaptic GABA receptors (Curtis and Watkins, 1960; Johnston et al., 1984) in the neuronal membrane. This results in an increased permeability of the membrane to chloride ions (Boistel and Fatt, 1958; Harris and Allen, 1985) and, in most cases, hyperpolarization of the neuron. GABA action is potentiated by benzodiazepines (Mohler and Okada, 1976; Tallman and Gallagher, 1985) or by barbiturates (Johnston and Willow, 1982) and it is selectively blocked by a naturally-occurring alkaloid bicuculline (Curtis et al., 1970). Apart from bicuculline-blocked, barbiturate- and benzodiazepine-potentiated (GABA$_A$) receptors, a second receptor type (GABA$_B$) sensitive to the muscle relaxant baclofen (a β-p-chlorophenyl derivative of GABA) and linked to Ca^{2+}-, rather than Cl^-- selective channels has been described (Bowery, 1982).

GABA receptors have been shown to be located not only post- but also pre-synaptically (Johnston and Mitchell, 1971) and this observation resulted in the formulation of the concept of a GABA "autoreceptor" (Snodgrass, 1978; Mitchell and Martin, 1978; Brennan et al., 1981) limiting the release of GABA by inhibiting the electrical activity of GABAergic terminals. Also, release of other transmitters may be influenced by GABA (Potashner, 1979; Johnston et al., 1980; Aloisi et al., 1983; Farkas et al., 1986).

Catabolism of GABA is mediated by 4-aminobutyrate-2-oxoglutarate aminotransferase (EC 2.6.1.19, GABA trans-aminase, GABA-T) an enzyme which has been extensively studied from the pharmacological point of view. There are several inhibitors of GABA-T which can be used to increase the levels of GABA in vitro (Metcalf, 1979).

GABA is removed from the extracellular synaptic environment by uptake into nerve terminals and neighboring glial cells (Iversen and Neal, 1968). Such uptake appears to limit the action of GABA and certain GABA agonist in vivo and may be involved in the inactivation of synaptically released GABA (Johnston, 1978; Lodge et al., 1978). The uptake of GABA by nerve terminals and glial cells appears to be mediated by high affinity transport systems with different substrate specificities with cis-3-aminocyclohexane carboxylic acid (ACHC) and β-alanine being preferential substrates for the neuronal and glial transport systems respectively (Schon and Kelly, 1975; Bowery et al., 1976). Nipecotic acid and L-2,4-diaminobutyric acid may also show some selectivity for the neuronal GABA transport system (Krogsgaard-Larsen and Johnston, 1975; Johnston et al., 1976). The high affinity uptake of GABA, ACHC, nipecotic acid and L-2,4-aminobutyric acid may be used as markers for GABAergic nerve terminals, but these substrates may also be taken up by other structures (e.g. astrocytes in culture take up ACHC; Larsson et al., 1983).

Synthesis, release, uptake and metabolism of GABA and experimental models for quantitative studies of GABA receptors in vitro are often referred to as neurochemical markers for GABAergic synaptic inhibitory systems. Attempts have been made to correlate the ontogenetic development of neurochemical markers of GABAergic systems with that of the morphological and functional characteristics of differentiating GABAergic neurons (Coyle, 1982; Wolff et al., 1984b) and in the present article we shall re-examine some of these correlations in the light of the hypothesis that, at some stage of the ontogenetic development, GABA may act as a trophic factor rather than a simple synaptic transmitter.

PRESENCE AND LOCATION OF GABA IN THE DEVELOPING CORTEX

Changes in the content of GABA in the embryonic and early postnatal brain were reviewed and discussed by Safarov and Sytinsky (1980). GABA is present in the embryonic rat brain as early as on E 15. The levels of GABA at that time are equivalent to about one-fifth of those in the adult tissue and, moreover, there is a large increase in GABA levels between E 16 and E 19 resulting in the values at birth as high as half of those in the adult brain (Carver et al., 1965; Coyle and Enna, 1976; Safarov and Sytinsky, 1980). In the rat, there are relatively large regional differences in GABA levels during the postnatal period (Cutler and Dudzinski, 1974), those in the cerebral cortex increasing approximately twofold between the birth and adulthood (Hedner et al., 1984).

At least a part of cortical GABA is present in neurons as evidenced by studies using antibodies against GABA fixed in the tissue (Miller, 1986b). GABA-immunoreactive neurons are found predominantly in the marginal zone at birth and as from the postnatal day 4 (P4), or perhaps even P2, there are GABA-immunoreactive neurons in all laminae (Miller, 1986b).

Thus GABA is present in the brain even before most of the presumptive GABAergic neurons have finished mitosis and migration. Furthermore, GABA reaches relatively high levels and becomes, at least in part, localized in neurons well before the majority of GABAergic synapses have been formed.

SYNTHESIS AND CATABOLISM OF GABA DURING DEVELOPMENT

The activity of GAD was one of the first GABA-related neurochemical markers studied during brain ontogeny (van den Berg et al., 1965; Simms and Pitts, 1970). It has since been measured in various parts of the developing CNS of several species and the general conclusion drawn from those studies was that it closely correlated with the development of GABAergic synaptic endings (Safarov and Sytinsky, 1980). However, this is not born out by a more detailed examination of the data, for example of those in the rat cortex (Coyle and Enna, 1976; Wong and McGeer 1981; Wolff et al., 1984b). There is a detectable GAD activity in the embryonic cortex, well before the appearance of any GABAergic synapses and the largest increase in GAD activity takes place during the second postnatal week thus preceding the maximum rate of growth of GABAergic synapses by several days (Wolff et al., 1984b; Bahr and Wolff, 1985). In fact, immunohistochemical studies indicated that, in the rat cerebellum, GAD is present in growing axons during the development of Purkinje and Golgi cells and only in the adult tissue it becomes preferentially associated with synaptic nerve terminals (McLaughlin et al., 1975). Similar results were obtained in the cerebral cortex (Wolff et al., 1984a). In this context, it is interesting to note that an important factor regulating the GAD activity and the production of GAD molecules appears to be GABA itself (repression of the enzyme synthesis by its product, Sze, 1970; Tunnicliff and Ngo, 1986).

GAD activity in vitro is significantly increased by the presence of the non-polar detergent Triton X-100 which is thought to liberate additional GAD from occluded GAD pools (van Kampen et al., 1965). Although it was claimed that there were no differences between the early postnatal and adult tissue with respect to the activation by Triton X-100 (van den Berg et al., 1965), more detailed studies suggest that from about the third postnatal week, there may be an additional pool of GAD in the cortical tissue, which requires a higher (0.5% as compared to 0.1%) concentration of Triton X-100 to be activated (Zetzsche et al., 1985; Table 1). This pool of GAD increases during the third and second postnatal week and it could represent the part of GAD associated with the active GABAergic synapses.

There are other differences between the activities of neonatal and adult GAD. For example, GAD in the rat cortex at birth is less sensitive than that in the adult to the inhibition by hydroxamates of aspartate (Wolff et al., 1984b). Since hydroxamates of aspartate act presumably by interfering with the GAD coenzyme pyridoxal phosphate (Taberner et al., 1977) it is possible that the neonatal and adult GAD differ in their relationship to pyridoxal phosphate.

Available experimental data suggest that the alternative synthetic route to GABA, using polyamines as precursors, is not quantitatively very important in the developing central nervous tissue (Seiler and Sarhan, 1983).

Ontogenic development of GABA-T does not differ substantially from that of GAD (Simms and Pitts, 1970) and GABA levels in the developing brain can be manipulated by GABA-T inhibitors in vivo (Hedner et al., 1984; Sykes and Horton, 1986).

The levels of GABA and the activities of GABA-metabolizing enzymes have also been measured in developing cultured neurons (Hauser et al., 1980; Schousboe and Hertz, 1986). The developmental profiles are similar to those observed when the tissue is allowed to develop in vivo and there are no obvious direct relationships to the presence of synapses in culture.

Table 1. GAD Activity in Developing Rat Cortex

Concentration of Triton X-100:	0.1%	0.5%

(a) Frontal Cortex

P 6	2.47 + 0.27 (4)	2.40 + 0.17 (4)
P 10	6.01 ∓ 0.32 (3)	6.01 ∓ 0.66 (4)
P 15	13.55 ∓ 0.93 (3)	15.34 ∓ 0.64 (4)
P 17	14.00 ∓ 0.84 (8)	16.89 ∓ 0.70 (7)[*]
Adult	17.00 ∓ 1.45 (4)	21.21 ∓ 1.84 (4)[*]

(b) Occipital Cortex

P 6	2.12 + 0.13 (4)	2.36 + 0.18 (4)
P 10	5.02 ∓ 0.25 (4)	4.31 ∓ 0.38 (4)
P 16	10.73 ∓ 1.13 (4)	12.63 ∓ 0.69 (4)
P 17	10.92 ∓ 0.51 (8)	14.18 ∓ 0.40 (8)[*]
Adult	15.18 ∓ 1.48 (4)	21.65 ∓ 1.53 (4)[*]

GAD activity (nmol/mg tissue/hour, mean + S.D. of the number of determinations shown in brackets) was measured by the method of Wilson et al. (1972). The asterisks mark statistically significant (P < 0.02) differences between the preparations treated with 0.1% and 0.5% Triton X-100, respectively. P 6, P 10, = Postnatal day 6, 10, etc.

UPTAKE AND RELEASE OF GABA IN THE DEVELOPING RAT CEREBRAL CORTEX

High affinity uptake of GABA (Iversen and Johnston, 1971) exists in the rat cerebral cortex at birth (Johnston and Davies, 1974) and develops at a rapid rate (Coyle and Enna, 1976). Experiments with synaptosomal preparations indicated that the potency of GABA uptake (V_{max}) during the second postnatal week was higher than that in the adult cortex (Redburn et al., 1978). This maximum, which was not observed in the experiments with brain slices (Johnston and Davies, 1974) may have, to some extent, resulted from expressing the results per amount of protein rather than per wet weight of tissue as when using the brain slices. On one hand, this could have artificially increased the values of GABA uptake during the early postnatal period when the content of protein in the tissue is relatively low (Safarov and Sytinsky, 1980) but, on the other hand, the values obtained from studies with brain slices may have been underestimated as a result of the damage to the tissue caused by the experimental procedure (Iversen and Neal, 1968). Preliminary investigations (Balcar, unpublished) indicated that, while this damage was negligible in tissue slices prepared from the adult tissue, it may have reduced the GABA uptake observed in the slices of early postnatal cortex by more than 50%. Consequently, it seems that the potency of high affinity uptake of GABA in the rat cortex indeed passes through a maximum during the second postnatal week, perhaps because of a transiently high density of GABA-accumulating structures. The precise nature of these structures is not known. It is improbable that they are GABAergic synaptic terminals (Wolff et al., 1984b; Bahr and Wolff, 1985) and, in fact, the substrate specificity of GABA uptake in young cortical tissue would seem to suggest that at least a part of GABA uptake system at that developmental stage is localized in glial cells (Wong and McGeer, 1981; Wolff et al., 1984b). However, [^{3}H]β-alanine used in the experiments of Wong and McGeer (1981) to mark the GABA-accumulating compartment in glial cells, may not be the ideal substrate for this purpose (Balcar and Chronwall, 1981; Larsson et al., 1986) and, furthermore, the structural requirements of the binding site on the GABA uptake carrier may undergo changes during the differentiation (Balcar et al., 1979; Balcar and Hauser, 1982).

Kelly et al. (1974) studied the locus of GABA uptake in the developing brain tissue by an alternative experimental approach based on subcellular fractionation of cortical slices preloaded with [^{3}H]GABA. The results indicated that GABA uptake into cell bodies, but not that into nerve terminals, was greater in immature as compared to mature brain tissue. However, this technique involves homogenization of the tissue under Na^+- free conditions and, since GABA uptake is strongly dependent on extracellular concentrations of Na^+ (Martin, 1976) this may have lead to leakage of radioactivity from structures containing [^{3}H]GABA. Consequently, the observed differences may reflect different sensitivities of GABA uptake to external Na^+ in immature and adult tissue, respectively. In fact, it has been demonstrated that the relationship between GABA uptake and extracellular concentrations of Na^+ changes during the development, both in vivo (Vanker, 1979) and in cultured neurons (Schousboe and Hertz, 1986).

Potassium-stimulated, Ca^{2+}-dependent release of [^{3}H]GABA was demonstrated in the slices of neonatal developing rat cortex (Davies et al., 1975) i.e. at a developmental stage when most of the cortical synapses have not yet been formed. In contrast, according to studies on cortical synaptosomes, Ca^{2+} -dependent release of GABA did not develop significantly before the third postnatal week (Redburn et al., 1978). More recent studies (Balcar et al., 1983; 1986b) indicated that, in the rat cortex, development of GABA-releasing mechanism preceded the formation of synapses by about 10 days and, moreover, a large part of the stimulus-coupled release of GABA in the early postnatal cortex was Ca^{2+}-independent. It is interesting that the development of GABA release was found to precede the GABAergic synaptogenesis even when a very different experimental model – evoked release of endogenous GABA from the cortex of anaesthetized kittens – was used (Hicks et al., 1986). While the appearance and development of Ca^{2+} -dependent release of GABA in rat cortex may correlate with the formation and maturation of GABAergic synapses, the non-synaptic, less Ca^{2+}-dependent release observed during first two postnatal weeks may represent the release from axonal growth cones (Gordon-Weeks et al, 1984) some of which may eventually develop into GABAergic synapses (Bahr and Woltt, 1985).

GABA RECEPTORS AND ENDOGENOUS INHIBITORS

The proposed mechanism of the trophic action of GABA would involve changes in the average potential of the neuronal membrane (Wolff, 1981). Such changes would presumably be brought about by interactions of GABA with GABA receptor-ionophore complexes. In fact, GABA receptor-binding sites appear very early in the ontogeny (Coyle and Enna, 1976), well before the GABAergic synapses are present in any significant number. In the developing rat cerebral cortex, there is a steady increase in the density of GABA binding sites but their gross characteristics, such as relative proportions of $GABA_A$ and $GABA_B$ sites, do not change significantly with age (Balcar et al., 1986a). Both high and low affinity components of $GABA_A$ binding sites (Skeritt and Johnston, 1982) are present at birth (Aldinio et al., 1980) even though the affinity of $GABA_B$ sites seems to decrease somewhat with age (Horton and Sykes, 1982).

The kinetic parameters of GABA binding sites in brain membranes are dependent on the methods used to prepare the membranes; for example, increases in affinity and/or number of binding sites following detergent treatment or freeze-thaw regimes (Enna and Snyder, 1977; Johnston and Kennedy, 1978; Chiu and Rosenberg, 1979). Exposure of these 'latent' binding sites is due to the removal of substances that inhibit GABA binding and which are normally incorporated into the membranes (Johnston and Kennedy, 1978). A variety of such endogenous inhibitors exist and they have been called collectively GABARINS (GABA Receptor Inhibitors) (Johnston et al., 1982). GABARINS are likely to be involved in many aspects of the function of GABA as a major inhibitory transmitter, controlling the affinity and availability of certain receptors, e.g. in supersensitivity or desensitization phenomena. Peptides, phospholipids, proteins, purines and steroids may function as GABARINS. Ontogenetic studies indicate that there is greater endogenous inhibition of GABA binding sites in neonatal rat brain than in the adult suggesting that decreases in endogenous inhibitor levels during maturation may be related to neuronal development (Skerritt and Johnston, 1982). The presence of endogenous inhibitors of GABA binding in rat forebrain and cerebellum before most synapses have been formed may suggest that these inhibitors function to make 'non-synaptic' GABA binding sites less sensitive to GABA until they are activated by the presence of GABAergic structures.

The existence of receptor-associated phenomena, such as denervation supersensitivity or receptor desensitization would seem to suggest that the GABA receptor and its endogenous inhibitors could be the most flexible link in the chain of events constituting the trophic action of GABA. Several recent experimental studies support this notion but the findings are somewhat paradoxical. Introduction of exogeneous GABA or (artificial) elevation of the levels of endogeneous GABA seems to increase the number of GABA receptor-binding sites, i.e. presumably they sensitize, rather than desensitize, the neuronal membrane to GABA. This result has been obtained with a wide variety of experimental models both in the adult and early postnatal brain tissue and also in cultured neurons (Madtes and Redburn, 1983; Meier et al., 1983; 1984; Sykes et al., 1984; Beart et al., 1985; Sykes and Horton, 1986). It seems to be mediated by high affinity GABA receptors (Meier et al., 1985; Belhage et al., 1986) and studies with retina suggest that there is a sensitive time-period during which the effect is particularly strong (Madtes and Bashir-Elahi, 1986).

This raises some interesting questions which may have significant implications for the studies of the mechanism of the trophic action of GABA on the molecular level. For example, can barbiturates, which interact preferentially with the high affinity component of GABA binding, influence the GABA-dependent aspects of neuronal development? Is the period of increased in vivo sensitivity to the trophic action of GABA related to the greater effect of endogeneous GABA-inhibitory factors (GABARINS) observed in neonatal brain? Does the increased density of GABA-binding sites indeed reflect a more potent effect of GABA on Cl^--permeability of the neuronal membrane?

CONCLUSIONS

The available experimental data suggest that the neurochemical functions of GABAergic neurons undergo a set of distinct changes which may be quite complex in nature. In particular, the presence of synthesis, catabolism, stimulus-coupled release, neuronal receptors, endogeneous inhibitors and specific uptake, of GABA, respectively, in the pre-natal or early post-natal nervous tissue and the fact that the process of neurochemical maturation precedes, rather than follows, the GABAergic synaptogenesis, is in accordance with the proposition that GABA acts as a trophic factor in the neuronal development.

ACKNOWLEDGEMENTS

The authors are grateful to the Australian National Health and Medical Research Council for financial support.

REFERENCES

Aghajanian GK, Bloom FE (1967): The formation of synaptic junctions in developing rat brain: a quantitative electron microscopic study. Brain Res 6:716-727.

Aldinio C, Balzano MA, Toffano G (1980): Onto-genetic development of GABA recognition sites in different brain areas. Pharmacol Res C 12:495-500.

Aloisi F, Gallo V, Levi G (1983): Substrate specificity and development aspects of a presynaptic GABA receptor regulating glutamate release in the rat cerebellum. J Neurosci Res 10:141-149.

Bahr S, Wolff JR (1985): Postnatal development of axosomatic synapses in the rat visual cortex: morphogenesis and quantitative evaluation. J Comp Neurol 233:405-420.

Balcar VJ, Mark J, Borg J, Mandel P (1979): High affinity uptake of gamma-aminobutyric acid in cultured glial and neuronal cells. Neurochem Res 4:339-354.

Balcar VJ, Chronwall BM (1981): High affinity uptake of taurine and beta-alanine - A mechanism involved in neuronal differentiation In DeFeudis FV, Mandel P: "Amino Acid Neurotransmitters". Advances in Biochemical Pharmacology Vol. 29, New York: Raven Press, pp 151-160.

Balcar VJ, Hauser KL (1982): Development of uptake of gamma-aminobutyrate in cultured neurons. In "Abstracts of XIIth International Congress of Biochemistry". Perth, WA, p 95.

Balcar VJ, Dammasch I, Wolff JR (1983): Is there a non-synaptic component in the K^+-stimulated release of GABA in the developing rat cortex? Dev Brain Res 10:309-311.

Balcar VJ, Joo F, Kasa P, Dammasch IE, Wolff JR (1986a):

GABA receptor binding in rat cerebral cortex and superior cervical ganglion in the absence of GABAergic synapses. Neurosci Lett 66:269-274.

Balcar VJ, Damm S, Wolff JR (1986b): Ontogeny of K⁺-stimulated release of [³H]GABA in rat cerebral cortex studied by a simple technique in vitro. Neurochem Int 89:573-580.

Beart PM, Scatton B, Lloyd KG (1985): Sub-chronic administration of GABAergic agonists elevates [³H]GABA binding and produces tolerance in striatal dopamine catabolism. Brain Res 335:169-173.

Belhage B, Meier E, Schousboe A (1986): GABA agonists induce the formation of low-affinity GABA receptors on cultured cerebellar granule cells via preexisting high affinity GABA receptors. Neurochem Res 11:599-606.

Berry M, Rogers AW (1965): The migration of neuroblasts in the developing cerebral cortex. J Anat 99:691-709.

Blue M, Parnavelas JG (1983): The formation and maturation of synapses in the visual cortex of the rat. II. Quantitative analysis. J Neurocytol 12:697-712.

Boistel J, Fatt P (1958): Membrane permeability change during inhibitory transmitter action. J Physiol (Lond) 144:176-191.

Bowery NG (1982): Baclofen, 10 years on. Trends Pharm Sci 3:400-403.

Bowery NG, Jones GP, Neal MJ (1976): Selective inhibition of neuronal GABA uptake by cis-1,3-aminocyclohexane carboxylic acid. Nature 264:281-284.

Brennan MJW, Cantrill RC, Krogsgaard-Larssen P (1981): GABA autoreceptors: Structure-Activity Relationships for Agonists. In Costa E, DiChiara G, Gessa GL (eds): "GABA and Benzodiazepine Receptors". New York: Raven Press, pp 151-167.

Carver MJ, Copenhaver JH, Serpan RA (1965): Free amino acids in fetal rat brain. Influence of L-phenylalanine. J Neurochem 12:857-861.

Chiu TH, Rosenberg HC (1979): Differential effects of Triton X-100 on benzodiazepine and GABA binding in a freeze-thawed synaptosomal fraction of rat brain. Eur J Pharmac 58:335-338.

Chronwall BM, Wolff JR (1980): Prenatal and postnatal development of GABA accumulating cells in the occipital neocortex of rat. J Comp Neurol 190:187-208.

Coyle JT (1982): Development of neurotransmitters in the neocortex. In Rakic P, Goldman PS (eds): "Development and Modifiability of the Cerebral Cortex". Neurosci Res

Progr Bull 20:479–492.

Coyle JT, Enna SJ (1976): Neurochemical aspects of the ontogenesis of GABAergic neurons in the rat brain. Brain Res 111:119–133.

Curtis DR, Duggan AW, Felix D, Johnston GAR (1970): GABA, bicuculline and central inhibition. Nature 226:1227–1224.

Curtis DR, Watkins JC (1960): The excitation and depression of spinal neurons by structurally related amino acids. J Neurochem 6:117–141.

Cutler RWP, Dudzinski DS (1974): Regional changes in amino acid content in developing rat brain. J Neurochem 23:1005–1009.

Dames W, Joo F, Feher O, Toldi J, Wolff JR (1985): Gamma-aminobutyric acid enables synaptogenesis in the intact superior cervical ganglion of the adult rat. Neurosci Lett 54:159–164.

Davies LP, Johnston GAR, Stephanson AL (1975): Postnatal changes in the potassium stimulated calcium-dependent release of radioactive GABA and glycine from slices of rat cerebral nervous tissue. J Neurochem 25:387–392.

Emson PC, Hunt SP (1981): Anatomical chemistry of the cerebral cortex. In Schmitt FO, Worden FG, Adelman G, Dennis SG (eds): "The Organization of Cerebral Cortex". Cambridge, Mass. and London, England: MIT-Press, pp 325–345.

Enna SJ, Snyder SH (1977): Influences of ions, enzymes and detergents on gamma-aminobutyric acid receptor binding. Mol Pharmac 13:442–453.

Farkas Z, Kasa P, Balcar VJ, Joo F, Wolff JR (1986): Type A and B GABA receptors mediate inhibition of acetylcholine release from cholinergic nerve terminals in the superior cervical ganglion of rat. Neurochem Int 8:565–572.

Fonnum F (1968): The distribution of glutamate decarboxylase and aspartate transaminase in subcellular fractions of rat and guinea-pig brain. Biochem J 106:401–412.

Gordon-Weeks PR, Lockerbie RO, Pearce BR (1984): Uptake and release of [^{3}H]GABA by growth cones isolated from neonatal rat brain. Neurosci Lett 52:205–210.

Harris AR, Allen AM (1985): Functional coupling of gamma-aminobutyric acid receptors to chloride channels in brain membrane. Science 228:1108–1110.

Hauser KL, Balcar VJ, Bernasconi R (1980): Development of GABA neurons in dissociated cell cultures of rat cerebral cortex. In Lal H et al (eds): "GABA Neurotransmitters" Brain Res Bull (Suppl) 5:37–41.

Hansen GH, Meier E, Schousboe A (1984): GABA influences the ultrastructure composition of cerebellar granule cells during development in culture. Int J Dev Neurosci 2:247–257.

Hedner T, Iversen K, Lundberg P (1984): Central GABA mechanisms during postnatal development in the rat: neurochemical characteristics. J Neural Transmission 59:105–118.

Hicks TP, Ruwe WD, Veale WL (1986): Release of gamma–aminobutyric acid from the visual cortex of young kittens. Dev Brain Res 24:299–304.

Horton RW, Sykes CC (1982): Development of GABA-B binding sites in the cerebral cortex and cerebellum of the rat. Br J Pharmacol 77:498P.

Iversen LL, Neal MJ (1968): The uptake of $[^3H]$GABA by slices of cerebral cortex. J Neurochem 15:1141–1149.

Iversen LL, Johnston GAR (1971): GABA uptake in rat cerebral nervous system: comparison of uptake in slices and homogenates and the effect of some inhibitors. J Neurochem 18:1939–1950.

Jacobson M (1978): "Developmental Neurobiology". New York: Plenum Press.

Jaffe EH, Cuello AC (1980): Release of gamma–aminobutyrate from the external plexiform layer of the rat olfactory bulb: possible dendritic involvement. Neuroscience 5:1859–1869.

Johnston GAR (1977): Effects of calcium on the potassium–stimulated release of radioactive beta–alanine and gamma–aminobutyric acid from slices of rat cerebral cortex and spinal cord. Brain Res 121:119–121.

Johnston GAR (1978): Transmitter inactivation processes. Proc Aust Physiol Pharmac Soc 9:94–98.

Johnston GAR, Mitchell JF (1971): The effect of bicuculline, metrazole, picrotoxin and strychnine on the release of $[^3H]$GABA from rat brain slices. J Neurochem 18:2441–2446.

Johnston GAR, Davies LP (1974): Postnatal changes in the high affinity uptake of glycine and GABA in the rat central nervous system. J Neurochem 22:101–105.

Johnston GAR, Krogsgaard–Larsen P, Stephanson AL, Twitchin B (1976): Inhibition of the uptake of GABA and related amino acids in rat brain slices by the optical isomers of nipecotic acid. J Neurochem 26:1029–1033.

Johnston GAR, Kennedy SME (1978): GABA receptors and

phospholipids. In Fonnum F (eds): "Amino Acids as Chemical Transmitters" Plenum Press, New York: pp 507-516.

Johnston GAR, Willow M (1982): GABA and barbiturate receptors. Trends Pharmac Sci 3:328-330.

Johnston GAR, Hailstone MH, Freeman CG (1980): Baclofen: Stereoselective inhibitor of excitant amino acid release. J Pharm Pharmacol 32:230-231.

Johnston GAR, Skerritt JH, Willow W (1982): Endogenous inhibitors of GABA receptors: developmental, drug and environmental aspects. In Okada A, Roberts E (eds): "Problems in GABA Research" Excerpta Medica pp 293-301.

Johnston GAR, Allan RD, Skerritt JH (1984): GABA receptors. In Lajtha A (ed): "Handbook of Neurochemistry" New York: Plenum Press, pp 213-237.

Johnston MV, Coyle JT (1980): Ontogeny of neurochemical markers for noradrenergic, GABAergic and cholinergic neurons in neocotex lesioned with methylazoxymethanol acetate. J Neurochem 34:1429-1441.

Kasematsu T, Pettigrew JD (1976): Depletion of brain catecholamines: failure of ocular dominance shift after monocular occlusion in kittens. Science 194:206-209.

Kelly P, Luttges M, Johnston T, Grove W (1974): Maturation-dependent compartmentalization in neural tissue in vitro. Brain Res 68:267-280.

Krogsgaard-Larsen P, Johnston GAR (1975): Inhibition of GABA uptake in rat brain slices by nipecotic acid, various isoxazoles and related compounds. J Neurochem 25:797-802.

Larsson OM, Johnston GAR, Schousboe A (1983): Differences in uptake kinetics of cis-3-aminocyclohexane carboxylic acid into neurons and astrocytes in primary cultures. Brain Res 260:279-285.

Larsson OM, Griffiths R, Allen IC, Schousboe A (1986): Mutual inhibition kinetic analysis of gamma-aminobutyric acid, taurine and beta-alanine high-affinity transport into neurons and astrocytes: Evidence for similarity between the taurine and beta-alanine carriers in both cell types. J Neurochem 47:426-432.

Levy WB, Redburn DA, Cotman CW (1973): Stimulus-coupled secretion of gamma-aminobutyric acid from rat brain synaptosomes. Science 181:676-678.

Lodge D, Curtis DR, Johnston GAR (1978): Does uptake limit the action of GABA agonists in vivo Experiments with muscimol, isoguvacine and THIP in cat spinal cord. J Neurochem 31:1525-1528.

Madtes P Jr, Redburn DA (1983): GABA as a trophic factor during development. Life Sci 33:979-984.

Madtes P Jr, Bashir-Elahi R (1986): GABA receptor binding site "induction" in rabbit retina after nipecotic acid treatment: changes during postnatal development. Neurochem Res 11:55-61.

Martin DL (1976): Carrier-mediated transport removal of GABA from synaptic regions. In Roberts E, Chase TN, Tower DB (eds): "GABA in Nervous System Function" New York: Raven Press, pp 347-386.

McLaughlin BJ, Wood JG, Saito K, Roberts E, Wu JY (1975): The fine structural localization of glutamic acid decarboxylase in developing axonal processes and pre-synaptic terminals of rodent cerebellum. Brain Res 85:355-371.

Meier E, Drejer J, Schousboe A (1983): Trophic actions of GABA on the development of physiologically active GABA receptors. In Mandel P, DeFeudis (eds): "CNS Receptors - From Molecular Pharmacology to Behavior". New York: Raven Press, pp 47-58.

Meier E, Drejer J, Schousboe A (1984): GABA induces functionally active low-affinity GABA receptors in cultured cerebellar granule cells. J Neurochem 43:1737-1744.

Meier E, Hansen GH, Schousboe A (1985): The trophic effect of GABA on cerebellar granule cells is mediated by GABA-receptors. Int J Dev Neurosci 3:401-407.

Meier E, Jorgensen OS (1986): Gamma-aminobutyric acid affects the developmental expression of neuron-associated proteins in cerebellar granule cells. J Neurochem 46:1256-1262.

Metcalf BW (1979): Inhibitions of GABA metabolism. Biochem Pharmacol 28:1705-1712.

Miller MW (1986a): Maturation of rat visual cortex III. Postnatal morphogenesis and synaptogenesis of local circuit neurons. Dev Brain Res 25:271-285.

Miller MW (1986b): The migration and neurochemical differentiation of gamma-aminobutyric acid (GABA) - immunoreactive neurons in rat visual cortex as demonstrated by a combined immunochemical-autoradiographic technique. Dev Brain Res 28:41-46.

Minchin MCW, Iversen LL (1974): Release of [^{3}H]gamma-aminobutyric acid from glial cells in rat dorsal root ganglia. J Neurochem 23:535-540.

Mitchell PR, Martin IL (1978): Is GABA release modulated by presynaptic receptor Nature 271:901 905.

Mohler H, Okada T (1977): Benzodiazepine receptor: Demonstration in the central nervous system. Science 198:849–851.

Potashner SJ (1979): Baclofen effects on amino acid release and metabolism in slices of guinea pig cerebral cortex. J Neurochem 32:103–109.

Redburn DA, Broome D, Ferkany J, Enna SJ (1978): Development of rat brain uptake and calcium–dependent release of GABA. Brain Res 152:511–519.

Ribak CE (1978): Aspinous and sparsely spinous stellate neurons in the visual cortex of rat contain glutamic acid decarboxylase. J Neurocytol 7:461–478.

Rickman M, Chronwall BM, Wolff JR (1977): On the development of non-pyramidal neurons and axons outside the cortical plate: the early marginal zone as a pallial anlage. Anat Embryol 151:285–307.

Roberts PJ (1974): Amino acid release from isolated rat dorsal root ganglia. Brain Res 74:327–332.

Roberts E, Frankel S (1951): Further studies of glutamic acid in brain. J Biol Chem 190:505–512.

Safarov MI, Sytinsky IA (1980) "Gamma–aminobutyric acid in the developing brain". Baku, ASSR: Publishing House "Elm", pp 10–22.

Schon F, Kelly JS (1975): Selective uptake of ^{3}H–beta–alanine by glia: association with glial uptake system for GABA. Brain Res 86:243–247.

Schousboe A, Hertz L (1986): Primary cultures of GABAergic and glutamatergic neurons as model systems to study neurotransmitter functions. In Vernadakis A, Giacobini E (eds): "Model Systems of Development and Aging of the Nervous System" Boston: M Nijhoff Publ, in press.

Seiler N (1981): Polyamine metabolism and function in brain. Neurochem Int 3:95–110.

Seiler N, Sarhan S (1983): Metabolic routes of GABA formation in chicken embryo brain. Neurochem Int 5:525–633.

Sims KL, Pitts FN Jr (1970): Brain glutamate decarboxylase: changes in the developing rat brain. J Neurochem 17:1607–1612.

Skerritt JH, Johnston GAR (1982): Postnatal development of GABA binding sites and their endogenous inhibitors in rat brain. Devel Neurosci 5:189–197.

Snodgrass SR (1978): Use of ^{3}H–muscimol for GABA receptor studies. Nature 273:392–394.

Spoerri PE, Wolff JR (1981): Effect of GABA administration on murine neuroblastoma cells in culture cell. Cell

Tiss Res 218:567-579.

Srinivasan V, Neal MJ, Mitchell JF (1969): The effect of electrical stimulation and high potassium concentration on efflux of [^{3}H]gamma-aminobutyric acid from brain slices. J Neurochem 16:1235-1244.

Sykes CC, Prestwich S, Horton R (1984): Chronic admini stration of the GABA-transaminase inhibitor ethanola-mine-O-sulphate leads to up-regulation of GABA binding sites. Biochem Pharmacol 33:387-393.

Sykes CC, Horton RW (1986): Development of the gamma-aminobutyric acid neurotransmitter system in the rat cerebral cortex during repeated administration of the GABA-transaminase inhibitor, ethanolamine-O-sul-phate. J Neurochem 46:213-217.

Sze PY (1970): Possible repression of L-glutamic acid decarboxylase by gamma-aminobutyric acid in developing mouse brain. Brain Res 19:322-325.

Taberner PV, Pearce MJ, Watkins JC (1977): The inhibition of mouse brain glutamate decarboxylase by some structural analogues of L-glutamic acid. Biochem Pharmacol 26:345-349.

Tallman JW, Gallagher DW (1985): The GABAergic system. A locus of benzodiazepine action. Ann Rev Neurosci 8:21-24.

Tunnicliff G, Ngo TT (1986): Commentary: regulation of gamma-aminobutyric acid synthesis in the vertebrate nervous system. Neurochem Int 8:287-297.

Vanker AD (1979): Effects of temperature and sodium on ^{14}C-GABA transport into adult and neonatal rat brain crude synaptosomal fractions. Dev Neurosci 2:86-93.

van den Berg CJ, van Kampen GMJ, Schade JP, Veldstra M (1965): Levels and intracellular localization of glutamate decarboxylase and other enzymes during the development of the brain. J Neurochem 12:863-869.

van Kampen GMJ, van den Berg CJ, van der Helm HJ, Veldstra H (1965): Intracellular localization of glutamate decarboxylase, gamma-aminobutyric transaminase and some other enzymes in brain tissue. J Neurochem 12:581-588.

Wilson SH, Schrier BK, Farber JL, Thompson EJ, Rosenberg RN, Blume AJ, Nirenberg MW (1972): Markers for gene expression in cultured cells from the nervous system. J Biol Chem 247:3159-3169.

Wolff JR (1981): Evidence for a dual role of GABA as a synaptic transmitter and a promoter of synaptogenesis. In DeFeudis FV, Mandel P (eds): "Amino Acid Neurotransmitters", Adv Biochem Psychopharmacol 29. New

York: Raven Press, pp 125-239.

Wolff JR, Joo F, Dames W (1978): Plasticity in dendrites shown by continuous GABA administration in superior cervical ganglion of adult rat. Nature 274:72-74.

Wolff JR, Bottcher H, Zetzsche T, Oertel WH, Chronwall BM (1984a): Development of GABAergic neurons in rat visual cortex as identified by glutamate decarboxylase-like immunoreactivity. Neurosci Lett 47:207-212.

Wolff JR, Balcar VJ, Zetzsche T, Bottcher H, Schmechel DE, Chronwall BM (1984b): Development of GABAergic system in rat visual cortex. In Lauder JM, Nelson PG (eds): "Gene Expression and Cell-Cell Interactions in the Developing Nervous System". New York: Plenum Press, pp 121-239.

Wong PT, McGeer EG (1981): Postnatal changes of GABAergic and glutamatergic parameters. Dev Brain Res 1:519-530.

Zetzsche T, Balcar VJ, Wolff JR (1985): Comparison of GAD in early postnatal and adult cortex. J Neurochem 44:S128B.

Neurotrophic Activity of GABA During Development, pages 79–108
© **1987 Alan R. Liss, Inc.**

DEVELOPMENTAL ALTERATIONS IN RETINAL GABAERGIC NEURONS

Dianna A. Redburn and M. Elizabeth Keith

Department of Neurobiology and Anatomy
University of Texas Medical School
Houston, Texas 77025

INTRODUCTION

The preceding chapters of this volume have provided an extensive and thorough review of the general characteristics of the GABAergic system and its development in the nervous system. We have focused on one specific CNS structure, the retina, in a careful examination of the postnatal development of its GABAergic pathways. Our results have revealed a highly complex, neonatal pattern, associated with certain cell populations whose anatomical relationships and time of appearance suggest an important, perhaps pioneering role in retinal development. Our aim in this chapter is to review morphological data from our studies of the neonatal rabbit retina and evaluate these results in terms of support for the hypothesis that pioneering GABAergic cells may provide structural and/or chemical (trophic) influences important in retinal synaptogenesis. Subsequent chapters in this volume describe more direct experimental tests of the possible trophic actions of GABA in retina (Madtes, this volume) and other tissues in situ or in culture. Our studies per se do not directly test this hypothesis, rather they provide circumstantial evidence for the importance of GABAergic neurons and they offer an indepth analysis of developing relationships, in the hope that more specific and discrete predictions and hypotheses might be developed. Before presenting data from our own laboratory, we provide below, a brief review of retinal development.

The vertebrate retina provides a highly appropriate CNS tissue for developmental analysis. The structure-function relationships of retinal neurons have been intensely studied for almost a hundred years (Ramon y Cajal, 1893), and the resulting body of knowledge makes the retina one of the best understood areas of the CNS. Major cell types are clearly recognizable and major functional circuits have been defined (Kolb and Nelson, 1985; Sterling et al., 1986). Patterns of light and darkness within the visual field create a visual mosaic which is transduced by photoreceptors and transmitted to higher centers via the "straight-through" retinal pathway. This rigorously studied pathway consists of projections from photoreceptor to bipolar to ganglion cells. Interestingly, all three of these cell types probably use glutamate as their neurotransmitter (Brecha, 1983).

Structural studies have established some broad principles which may govern the development of the straight-through pathway. ^{3}H-Thymidine studies have determined specific dates at which cell populations undergo their final mitotic division, thus establishing birthdays for major morphological cell types. Ganglion cells are produced first, then bipolar cells in the inner nuclear layer and finally photoreceptors (Carter-Dawson and LaVail, 1979; Rapaport and Stone, 1983; Walsh and Polley, 1985). However, synapses between these cell types mature in a different sequence. Ganglion cell dendrites and photoreceptor terminals, which appear first, are subsequently linked by the insertion of bipolar axons and dendrites, which appear later (Blanks et al., 1974; McArdle et al., 1977; Maslim and Stone, 1986).

Developmental cues responsible for establishing the arrangement of the straight-through pathway can be explained theoretically with fairly simple principles (Sidman, 1961; Sidman and Rakic, 1973). Cell division is primarily restricted to the germinal layer at the ventricular surface of the optic lobe in the developing diencephalon. Cells undergo interkinetic migration to the outer retinal surface during interphase and they drop out of the mitotic cycle at the most distant point in their migration. Ganglion cells drop out first and are therefore located at the furthest point from the germinal layer, appropriately named the ganglion cell layer. Large numbers of ganglion cells are present initially. Cell death pares down the final number substantially (Sengelaub and Finlay, 1982; Young, 1984). Bipolar cells are produced in a like manner and are layered immediately adjacent to the ganglion cell population. Finally, photoreceptors leave the mitotic cycle and form the largest population of cells in the retina. Simple competition could establish a mosaic arrangement and ensure uniform cell density based on the minimum nearest-neighbor distance which would be consistant with cell viability. Their common use of glutamate might suggest other similarities among these cell populations.

The development of synaptic connections could simply reflect the birthday sequence of cell types, coupled with temporal as well as spatial competition. Ganglion and photoreceptor cell bodies lie directly adjacent to the synaptic layer to which their respective dendrites and axons project. Since these processes extend relatively short distances from the parent cell body, they would be the first to appear during development. On the other hand, bipolar cell bodies lie in the middle of the inner plexiform layer and their processes must extend relatively longer distances to the synaptic layers from the cell body, which could explain why they are observed to synapse with photoreceptor and ganglion cell processes already in place.

This highly simplistic hypothesis addresses only the major classes of cells in the straight-through pathway. It does not take into account the different subclasses of photoreceptor, bipolar and ganglion cells and how they may sort themselves out into correct visual circuits. However, it serves to illustrate the point that general principles may be developed to offer a simplistic explanation of developmental events governing the straight-through pathway.

The lateral pathways of the retina are a different matter. The two major classes of laterally arranged cells, horizontal and amacrine cells, are primarily involved in horizontal integration of information from the straight-through pathway (Dacheux and Miller, 1981a; Dacheux and Miller, 1981b). Thus, their primary functional organization relates to synaptic space across the retina rather than space within the visual field. Their processes are functionally organized perpendicular to the migration path of developing neurons along radial glia. In contrast to the straight-through neurons, the functional arrangement of lateral neurons cannot be explained, even at the most superficial level, by the order in which neurons leave the mitotic cycle or by formation of synaptic connections based on the growth rate of neurites. Lateral networks must select synaptic partners through a process which distinguishes among elements in the immediate surround and it seems unlikely that simple temporal or spatial competition could provide the necessary cues for the appropriate developmental arrangement of these cells.

Different classes of horizontal cells seek out synaptic connections within specific populations of cones or rods, or both (Dowling and Boycott, 1966; Stell, 1972). They provide inhibitory feedback surrounds for each mosaic unit of the straight-through pathway. Their function is linked to the fact that these cells remain electrically coupled to gap junctions even in the adult (Negishi and Drujan, 1979; Dowling, 1986). Perhaps these gap junctions provide a means during development for coordinated development of all the cells in a homogenous population. Horizontal cell bodies are arranged in functional layers; their synaptic connections follow a much more complex arrangement (Stell, 1967).

In contrast, amacrine cell bodies are not strictly arranged in functional layers; different functional classes of amacrines can be found side by side (Kolb and Nelson, 1985; Pourcho, 1980). Their terminals, however, are distinctly layered and form discrete horizontal bands throughout the inner plexiform layer. Disregarding possible differences in amacrine subclasses, many or most of these cells leave the mitotic cycle after ganglion cells but before bipolar cells. However, this inner-to-outer maturation gradient alone is not sufficient to explain the complex synaptic contacts and precisely arranged terminal fields of amacrine processes. Clearly synaptogenesis and neurite growth must follow some radically different set of developmental cues.

The inner plexiform layer represents a formatible challenge because the function of the majority of synaptic connections are not fully understood. Amacrine cell synapses are by far the largest component of this synaptic layer. Electrophysiological studies are beginning to elucidate the subtle functional effects of these cell types on higher order visual processing which are reflected in the complex field characteristics of established ganglion cells (Kolb and Nelson, 1985; Miller, 1979).

Interplexiform cells represent an additional class of retinal interneurons which were observed in early reports (Ramon y Cajal, 1893)) but only recently appreciated (Gallego, 1971; Oyster and Takahashi, 1977). These cells are thought to be primarily arranged with dendrites in the inner synaptic layer and axons in the outer plexiform layer. Emerging knowledge of their functional importance suggest they may feedback to control horizontal cells and thus participate in light adaptive responses (Dowling and Ehinger, 1978; Hedden and Dowling, 1978).

The identification of retinal neurotransmitters such as GABA, has provided important tools for circuit analysis and hence developmental studies. Studies over the past decade have established the identity of the neurotransmitters used by approximately 75% of the amacrine cell population of which there are approximately 30 subclasses (Brecha, 1983; Massey and Redburn, 1987). Numerous GABAergic amacrine cells are present in the vertebrate retina, and they form complex circuits which are arranged in at least five different populations (Kolb and Nelson, 1985). GABAergic horizontal cells (H1) are found in nonmammalian (Stell, 1972; Marc et al., 1978) and neonatal mammalian vertebrates (Schnitzer and Rusoff, 1984; Redburn and Madtes, 1986; Osborne et al., 1986). However, most (Ehinger, 1970; Brandon et al., 1979) but not all investigators (Bolz and McGuire, 1985) fail to find GABAergic horizontal cells in adult mammalian species. GABAergic interplexiform cells have been described in adult retinas from several vertebrate species (Nakamura et al., 1980) and we describe them here, for the first time, in neonatal rabbit retina.

POSTNATAL DEVELOPMENT OF GABA IN RABBIT RETINA

Our interest in retinal development has centered on the role of neurotransmitters in the formation of functional visual circuits. We wish to determine the nature of directed outgrowth of neurotransmitter-specific neuronal processes and their eventual synaptic connections. For several reasons, we have focused primarily on cells which are GABAergic. First, we have studied GABAergic neurons and their related circuitry in the adult and thus have some general notions about the maturational end-point of the developmental process for these cells. Furthermore we are able to take advantage of a variety of cell markers for GABAergic cells as well as several useful GABA mimetics to alter GABAergic functions. We had hoped, rather naively as it turns out, that the documentation of GABAergic development could also help to simplify some of the confusion which exists concerning functional subclasses of GABAergic amacrine cells. We had hoped to follow the development of the rabbit retina from a relatively undifferentiated and simple state to the more complex adult state in which perhaps five different GABAergic amacrine cell populations exist. Furthermore we were hopeful that these five cell populations might develop at slightly different times so that we could differentiate among them in the immature retina if not in the adult. Our experimental results did not meet these early expectations. Rather we found the neonatal retina contains a more complex array of GABA-positive cells than does the adult. Thus it appears that post-natal retinal development does not involve sequential addition of specific GABAergic cell populations; rather, it involves a significant pearing down or subtraction of GABAergic cells, leaving only selected cells for formation of mature circuits. These conclusions are based on the findings which are summarized below and which have been previously published (Redburn et al., 1985); Redburn et al., 1982; Redburn et al., 1983; Redburn and Madtes, 1986; Moran et al., 1986; Keith and Redburn, 1987) or are currently in preparation (Keith and Redburn, in preparation; Moran et al., in preparation).

Methods

Litters of New Zealand white rabbits were obtained from a local supplier 1 and 5 days after birth. When necessary pups were housed with their mothers in the original breeding box. Animals were maintained on a 12-hour light/dark cycle and given food and water ad libitum. A minimum of three retinas were examined for each time point.

Autoradiography. At 1 and 5 days after birth, pups were decapitated and retinas were harvested for autoradiography. Isolated retinas were incubated at 37°C with 50 µCi of ^{3}H-GABA (80 µCi/mmol, specific activity, Amersham Corp.), in 0.5 ml of modified Ringer's buffer (Redburn and Madtes, 1986) in a shaking water bath. A steady stream of 95% O_2/5% CO_2 was supplied to the tissue during a 15 min incubation period. Selected samples were postincubated in label-free medium for 30 additional min. As previously reported (Hampton and Redburn, 1983), greater than 90% of the total radioactivity recovered after either of these procedures is still associated with authentic GABA as confirmed by thin-layer chromatography.

The tissue was rinsed, fixed in 2.5% glutaraldehyde in 0.05 M cacodylate buffer overnight at 4°C, post-fixed in 1% osmium tetroxide, dehydrated and embedded in epoxy resin. Vertically oriented sections were cut for light and electron microscopy and autoradiography. For light microscopic (LM) autoradiography the sections were coated with Kodak NBT-2 emulsion; Ilford L-4 emulsion. The emulsion was exposed to the tissue 2-4 weeks. Morphometric analysis of both LM autoradiography and the following immunocytochemistry was aided with a Zeiss Videoplan. Measurements of labeled cells were limited to sections taken from the mid-periphery of the eyecup.

Immunocytochemistry. At 1 and 5 days after birth the pups were decapitated and immediately pithed. The eyecups were hemisected and the posterior half emersed in 4% glutaraldehyde in 0.1 M phosphate buffer for 1 hour, followed by overnight fixation in 0.5% glutaraldehyde, 4% paraformaldehyde in 0.1 M phosphate buffer. Retinas were removed from their eyecups and cryopreserved in 30% sucrose. Frozen sections (20 µm) were cut and melted onto gelatin-coated slides. Sections were incubated in anti-sera (1:1000) overnight in a cold moist chamber. In order to visualize the immunoreactivity, the sections were washed briefly, exposed to goat anti-rabbit IgG conjugated to fluorescein for 1 hour and coverslipped for light microscopy.

The GABA anti-sera (Chemicon) obtained was tested for glutaraldehyde BSA-GSA specificity. Nitrocellulose paper activated with poly-L-lysine (100 µg/ml) was fixed for 1

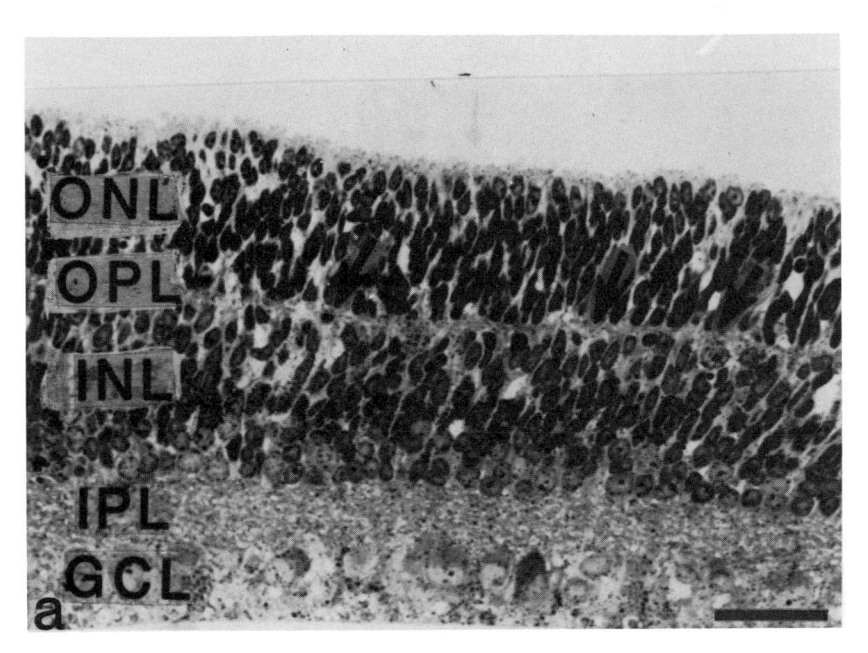

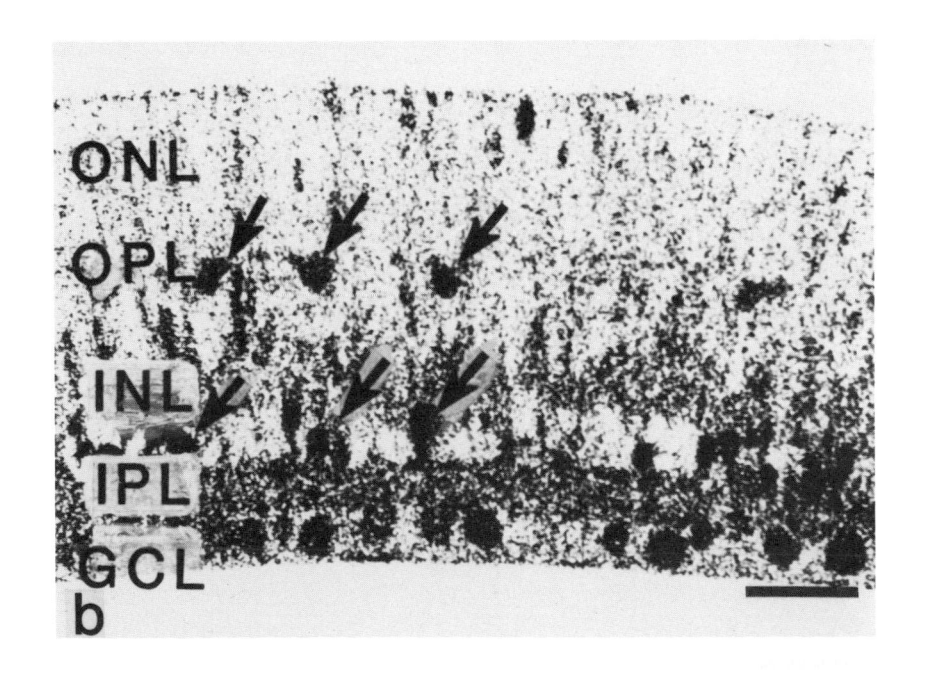

hour with 10% glutaraldehyde in NaOH/KCl buffer (0.2 M, pH 10.0). Amino acids having similar structural characteristics to GABA were chosen as test compounds. Test compounds were spotted onto strips of pre-treated nitrocellulose paper. The strips were incubated in GABA antisera (1:1000) overnight, washed, incubated in goat anti rabbit IgG (1:30), and treated with peroxidase - antiperoxidase. Following a second wash the immunoreactivity was visualized with diaminobenzidine tetrahydrochloride (0.05%) in Tris buffer (50 mM, pH 7.4) with 0.1% hydrogen peroxide added 5 minutes into the twenty minute incubation period.

RESULTS

General Morphology. A pronounced morphological maturation gradient, in the proximal to distal direction, is apparent in neonatal retina (Figs. 1a, b; Fig. 2a). At postnatal day 1, cell bodies in the ganglion cell layer

---

Figure 1. Autoradiograms of isolated retinas from 1-day-old rabbits. a) In general, an inner-to-outer maturation gradient is observed for most retinal cell bodies. Cells in the ganglion cell layer (GCL) and the innermost portion of the inner nuclear layer (INL) have a more mature appearance with larger, more spherical-shaped cell bodies and pale-staining nuclei. In contrast, those in the outer nuclear layer (ONL) and the outermost portion of the INL contain cells with immature morphology, i.e., elongated, darkly-stained nuclei. Likewise the inner plexiform layer (IPL) is well established while the outer plexiform layer (OPL) is poorly defined at this developmental stage. Bar = 40 μm. The most prominent feature of the OPL is a population of mature horizontal cells (arrows). Unstained autoradiogram demonstrates three cell populations which are heavily labeled by ^{3}H-GABA. All cells in the GCL are labeled, as are cells at the innermost (lower arrows) and outermost (upper arrows) extremes of the INL, corresponding to amacrine and horizontal cell layers respectively. Light labeling in the center of the INL may be attributed to developing Muller cells and/or interplexiform cells. Bar = 40 μm.

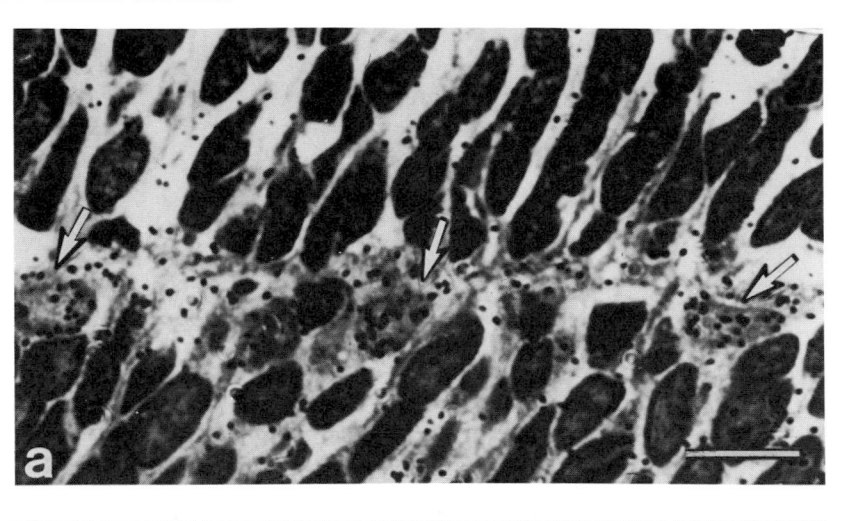

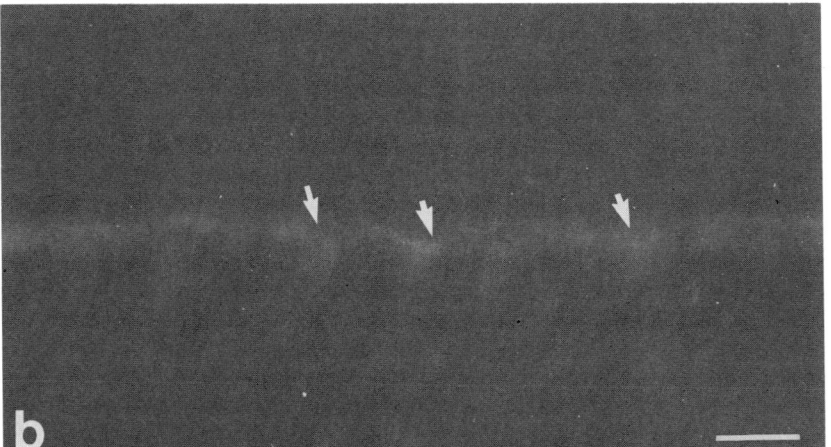

Figure 2. a) Stained autoradiogram of ^{3}H-GABA
accumulating horizontal cells in rabbit retina at one day
postnatal. Arrows denote labeled horizontal cells along
the innermost border of the emerging outer plexiform
layer. Bar = 10 μm. b) Horizontal cells (arrows) are
lightly immunoreactive to GABA anti-sera at this
developmental stage. The outline of fluorescent cell
somata and processes resembles that seen in the
autoradiogram above. Bar = 10 μm.

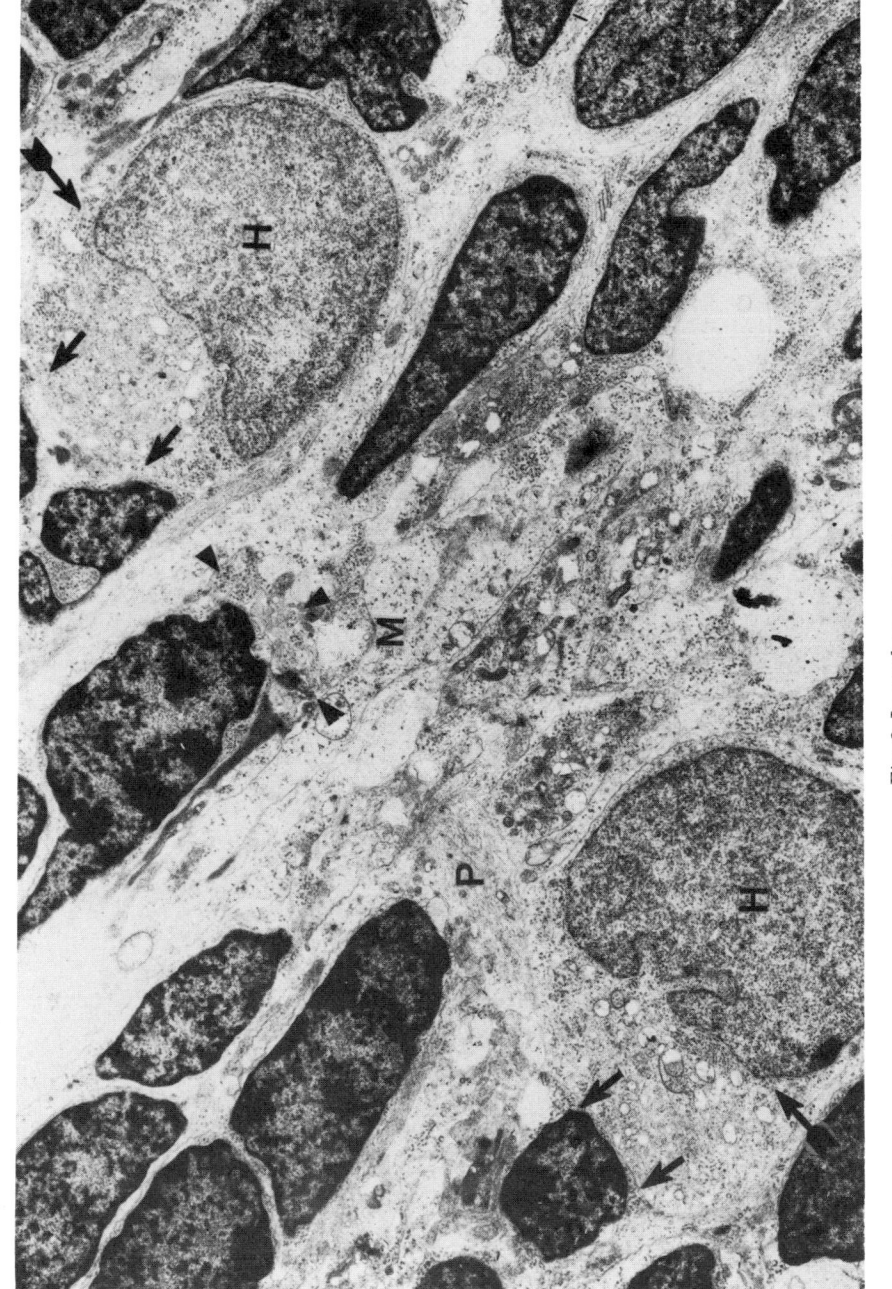

Fig. 3. Legend on next page

and in the innermost portion of the amacrine cell layer appear relatively mature and display large, round, pale-staining nuclei. A well-defined inner plexiform layer is present. In contrast, cell nuclei lying in the remaining outer portion of the retina have an immature appearance evidenced by small, dark-staining elongated profiles. One obvious exception to this gradient is the presence of a small population of large cells with a mature appearance located in the presumptive horizontal cell layer. Similar cells have been previously classified as horizontal cells in early postnatal rabbit retina (Ramon y Cajal, 1893).

EM analysis shows that neonatal horizontal cells are the first recognizable element to appear in the area of the outer plexiform layer (Fig. 3). The mature appearance of the horizontal cell is in sharp contrast to the immature cells surrounding it. Large, horizontally arranged processes project from the cell body, and come in close contact with other neighboring cells (Figs. 3, 4). Isolated patches of small-diameter profiles, possibly growth cones, are observed on the flattened distal surfaces of these processes. Immature photoreceptor terminals are observed in association with some of these patches (Fig. 3).

Neonatal horizontal cells form an extensive structure in the outer retina at birth. The cell bodies are roughly 12-15 μm in diameter and they appear to be arranged in a 90° grid pattern with a cell-to-cell spacing of

---

Figure 3. Horizontal cells of neonatal rabbit retina. The two horizontal cells (H) shown in this micrograph display large pale-staining nuclei with flat distal surfaces (large arrows). The plasma membranes of these cells (small arrows) often abut the plasma membrane of surrounding cells which have darkly-stained, elongated nuclei, characteristic of immature cells. Large lateral processes (P) from horizontal cells and patches of smaller-diameter profiles (arrowheads), represent the emerging outer plexiform layer and are the first elements to establish a horizontal orientation, contrasting with the vertically arranged processes which dominate the majority of the outer retina at this stage in development. X 53,000.

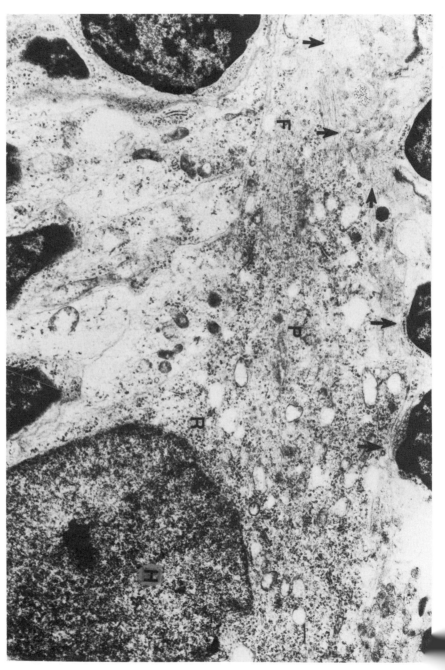

Fig. 4. Legend on next page

approximately 30 μm. The diameter of the lateral processes may be as large as 1/3rd the diameter of the cell body.

Retinas from 5-day-old rabbits show an advanced degree of maturation (Fig. 5a). Mature profiles are displayed by all cells in the inner retina, including cells of the ganglion cell layer and all cells of the inner nuclear layer. Elements of the outer plexiform layer are much more prominent and the layer is consistently present. Cell bodies in the outer nuclear layer still possess immature profiles with elongated, darkly staining nuclei, although the cell bodies do appear to have achieved some degree of columnar arrangement.

At the EM level, the outer plexiform layer at 5 days postnatal contains most of the cellular elements seen in the adult (Fig. 6), and a major portion of the proliferation of the outer plexiform layer has either been initiated or completed. Horizontal cell processes still dominate this layer; however, there is at this stage, a continuous layer of smaller diameter profiles and photoreceptor terminals along the distal surfaces of the processes.

Autoradiography. The autoradiographic pattern of ^{3}H-GABA-accumulating cells in the neonatal retina is complex and appears to become more restricted during development. At birth, heavy labeling is observed in at least three different cell populations, and each of these differs developmentally (Fig. 2b). All mature horizontal cells accumulate ^{3}H-GABA at birth; none do so after postnatal day 5 (Fig. 5b). Likewise, all cells in the ganglion cell layer accumulate ^{3}H-GABA at birth; however, a small population (some of which may be

---

Figure 4. Projection of a lateral process from a horizontal cell body is shown at higher magnification. At points closer to the nucleus (H), no other cellular elements are present between this cell and its neighbors (arrows). However, at points along the distal surface of the process (P), patches of smaller-diameter processes are seen (arrowheads). The cytoplasm contains rough endoplasmic reticulum (R) and filamentous structures (F). X 10,000.

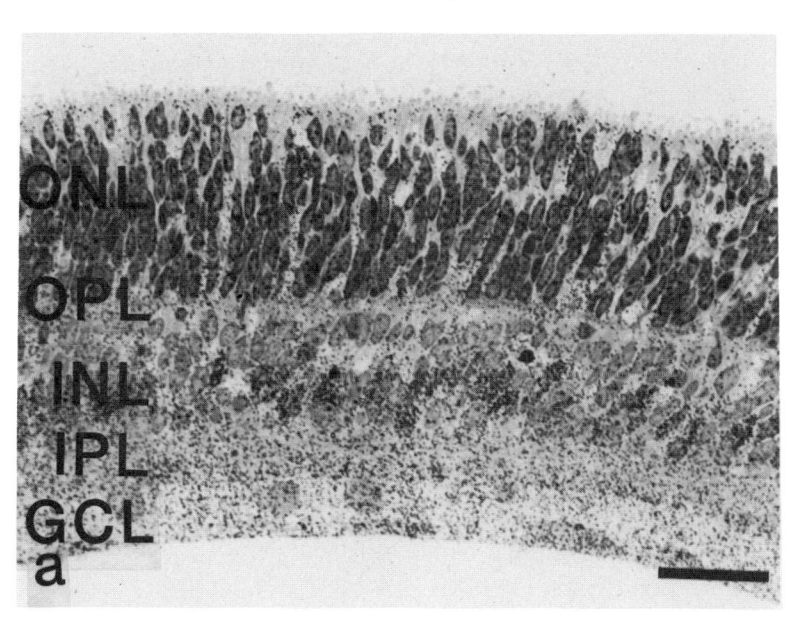

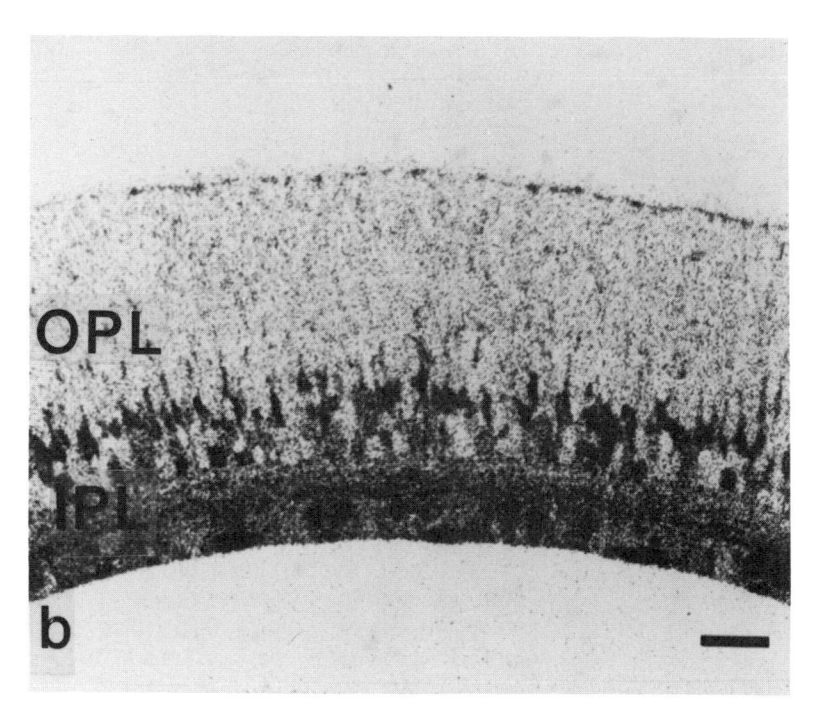

Fig. 5. Legend on next page

displaced amacrine cells) retain this ability in the adult (Redburn and Madtes, 1986). In contrast, little change is observed in amacrine cell labeling during postnatal development. Only selected amacrine cell populations are labeled at birth and they appear to remain relatively stable throughout development.

Muller cell uptake of ^{3}H-GABA at postnatal day one is questionable. Relatively low labeling of some cell bodies with vertical projections may denote uptake into presumptive Muller cells. However postincubation in label-free buffer, which is known to remove metabolically labile ^{3}H-GABA in Muller cells of adult retinas, fails to change the label distribution to any significant extent in 1-day-old animals (Redburn and Madtes, 1986). In light of our subsequent immunohistochemical data, this accumulation may in fact be attributed to interplexiform cells. By postnatal day five presumptive Muller cell labeling dominates the autoradiographic pattern and once again this pattern is unaltered following postincubation in label-free buffer. Heavy autoradiographic labeling of Muller cells after postnatal day 10 and through the adult, obscures amacrine cell accumulation under normal conditions; neuronal labeling is visible only after enhancement by a 30 min. postincubation in label-free buffer (Redburn and Madtes, 1986).

Figure 5. Autoradiograms of isolated retina from 5-day-old rabbit. a) In comparison to retinas from one-day-old rabbit, cells in the inner nuclear layer (INL) appear more mature and the outer plexiform layer (OPL) is much more distinct. No major changes in the inner plexiform layer (IPL) and ganglion cell layer (GCL) are observed at this level of magnification. Photoreceptor cell bodies in the outer nuclear layer still appear relatively immature; however, a columnar arrangement of these is emerging. Bar = 40 m. b) Unstained autoradiogram clearly demonstrates the lack of labeling in horizontal cell bodies or processes in the outer plexiform layer (OPL). Labeling of cell bodies in the amacrine and ganglion cell layers on either side of the innerplexiform layer (IPL) is presented. Labeling of vertically arranged processes (arrows) may be attributed to Muller or interplexiform cells. Bar = 40 m.

Immunocytochemistry. The GABA antisera were tested for cross reactivity with the structurally-related compounds, glutamine, glycine, taurine, glutamate and alanine. These compounds exhibited no detectable reactivity, as visualized with DAB, following incubation with GABA antisera. Only the sample containing GABA-antiGABA complex produced a positive brown precipitate following DAB incubation.

Retinas from all ages show intensely fluorescent labeling of elements in the inner plexiform layer (Figs. 6 and 7). In well-oriented sections, a distinct bilaminar pattern is observed roughly corresponding to sublamina 2 and 4. The middle area appears to be the least fluorescent region of the inner plexiform layer. The relative position of the two fluorescent bands in the inner plexiform layer is stable from day 1 through day 5. Cell bodies on either side of the inner plexiform layer are also labeled but with the much less intensity than that seen within the inner plexiform layer. Usually the fluorescence appears as a halo around a less fluorescent center, presumably corresponding to the nucleus. In the amacrine layer, large, oval-shaped immunoreactive cell bodies are located immediately adjacent to the inner plexiform layer. Large, round immunofluorescent cell bodies are also located in the ganglion cell layer in close proximity to the border of the inner plexiform layer. Morphometric analysis of these cell bodies reveal that there is a fifty percent decrease in the number of labeled GABAergic cell bodies in the ganglion cell layer and inner nuclear layer as the retina increases with age. This decrease appears to occur simultaneous with an increase in volume of the remaining GABAergic somata and a shift toward a more spherical cell shape.

Apparent in sections of 1-and 5-day-old retinas are pyramidal-shaped immunoreactive cell bodies just distal to amacrine cell layer (Figs. 6b and 7). In favorable sections a highly fluorescent distal process is observed to project from these cells to the level of the developing outer plexiform layer where it branches and sends long horizontal processes in register with the outer plexiform layer. These stained cell bodies and processes are observed with regularity in all sections; morphologically they are reminiscent of interplexiform cells.

With the exception of the distal processes from interplexiform-like cells, elements of the outer retina are not intensely reactive. The most prominent pattern is a band of diffuse staining associated with processes in the developing outer plexiform layer (Figs. 2b, 6b, 7). Our initial impression is that this continuous band of fluorescence is associated with one set of processes, possibly from horizontal cells, and that it is distinct from the immunoreactivity of the distal processes from the interplexiform-like cells in the retina. The large cell bodies we have previously characterized as ^{3}H-GABA accumulating horizontal cells are very lightly stained (Figs. 1b, 2b). In many cases, fluorescence appears to be specifically associated with these cell bodies in the microscope; however, the low level of reactivity was at

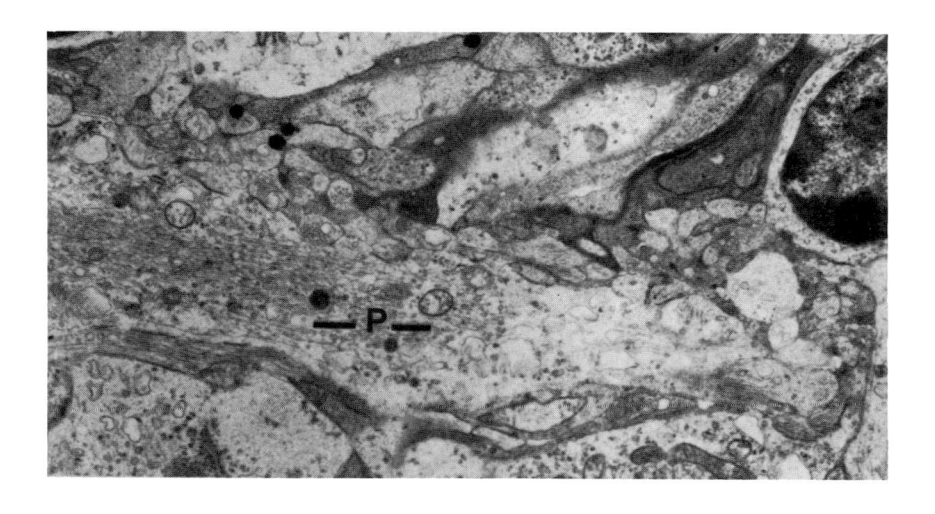

Figure 6. The outer plexiform layer from 5-day-old rabbit is dominated by lateral processes (P) from neonatal horizontal cells. The patches seen at one day postnatal, have expanded to form a continuous layer of processes which maintains its orientation along the distal surface of the horizontal cell processes. Thus it appears that most of the growth of the outer plexiform layer is confined to the region adjacent to this pioneer process. X 14,600.

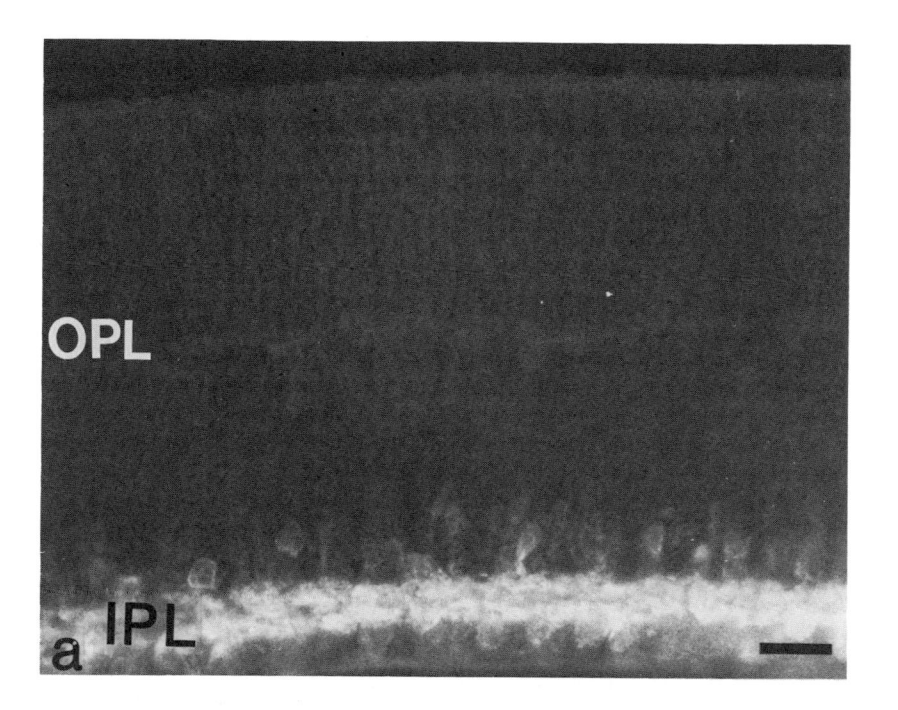

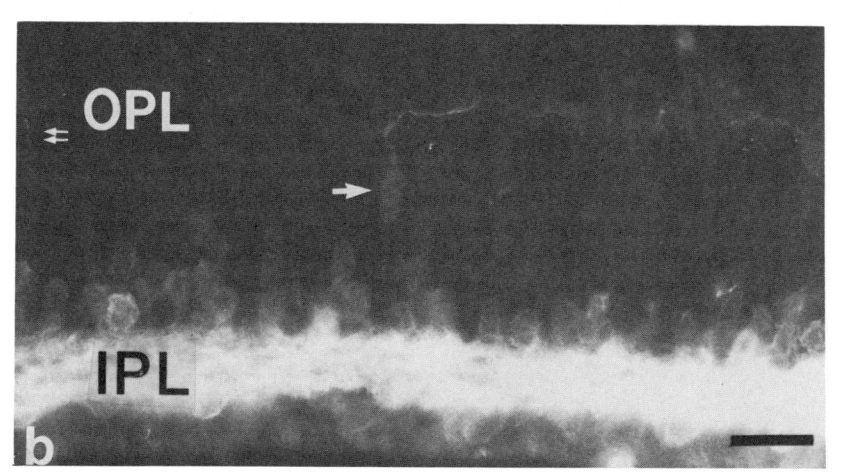

Fig. 7. Legend on next page

the limit of detectability under our photographic
conditions.

DISCUSSION

Our major findings are 1) there are at least two
exceptions to the inner-to-outer maturation gradient in
the neonatal retina. Horizontal cell and interplexiform
cell types display mature characteristics at birth even
though they are distally positioned to layers of immature
cell bodies. 2) Both of these cell types accumulate
^{3}H-GABA and are immunoreactive to GABA antisera. 3) All
cells in the ganglion cell layer and a relatively large
population of amacrine cells accumulate ^{3}H-GABA and
appear to be GABA-immunoreactive.

Horizontal cells. The developmental progression in
retina appears to be dictated at least in part by a

Figure 7. GABA immunoreactive cell bodies and fibers in
retina from 1-day-old rabbits. a) Highly immunoreactive
fibers presumably from amacrine (and perhaps
interplexiform) cells have a bilaminar labeling pattern
corresponding to sublamina 2 and 4 of the inner plexiform
layer (IPL). Large numbers of intensely immunoreactive
cell bodies are present on either side of the IPL. In
comparison, immunofluorescence in the outer plexiform
layer (OPL) is barely discernable under these photographic
conditions. This section is somewhat unusual in that it
is devoid of immunoreactive interplexiform-like cells (see
below), allowing a more valid comparison of staining in
horizontal cells vs (arrows) amacrine and ganglion cells.
Bar = 40 μm. b) In addition to the immunoreactive cells
described above, staining was also observed in
interplexiform-like cells. The arrow denotes a
GABA-positive, pyramidal-shaped cell whose soma lies in
the middle of the inner nuclear layer. Its distal process
is intensely fluorescent and projects to the outer retina,
where it branches and sends long horizontal processes in
register with the emerging outer plexiform layer. These
stained processes were observed with regularity in the
majority of sections examined. The double arrows mark
what is presumed to be a similar process arising from a
cell whose soma is out of the plane of section. Bar = 40
μm.

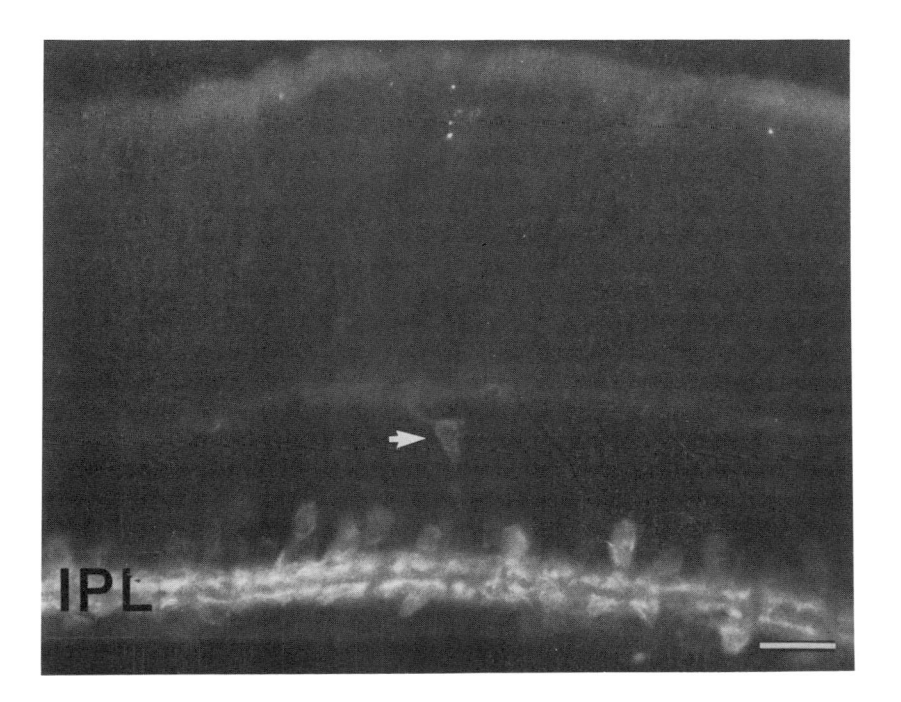

Figure 8. GABA immunoreactivity in 5-day-old rabbit retina. The immunoreactive bands in sublamina 2 and 4 of the inner plexiform layer (IPL) appear to be more distinct at this stage than at 1 day postnatal. Immunofluorescent cell bodies are present on either side of the inner plexiform layer; however, in contrast to 1 day postnatal retinas, morphometric analysis indicates that there is a 50% decrease in the number of stained cell bodies in these layers and the remaining cell bodies have assumed a more spherical shape. Interplexiform cells (arrow) are also observed. Bar = 40 μm.

pre-programmed dropout of cells from the mitotic cycle which ultimately results in the laminar separation of different classes of cells along a linear (inner-to-outer) gradient (Sidman, 1961). In general the first cells to become post-mitotic are ganglion cells; the last, are photoreceptors. However, some exceptions do exist. One such exception is a subclass of horizontal cells, first described by Ramon y Cajal (1893) in neonatal rabbit retina. These cells are located in the inner retina and they assume a mature appearance prior to the photoreceptor or bipolar cells which continue to undergo mitosis and interkinetic migration on either side of and between the mature-appearing horizontal cells. Two characteristics of these horizontal cells are of particular interest. First, they assume their mature position early in development, thus they appear to be the first component of the outer plexiform layer to be expressed. By their position, they establish the location of the developing outer plexiform layer. Second, they appear to have some influence in directing the subsequent growth of this synaptic layer since growing fibers appear first in patches and then as a continuous layer which remains closely associated with the flattened, distal surfaces of the horizontal cell processes. Postnatal growth of this plexiform layer is restricted to this area, and results in the trilaminar arrangement of this layer seen in the adult, with horizontal cell processes comprising the innermost border, photoreceptor terminals forming the outermost border, and many other smaller diameter processes, presumably from bipolar cells and other types of horizontal cells, filling in the middle layer. Both of these properties are similar to those described for pioneer or pathfinder cells in other parts of the CNS.

Weiss (1941) was perhaps the first to suggest the concept of a pioneer fiber which grows to the target area, and once there, begins to attract later growing fibers. Several developing neural systems have subsequently been shown to have cell processes with these attributes. Examples include pathfinding axons in the retina of Daphnia (Lopresti et al., 1973) and pioneer neurons in the developing innervation of rat diaphragm (Bennett and Pettigrew, 1974). Reviews by Edwards (1982) and Goodman (1982) also provide strong evidence for pioneer cells from their own work in the insect nervous system. Finally, Lauder and her associates (1986) find that GABA is one of the earliest neurotransmitters detected in the embryonic rat brain. Furthermore, GABA-immunoreactive fibers are part of the first contingent of cortical afferents to invade the telencephalic vesicle and thus they are associated with the stimulus for the beginning of neuronal differentiation in this region. It is suggested that these GABA-positive pioneer cells may have a trophic function in early development of the cortex.

One of the important properties of pioneer horizontal cells, precotious maturation, occurs for the most part, prenatally. Polley et al. (1985) have studied similar cells in cat retina and they show that in this population of horizontal cells (type A), neurogenesis was virtually complete by embryonic day 28, prior to any other cell type in the inner nuclear layer including amacrine cells. We have not studied prenatal development in rabbit retina and thus we have no information regarding the events associated with the early maturation of type A horizontal cells or their migration and alignment in the outer retina in rabbit. Pioneer cells in the other systems are believed to rely on extracellular matrix molecules as cues in their pathfinding role. Thus it is reasonable to suggest that similar mechanisms may also exist in retina. If such is the case, the isolation and growth of neonatal horizontal cells could be highly useful for future studies of process growth in an identified, CNS pathfinder cell.

The other important property of neonatal horizontal cells, namely their apparent influence on subsequent growth in the outer plexiform layer, is expressed within the first 5-10 days after birth. We have extensively examined retinas from this period and in addition to morphometric analysis of these cells, we have demonstrated that 1) they are immunoreactive to GABA antisera (Keith and Redburn, 1987; Keith and Redburn, in preparation, 2) they specifically accumulate ^{3}H-GABA (Redburn et al., 1985; Redburn and Madtes, 1986) and 3) they release it upon stimulation by depolarizing levels of potassium or by kainic acid (Moran et al., 1986; Moran et al., in preparation). These biochemical properties have been useful in a technical sense since they provide valuable markers for the horizontal cell population and thus have allowed a greater appreciation of specific maturation events. Perhaps more importantly, these findings raise the possibility that the GABAergic properties are more than coincidental. Given the evidence presented in the following chapters, it seems reasonable to suggest that GABA, produced from neonatal horizontal cells, acts as a trophic substance in retina, promoting and stimulating expansion of cell processes, synaptogenesis and expression of specific molecular components of synaptic transmission including its own receptor (Madtes and Redburn, 1983; Madtes, this volume).

In evaluating this hypothesis, several criteria might be considered. 1. If GABAergic horizontal cells act as pathfinders, they should be among the first to leave the mitotic cycle so they can provide early guidance for subsequently maturing neurons. 2. GABA positive processes should be present prior to the appearance of any other horizontally arranged process in the outer plexiform layer. Therefore, all processes in the outer plexiform layer should be GABA positive at the earliest time points in the development of this layer. 3. It also follows that the density of GABA-positive cells should be highest at birth than at any subsequent time. GABAergic cell density should decrease with age either by cell death, change of transmitter phenotype or dilution by addition of other non-GABAergic neurons. 4. Horizontal cells should establish a reference point for the further development of the plexiform layer. The position of the pioneering process should remain relatively constant while other growing processes emerge in reference to it.

Our morphological data suggests that the neonatal horizontal cells may in fact meet all four of these criteria. GABA-positive processes are present prior to any other markers for the outer plexiform layer and their position remains constant relative to the subsequent development of this synaptic layer and relative to the remaining retinal structure. Finally, the density of GABA-positive cells in the outer retina is without question, highest at birth, since no cells in the outer retina are GABA-positive in the adult. We cannot account for this loss by dilution from other cell types or by cell death, thus we are left with the possibility that type A horizontal cells change transmitter phenotype during postnatal development and utilize some other inhibitory neurotransmitter for their involvement in mature visual pathways.

GABA-immunoreactive interplexiform cells. Our more recent observations have added even more complexity to the hypothesis that GABA is involved in retinal development. We have observed the presence of a cell body in the middle region of the developing inner nuclear layer with what appears to be a single ascending and single descending process reminiscent of interplexiform cell morphology. The descending process joins the inner plexiform layer where it becomes indistinguishable among the large number of immunoreactive processes presumably from cell bodies in the amacrine and ganglion cell layers. The ascending process is more easily followed. It projects to the outer plexiform layer where it branches abruptly, forming a thinly branched, but widely distributed, dendritic arborization. The very distinct branching point of the ascending process is in register with the developing outer plexiform layer and the horizontal cell processes there, which generally show a lower level of immunofluorescence. Our current observations are limited to light microscopic histofluorescence and many important structural questions must await analysis at the EM level. How this presumptive interplexiform cell interacts specifically with the horizontal cell and other elements of the OPL are at present unclear, as is its possible role in development. However, its detection does establish that the inner plexiform layer and outer plexiform layer are linked at birth by processes from this cell. It has long been held that the two plexiform layers develop more or less independent of each other, only to be linked at the later stages of retinal development by bipolar cell dendrites and axons in the outer and inner plexiform layers respectively (Blanks et al., 1974; McArdle et al., 1977; Maslim and Stone, 1986). Since the GABA-positive interplexiform cell is present early in development and has a clearly-established mature profile, one must consider the possibility that the cell plays a role in retinal development and that GABAergic influences might be further implicated in retinal synaptogenesis. GABAergic interplexiform cells have not previously been reported in rabbit retina although they are present in adult retinas of closely related species (Nakamura et al., 1980). Thus it is not clear whether or not this cell has an adult counterpart.

GABA-labeled cells in amacrine and ganglion cell layers. Labeling in both the amacrine and ganglion cell layer, decreases during postnatal development. The developmental decrease in the density of GABA-labeled amacrine cells might be explained by a dilution effect resulting from the subsequent addition of non-GABAergic cells later in development. However, this is probably not the case for ganglion cells since ALL cells in the neonatal ganglion cell layer accumulate ^{3}H-GABA and are GABA-immunoreactive. Some of the labeling could be attributed to GABAergic displaced amacrine cells; however, most, if not all, ganglion cells are known to be present and post-mitotic at birth in rabbit retina and few, if any, are GABAergic in the adult rabbit retina (Ehinger, 1970; Redburn and Madtes, 1986). Thus, we are left with the possibility that some neonatal ganglion cells, like neonatal horizontal cells, transiently express GABAergic properties during development. Some cells in the ganglion cell layer die during development, but most or all that remain, must change their transmitter phenotype.

In summary, our studies have provided circumstantial evidence that GABA plays an important role in retinal development. These observations raise many questions regarding the transient expression of GABAergic properties by a large and diverse neonatal cell population, Our future goal is to utilize morphological analyses to establish morphometric criteria, amendable to quantitation. We will then use these as a basis for evaluating critical hypothesis regarding the production of GABA by pioneer cells and the trophic interactions which may establish retinal circuitry.

ACKNOWLEDGEMENTS

The authors are indebted to Dr. Paul Madtes who was instrumental in the early stages of this project; to Ms. Cheryl Mitchell for her patience and help in assembling this chapter; to Ms. Yvonne Blocker and Dr. Richard Wilkerson for technical assistance in producing the autoradiographs; to Ms. Diana Parker for typing the manuscript. This work was supported by NEI grant 1655-11 to D.A.R.

REFERENCES

Bennett MR, Pettigrew AG (1974). The formation of synapses in striated muscle during development. J Physiol Lond

241:515-545.

Blanks JC, Adinolfi AM, Lolley RN (1974). Synaptogenesis in the photoreceptor terminal of the mouse retina. J Comp Neurol 156:81-94.

Bolz J, McGuire BA (1985). GABA-like immunoreactivity in horizontal cells of the cat retina. Soc Neurosci Abstr 11:1215.

Brandon C, Lam DMK, Wu J-Y (1979). The γ-aminobutyric acid system in rabbit retina: Localization by immunocyto-chemistry and autoradiography. Proc Natn Acad Sci USA 76:3557-3561.

Brecha N (1983). Retinal neurotransmitters: Histochemical and biochemical studies. In PC Emson (ed): "Chemical Neuroanatomy," New York: Raven Press, pp 85-129.

Carter-Dawson LD, LaVail MM (1979). Rods and cones in the mouse retina. II. Autoradiographic analysis of cell generation using tritiated thymidine. J Comp Neurol 188:263-272.

Dacheux RF, Miller RF (1981a). An intracellular electro-physiological study of the ontogeny of functional synapses in the rabbit retina. I. Receptors, horizontal, and bipolar cells. J Comp Neurol 198:307-326.

Dacheux RF, Miller RF (1981b). An intracellular electro-physiological study of the ontogeny of functional synapses in the rabbit retina. II. Amacrine cells. J Comp Neurol 198:327-334.

Dowling JE (1986). Dopamine: A retinal neuromodulator. TINS 9: 236-240.

Dowling JE, Boycott BB (1966). Organization of the primate retina: Electron microscopy. Proc R Soc Lond B 116:80-111.

Dowling JE, Ehinger B (1978). The interplexiform cell system I. Synapses of dopaminergic neurons of the goldfish retina. Proc R Soc Lond B 201, 7-26.

Edwards JS (1982). Pioneer fibers. In N Spitzer (ed): "Neuronal Development," New York: Plenum Press, pp 255-266.

Ehinger B (1970). Autoradiographic identification of rabbit retinal neurons that take up GABA. Experientia Basel 26:1063.

Gallego A (1971). Horizontal and amacrine cells in the mammalian's retina. Vision Res Suppl 3:33-50.

Goodman CS (1982). Embryonic development of identified neurons in the grasshopper. In N Spitzer (ed): "Neuronal Development," New York: Plenum Press, pp 171-211.

Hampton CK, Redburn DA (1983). Autoradiographic analysis

of ^{3}H-glutamate, ^{3}H-dopamine, and ^{3}H-GABA accumulation in rabbit retina after kainic acid treatment. J Neurosci Res 9:239-251.

Hedden WL, Dowling J (1978). The interplexiform cell system II. Effects of dopamine on goldfish retinal neurons. Proc R Soc Lond B 201:27-55.

Keith ME, Redburn DA (1987). GABA-immunoreactivity in the developing rabbit retina. Invest Ophthalmol Vis Sci Suppl in press.

Keith ME, Redburn DA (In preparation). GABA-immunoreactive interplexiform-like cells link inner and outer synaptic layers in neonatal rabbit retina.

Kolb H, Nelson R (1985). Functional neurocircuitry of amacrine cells in the cat retina. In A Gallego, P Gouras P (eds): "Neurocircuitry of the Retina," New York: a Cajal Memorial, Elsevier Publ Co, Inc, pp 215-232.

Lauder JM, Han VKM, Henderson P, Vendoorn T, Towle AC (1986). Prenatal ontogeny of the GABAergic system in the rat brain: An immunocytochemical study. Neuroscience 19:465-493.

Lopresti V, Macagno ER, Levinthal C (1973). Structure and development of neuronal connections in isogenic organisms. Cellular interactions in the development of the optic lamina of Daphnia. Proc Nat Acad Sci, Wash 70:433-437.

Madtes P Jr, Redburn DA (1983). GABA as a trophic factor during development. Life Sci 33:979-984.

Marc RE, Stell WK, Bok D, Lam DMK (1978). GABAergic pathways in the goldfish retina. J Comp Neurol 182:221-246.

Maslim J, Stone J (1986). Synaptogenesis in the retina of the cat. Brain Res 373:35-48.

Massey SC, Redburn DA (1987). Transmitter circuits in the vertebrate retina. Prog Neurobiol 28:55-96.

McArdle CB, Dowling JE, Masland RH (1977). Development of outer segments and synapses in the rabbit retina. J Comp Neurol 175:253-274.

Miller RF (1979). The neuronal basis of ganglion cell receptive field organization and the physiology of amacrine cells. In FO Schmitt, FG Warden (eds): "The Neurosciences Fourth Program," Cambridge, MIT Press, pp 227-245.

Moran J, Pasantes-Morales H, Redburn DA (1986). Glutamate receptor agonists release ^{3}H-GABA preferentially from horizontal cells. Brain Res 398:276-287.

Moran J, Pasantes-Morales H, Redburn DA (In preparation). ^{3}H-GABA release from kainic acid-sensitive horizontal cells in neonatal rabbit retina.

Nakamura Y, McGuire BA, Sterling P (1980). Interplexiform cells in cat retina: Identification by uptake of $-^3$H aminobutyric acid and serial reconstruction. Proc Natn Acad Sci USA 77:658-661.

Negishi K, Drujan BD (1979). Effects of some amino acids on horizontal cells in the fish retina. J Neurosci Res 4:351-363.

Osborne NN, Patel S, Beaton DW, Neuhoff V (1986). GABA neurons in retinas of different species and their postnatal development in situ and in culture in the rabbit retina. Cel Tissue Res 243:117-123.

Oyster CW, Takahashi ES (1977). Interplexiform cells in rabbit retina. Proc R Soc Lond B 197:477-484.

Polley EH, Zimmerman RP, Fortney RL (1985). Development of the outer plexiform layer (OPL) of the cat retina. Soc Neurosci Abstr 11:14.

Pourcho RG (1980). Uptake of ^{3}H-glycine and ^{3}H-GABA by amacrine cells in the cat retina. Brain Res 198:333-346.

Ramon y Cajal S (1983). La retine des vertebres Translated in The Vertebrate Retina, RW Rodieck, WH Freeman and Co, San Francisco, pp 777-904.

Rapaport DH, Stone J (1983). Time course of the morphological differentiation of cat retinal ganglion cells: influences on cell size. J Comp Neurol 221:42-52.

Redburn DA, Madtes P Jr (1986). Postnatal development of ^{3}H-GABA accumulating cells in rabbit retina. J Comp Neurol 243:41-57.

Redburn DA, Blocker Y, Madtes PM (1985). ^{3}H-GABA-accumulating horizontal cells on neonatal rabbit retina. Invest. Ophthalmol. Vis. Sci. Suppl. 26:95.

Redburn DA, Massey SC, Madtes P (1983). The GABA uptake system in rabbit retina. In L Hertz, E Kvamme, EG McGeer, A Schousboe (eds): "Glutamine, Glutamate, and GABA in the Central Nervous System," New York: Alan R Liss, pp 273-286.

Redburn DA, Mitchell CK, Hampton CK (1982). Developmental analysis of neurotransmitter systems in rabbit retina. In HF Bradford (ed): "Neurotransmitter Interaction and Compartmentation," New York: Plenum Press, pp 79-97.

Schnitzer M, Rusoff AC (1984). Horizontal cells of the mouse retina contain glutamic acid decarboxylase-like immunoreactivity during early developmental stages. J Neurosci 4:2948-2955.

Sengelaub DR, Finlay BL (1982). Cell death in the mammalian visual system during normal development. I. Retinal ganglion cells. J Comp Neurol 204:311-317.

Sidman RL (1961). Histogenesis of mouse retina studied with thymidine-^{3}H. in GK Smelser (ed): "Structure of the Eye," New York: Academic Press, pp 487-492.

Sidman RL, Rakic P (1973). Neuronal migration, with special reference to developing human brain: a review. Brain Res 62:1-35.

Stell WK (1967). The structure and relationships of horizontal cells and photoreceptor-bipolar synaptic complexes in goldfish retina. Am J Anat 121:401-424.

Stell WK (1972). The morphological organization of the vertebrate retina. In MGF Fuortes (ed): "Handbook of Sensory Physiology," Berlin: Springer-Verlag, pp 111-213.

Sterling P, Freed M, Smith RG (1986). Microcircuitry and functional architecture of the cat retina. Elsevier Sci Publ, pp 186-192.

Walsh C, Polley EH (1985). The topography of ganglion cell production in the cat's retina. J Neurosci 5:741-750.

Weiss P (1941). Nerve patterns: mechanics of nerve growth. Growth 5:163-203.

Young RW (1984). Cell death during differentiation of the retina in the mouse. J Comp Neurol 229:362-363.

Neurotrophic Activity of GABA During Development, pages 109–138
© 1987 Alan R. Liss, Inc.

TROPHIC EFFECTS OF GABA ON CEREBELLAR GRANULE CELLS IN CULTURE

Gert H. Hansen, Eddi Meier[1], Jens Abraham and Arne Schousboe
Department of Biochemistry A, Pannum Institute
University of Copenhagen
DK-2200 Copenhagen, Denmark

INTRODUCTION

The possibility that GABA in addition to its role as an inhibitory neurotransmitter (cf. Seiler and Lajtha, this volume) may exert other functions in the central nervous system (CNS) was suggested by Campbell et al. (1966). They showed that GABA stimulated the incorporation of amino acids into proteins in cell-free microsomal systems from the brain. These results were subsequently confirmed by studies in which the incorporation of different radioactively labelled amino acids into proteins in cell-free systems as well as in slices and homogenates of the brain was investigated (Tewari and Baxter, 1969; Snodgrass, 1973; Goertz, 1979). These findings indicate that GABA might have a regulatory role in brain protein synthesis and hence, it may play a role in processes responsible for development and differentiation of the CNS.

However more than 10 years elapsed since the stimulating effect of GABA on protein synthesis was reported (Campbell et al., 1966) before it was shown that GABA in vivo affects neuronal development and differentiation in superior cervical ganglia and cerebral cortex

1 Present address:
  Department of Pharmacology
  H. Lundbeck and Co.
  DK-2500 Valby, Denmark

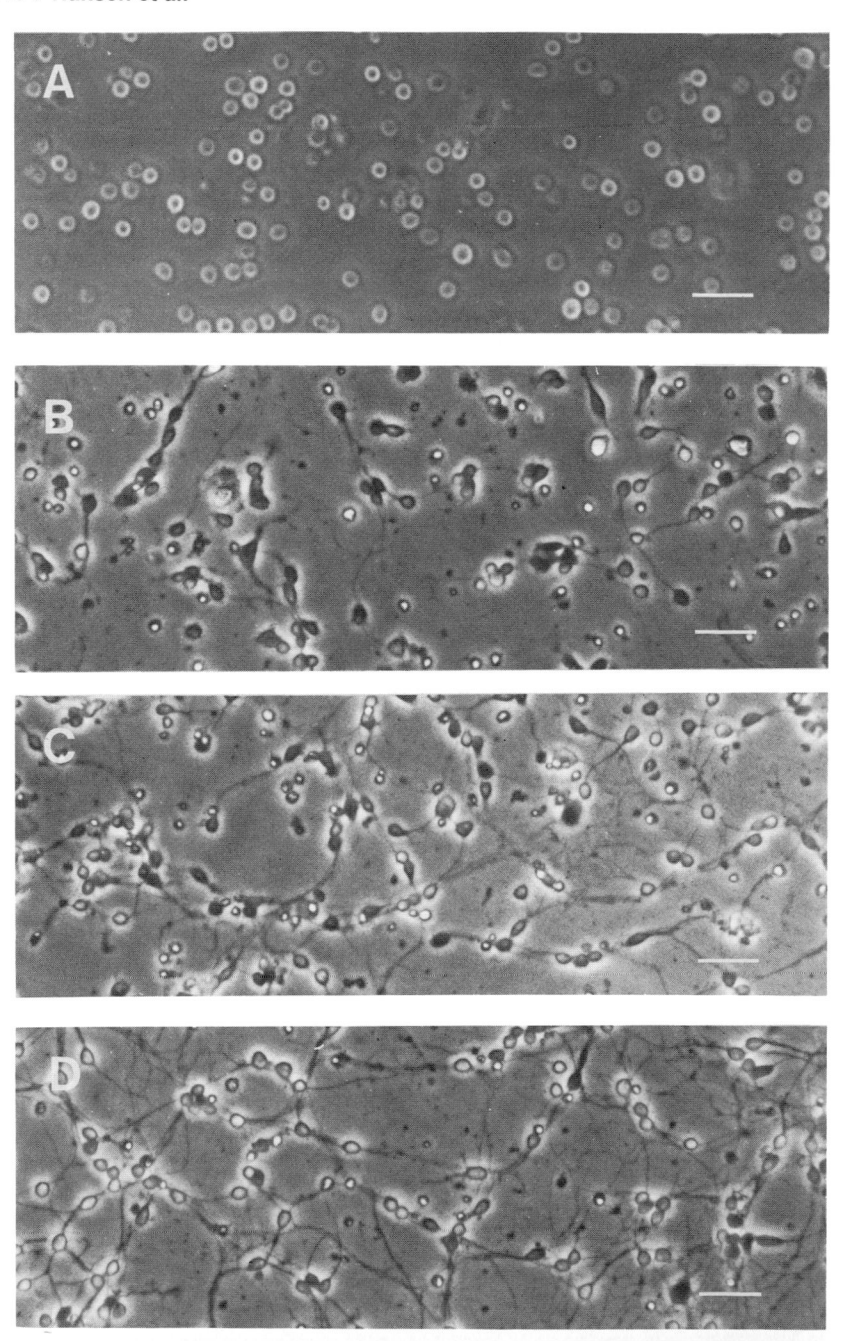

(Wolff et al., 1978; 1979). Recently, studies on the effect of GABA and GABA receptor agonists and antagonists performed on retina (Madtes and Redburn, 1983a, b; Redburn and Madtes, 1986; Madtes and Bashir-Elahi, 1986) and different types of cultured neurons such as neuroblastoma cells (Spoerri and Wolff, 1981; Eins et al., 1983), retinal and cortical neurons (Spoerri, 1986), tectal neurons (Michler-Stuke and Wolff, 1986) and cerebellar granule cells (Meier et al., 1983; 1984; 1985; Hansen et al., 1984; 1987; Schousboe et al., 1985b; 1987; Belhage et al., 1986) have established conclusive evidence that GABA plays a major role in the functional development and differentiation of at least certain types of neurons in the CNS.

The present chapter shall deal primarily with the effect of GABA on the morphological development of cerebellar granule cells in culture. Furthermore, the possible mechanism by which GABA mediates the neurotrophic effects will be discussed.

ANATOMY AND MORPHOLOGY OF CEREBELLAR GRANULE CELLS

Anatomy

The cell bodies of the cerebellar granule cells are situated in the granule layer of the cerebellar cortex. Each granule cell sends an axon to the molecular layer of the cerebellar cortex, where it bifurcates into a T-shaped axon running for long distances parallel to the cerebellar

---

Figure 1. Phase contrast micrographs of cerebellar granule cells cultured for 1h (A), 20 h (B), 48 h (C), and 4 days (D). Cells were prepared as described and seeded in tissue culture flasks at a concentration of 8×10^5 cells/ml. Bars indicate 10 μm.
A. The cells have a homogeneous globular appearance.
B. Due to varying stages of differentiation of the cells the culture has a heterogeneous appearance. The majority of the cells have extended neurites.
C. The density of neurites and groups of cells has increased compared to B.
D. Virtually all cells have extended neurites and they constitute an extensive network of processes.
Unpublished results of J. Abraham and G.H. Hansen.

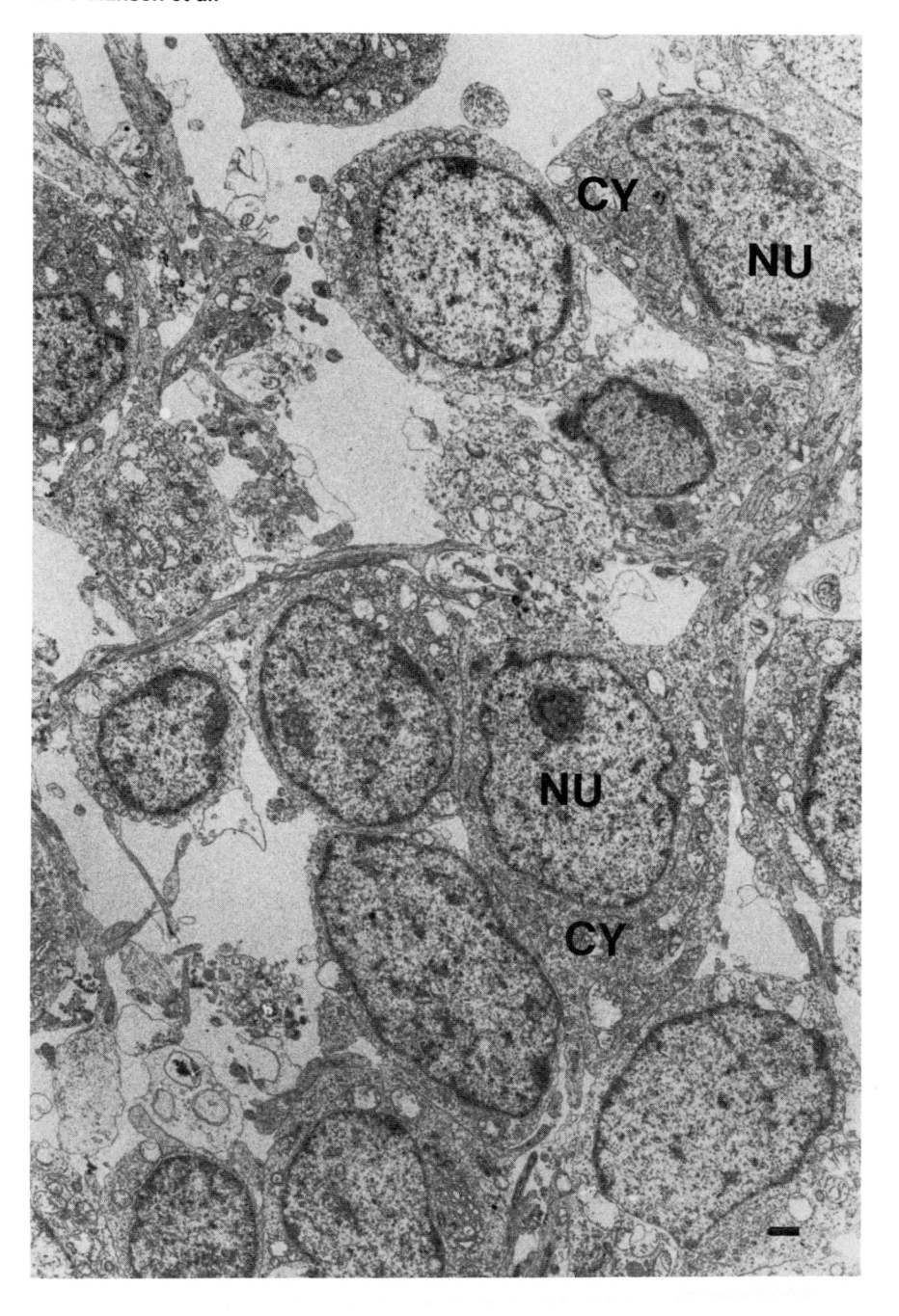

surface. Consequently, these axons are called parallel fibers and traverse the arborization of the Purkinje cells at right angles and make numerous synaptic contacts. The short numerous dendrites of the granule cells in the granule layer receive input from the Mossy fibers constituting the so-called glomeruli (cf. Palay, 1982).

Cell culture

The studies discussed in the present review have been preformed entirely on primary cultures of cerebellar granule cells which were derived from 7-day-old rats according to Messer (1977) and Hansen et al. (1984). Briefly, the cultures were prepared as follows. The tissue was minced, trypsinized for 15 min at 37°C (0.025%, w/v trypsin) and subsequently triturated in a DNAse solution (0.004%, w/v) containing a trypsin inhibitor (0.03%, w/v) and centrifuged (900 x g; 10 min). The pelleted cells were resuspended (1.5 x 10^6 cells/ml) in a modified Dulbecco's minimum essential medium (Hertz et al., 1982; Hansen et al., 1984) containing 10% (v/v) inactivated fetal calf serum and seeded in tissue culture dishes.

The use of primary cultures for studies of effects of epigenetic factors on cell morphology, development and differentiation has several advantages as compared to the use of complex in vivo systems due to the fact that the cellular environment can easily be controlled. Since cultured cerebellar granule cells are devoid of machinery necessary for synthesis and release of GABA (Oertel et al., 1981; Gallo et al., 1982) it is possible to test the

---

Figure 2. A low magnification electron micrograph of cerebellar granule cells cultured for 4 days. Note the prominent nuclei (nu) which occupy most of the perikaryon and characterize the cerebellar granule cells. Cytoplasma (cy). Bar indicates 1 μm. Cells were fixed in glutaraldehyde, postfixed in osmium tetroxide and blockstained in uranyl acetate. They were subsequently dehydrated in ethanol and methacrylic acid-2-hydroxy-propylester and embedded in Epon. Thin sections (75 nm) were stained in lead citrate and examined in a Philips electron microscope 201 C. Unpublished material of G.H. Hansen.

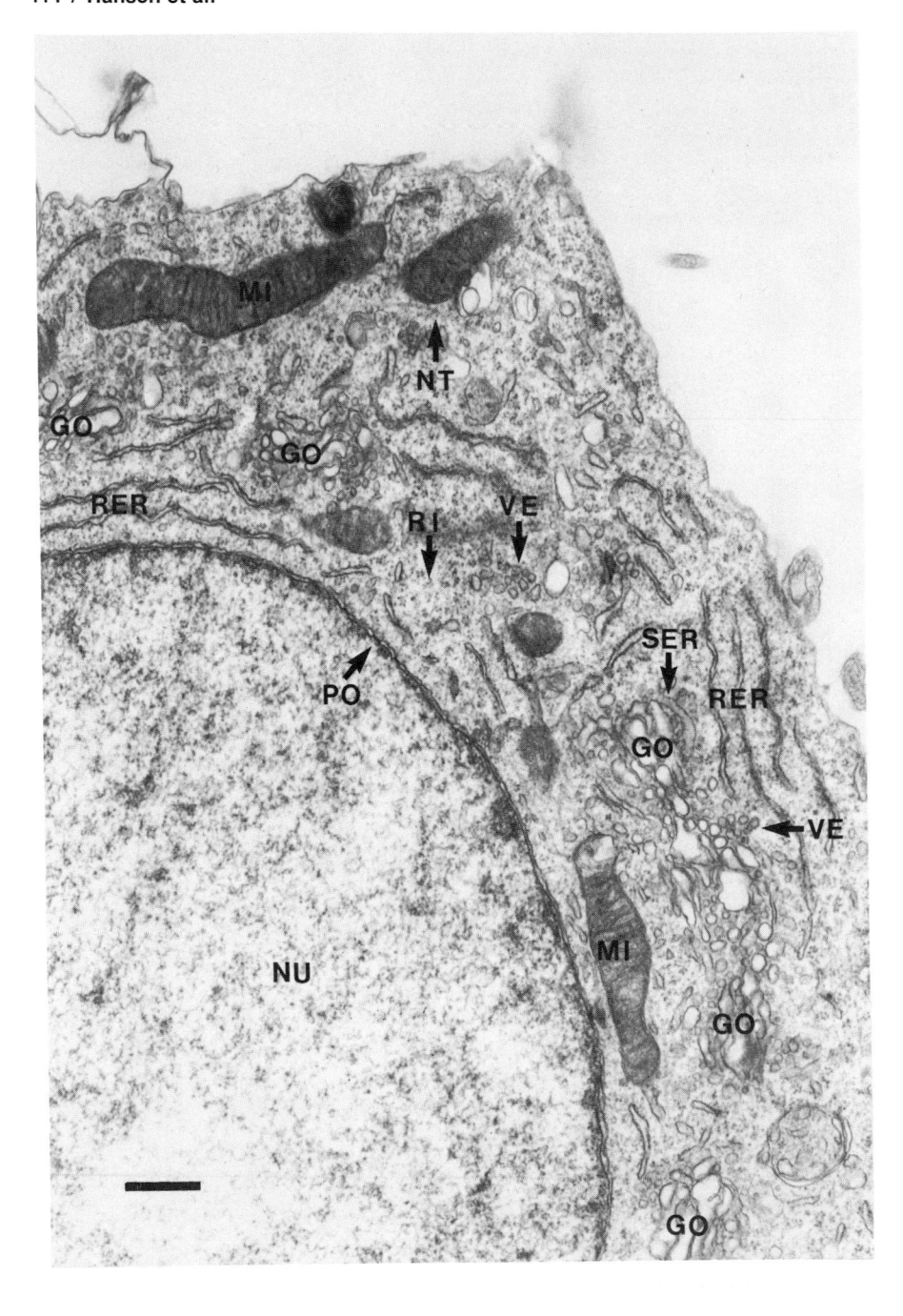

morphological and biochemical responses of the cells to administration of GABA and GABA receptor agonists and antagonists.

Morphology

Primary cultures of cerebellar granule cells exhibit a typical "neuron-like" structure when investigated by phase contrast light microscopy. A characteristic round to oval cell body (perikaryon or soma) is observed from which normally one-two processes are seen (Fig. 1C,D). The temporal development of the cells in culture is illustrated in Fig. 1A-D which shows that the cells possess neurites already after 20 hours in culture. The morphological appearance of the cells after 4 days in culture is very similar to that of older cultures (cf. Hansen et al., 1984). At the electron microscope level it can be seen that the granule cells are characterized by prominent nuclei, which occupy most of the perikaryon (Fig. 2). This is in agreement with the ultrastructure of granule cells observed by Seil (1979). In the perikaryon the nucleus is surrounded by the cytoplasm in which the different organelles involved in synthesis, intracellular transport, metabolism and degradation of macromolecules are located (Fig. 3). In the axon, however, most of the organelles are absent and only neurotubules, vesicles, coated vesicles and mitochondria are observed (Fig. 4A,B).

Ribosomes are scattered all over the perikaryon (Fig. 5A) but are never observed in the axon (Fig. 4A,B). Ribosomes are either located free in the cytoplasm or attached to the endoplasmic reticulum, constituting the rough endoplasmic reticulum (Fig. 5A). The smooth endoplasmic reticulum (Fig. 5B) is devoid of ribosomes.

The Golgi apparatus is mainly situated near the

Figure 3. Electron micrograph of a cerebellar granule cell illustrating the different organelles. A prominent nucleus (nu) and nuclear pores (po) are observed. In the cytoplasm, ribosomes (ri), rough endoplasmic reticulum (rer), smooth endoplasmic reticulum (ser), Golgi apparatus (go), mitochondria (mi), vesicles (ve) and neurotubules (nt) are seen. The bar indicates 500 nm.
Unpublished material of G.H. Hansen.

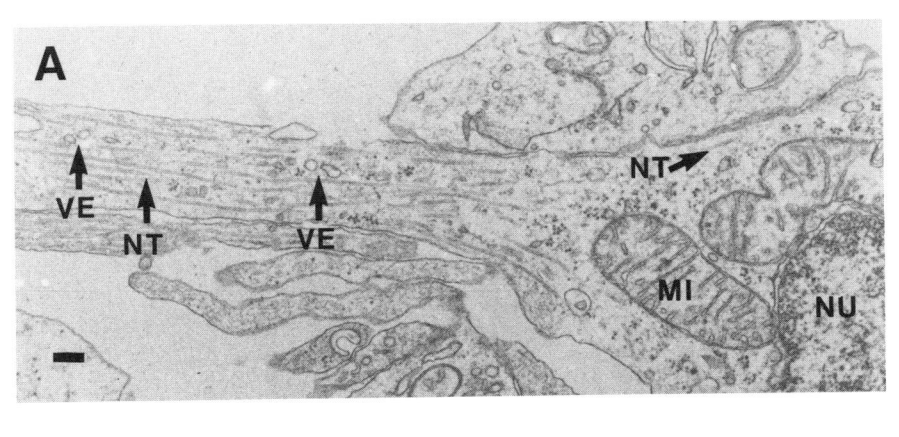

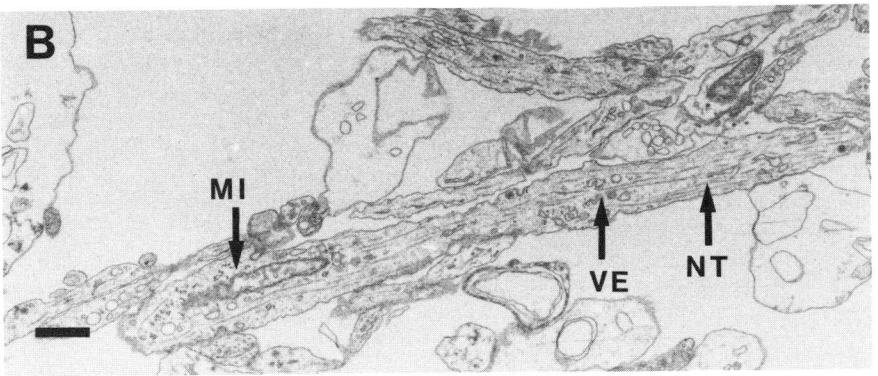

Figure 4. Electron micrograph of a cerebellar granule
cell from which an axon is extending (A). Note the
prominently developed neurotubules (nt) in the axon in
comparison with only few neurotubules in the perikaryon.
Nucleus (nu), mitochondria (mi) and vesicles (ve). The
bar indicates 200 nm (B). Electron micrograph showing
prominently developed neurotubules in the axon. Note that
mitochondria as well as vesicles are present in the axon.
The bar indicates 500 nm. Unpublished material of G.H.
Hansen.

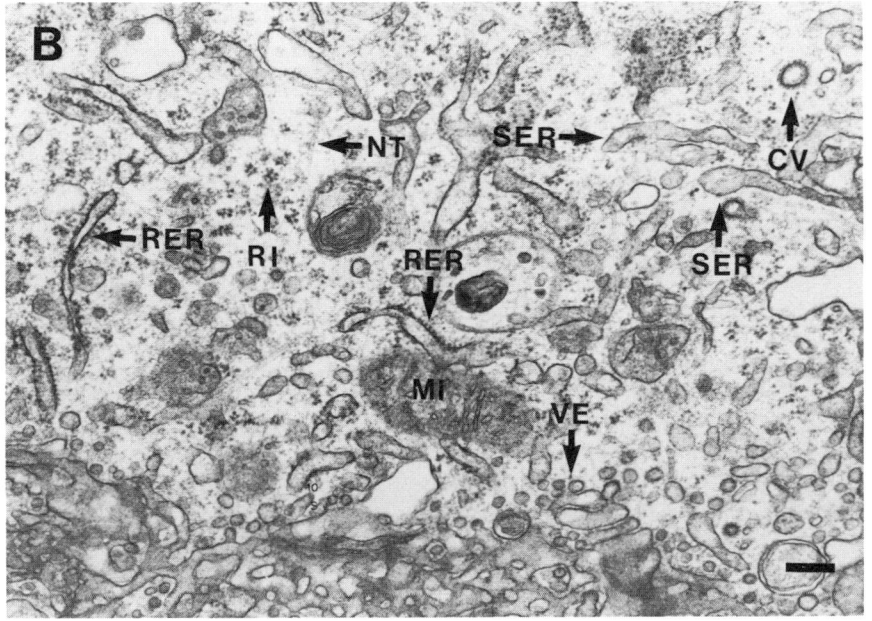

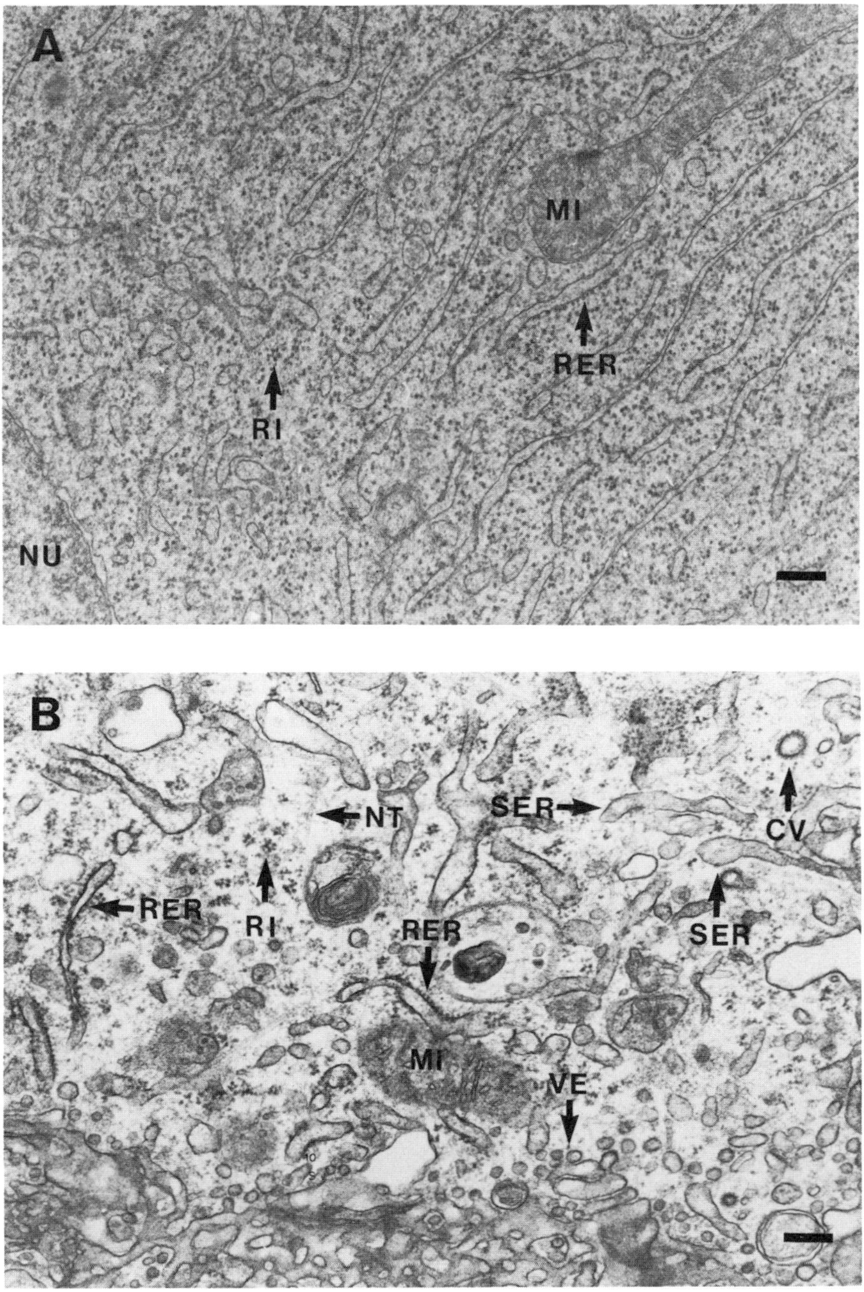

Fig. 5. Legend on next page

nucleus (Fig. 6A) and is usually divided into a convex
cis-face lying close to the nucleus and a concave
trans-face directed away from the nucleus (Fig. 6B).
Different types of vesicles are found both in the
perikaryon and the axon (Fig. 7 and Fig. 4A,B) accounting
for a prominent part of the cytoplasmic density. Coated
vesicles (Fig. 8A,B,C) are particularly densely located in
the Golgi region where occasionally budding or fusion is
observed (Fig. 8A). Close to the plasma membrane coated
pits and coated vesicles are frequently seen (Fig. 8B,C).
Neurotubules are seen in the perikaryon (Fig. 4A) but are
especially well developed in the axon (Fig. 4A,B).
Mitochondria are prominent in both the perikaryon (Fig. 7)
and the axon (Fig. 4B). Lysosomes (Fig. 9A) and
multivesicular bodies (Fig. 9B) are observed in the
perikaryon.

NEUROTROPHIC ACTION OF GABA AND GABA AGONISTS ON
CEREBELLAR GRANULE CELLS

Effects on morphology

Primary cultures of cerebellar granule cells were
prepared as described above and grown for 7 days in the
presence or absence of GABA. The morphological appearance
of the cultures was investigated using phase contrast
light microscopy. Micrographs were taken randomly and
scored double blind for neurite extending cells and
colonies of neuronal cell bodies (cf. Fig. 1). This
showed significant differences between granule cells grown
in the presence of 50 μM GABA and cells grown under
standard conditions (Table I). In addition to this, Table
I shows that the neurotrophic action of GABA or the GABA
analogue THIP (4,5,6,7-tetrahydroisoxazolo[5,4-c]pyridin-

Figure 5. Electron micrograph showing rough endoplamic
reticulum (rer) in a cerebellar granule cell (A).
Ribosomes (ri) are either free or attached to the
endoplasmic reticulum (rer). Nucleus (nu) and
mitochondria (mi). B. Electron micrograph showing smooth
endoplasmic reticulum (ser). Note that the smooth
endoplasmic reticulum is devoid of ribosomes.
Mitochondria, rough endoplasmic reticulum, vesicles (ve),
coated vesicles (cv) and neurotubules (nt). Bars
indicates 200 nm. Unpublished material of G.H. Hansen.

TABLE I. Effect of GABA or THIP on formation of neurites and neuronal colonies in granule cell cultures

Culture condition	Neurite-ext. cells per mm²		Colonies per mm²
	4-days-in culture	7-days-in culture	7-days-in culture
Control	1804 + 90	629 + 33	19 + 4
+ GABA (50 μM) or THIP (150 μM)	2160 + 104*	931 + 82**	43 + 7**

Cerebellar granule cells were cultured for 4 or 7 days in the absence or presence of 150 μM THIP (4 days) or 50 μM GABA (7 days) and phase contrast micrographs were taken randomly and scored double blind for neurite-extending cells and colonies of neuronal cell bodies. Results are averages of 6–12 micrographs taken of 2–3 cultures of each group. Asterisks indicate statistically significant differences from cells grown under standard conditions (* P < 0.025, Mann-Whitney test; ** P < 0.01, t-test). From Hansen et al., (1984) or unpublished results of J. Abraham, G.H. Hansen and A. Schousboe.

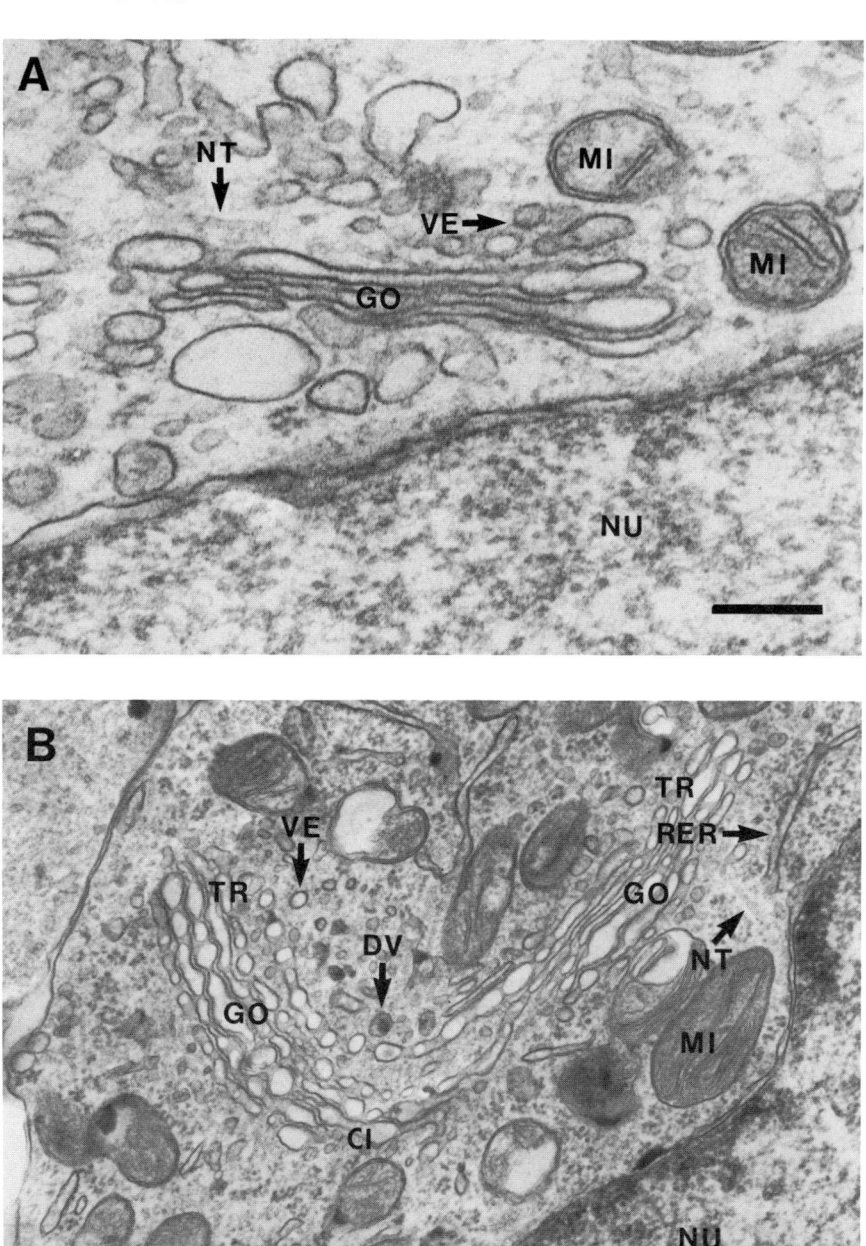

3-ol) could be observed also after 4 days in culture, since exposure of the cells to 150 µM THIP for this period of time leads to a statistically significant increase in the number of neurite extending cells per culture area.

Effects of ultrastructure

The light microscope demonstration of a neurotrophic effect of GABA was subsequently investigated at the electron microscope level. Granule cells were cultured for respectively 1, 2, 4 and 7 days in the presence or absence of 50 µM GABA, prepared for electron microscopy according to standard procedure and subjected to morphometric analyses (cf, Hansen et al., 1984; Meier et al., 1985). The ultrastructural analysis which included the organelles shown in Fig. 3-8 was performed double blind, i.e. the samples were randomized with regard to culture periods as well as conditions. The cytoplasmic density of rough endoplasmic reticulum, smooth endoplasmic reticulum, vesicles and coated vesicles was increased with the culturing period as exemplified in Fig. 10. On the other hand, the cytoplasmic density of the Golgi apparatus as well as mitochondria was unaffected by the culture period and the cytoplasmic density of free ribosomes was found to decrease (Hansen et al., 1984).

Addition of 50 µM GABA to the culture media led to pronounced changes in the ultrastructural composition of the cerebellar granule cells. The neurotrophic effect of GABA was obvious already after treatment with GABA for 1 day although the difference between cells grown in the presence of GABA or under standard conditions was much more pronounced after longer periods of culturing (Hansen et al., 1984). It is seen (Table II) that the cytoplasmic density of the Golgi apparatus, neurotubules, rough

---

Figure 6. Electron micrograph of a Golgi apparatus (go) located near the nucleus (nu) in a cerebellar granule cell (A). Mitochondria (mi), vesicles (ve) and neurotubules (nt). B. Electron micrograph illustrating the characteristic convex or cis-face (ci) and concave or trans-face (tr) of a Golgi apparatus. Nucleus, mitochondria, rough endoplasmic reticulum (rer), dense core vesicle (dv), vesicles (ve) and neurotubules. Bars indicate 200 nm. Unpublished materal of G.H. Hansen.

endoplasmic reticulum, vesicles and coated vesicles, was increased whereas no difference was found in the density of mitochondria, smooth endoplasmic reticulum and ribosomes (Hansen et al., 1984). These findings have recently been confirmed in studies on the effect of GABA on retinal and cerebral cortical neurons in culture (Spoerri, 1986).

Mechanism for the trophic action

The light and electron microscopic observations of the effects of GABA only allow the conclusion that GABA enhances growth and differentiation of cerebellar granule cells. Accordingly, these studies give no information about possible mechanisms by which the neurotrophic effect of GABA is mediated. Theoretically it could be mediated by an intracellular action of GABA since the plasma membrane of cerebellar granule cells is permeable to GABA

TABLE II. Summary of effects of GABA on the ultrastructure of cerebellar granule cells

Organelle	Effect of GABA	
Mitochondria	none	–
Golgi apparatus	increased	$p < 0.0005$
Neurotubules	increased	$p < 0.025$
Ribosomes	none	–
Rough endoplasmic reticulum	increased	$p < 0.025$
Smooth endoplasmic reticulum	none	–
Coated vesicles	increased	$p < 0.05$
Other vesicles	increased	$p < 0.05$

Cerebellar granule cells were cultured for 1–7 days in the absence or presence of 50 μM GABA and the temporal development of the cytoplasmic densities of the different organelles was followed as exemplified in Fig. 10. Electron micrographs (cf. Figs. 3–8) were taken at random and the densities of the structures were determined double-blind using the point method for morphometric analysis. Summary from Hansen et al. (1984).

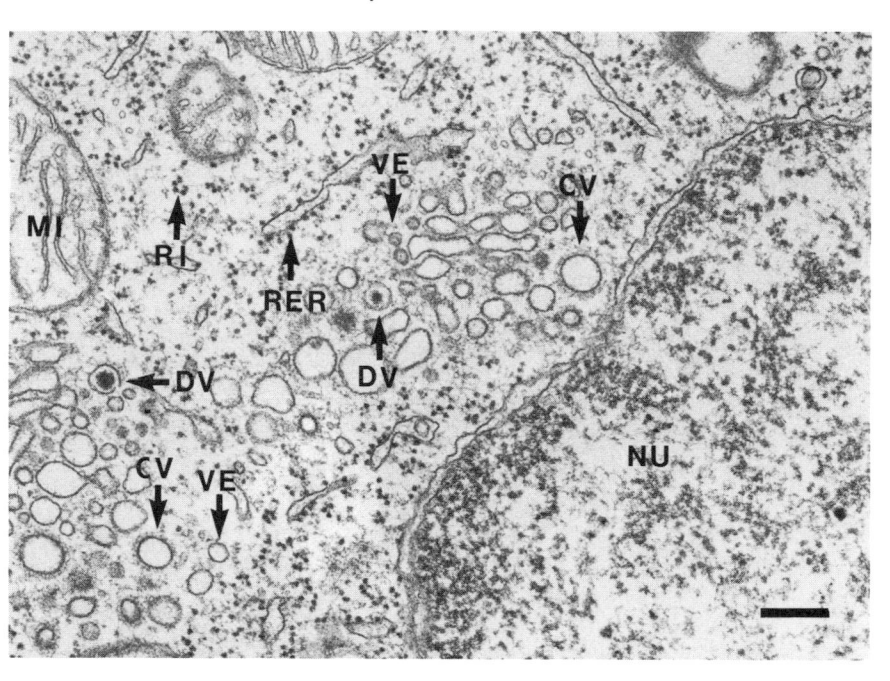

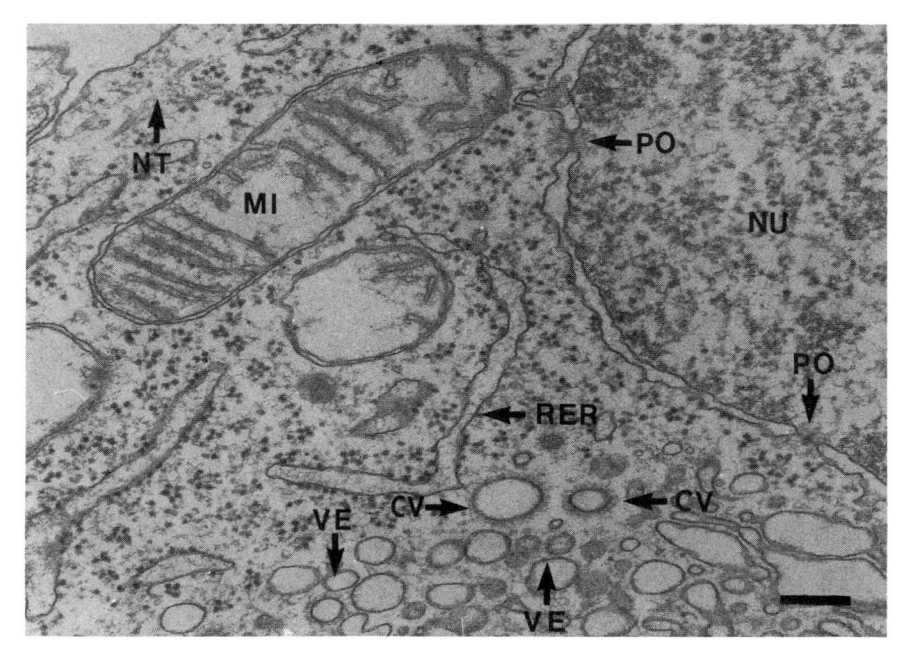

Fig. 7. Legend on next page

(Yu and Hertz, 1982). Alternatively, GABA could act via GABA receptors present in the plasma membrane of the cerebellar granule cells which are known to be particularly rich in GABA receptors (Simantov et al., 1976; Olsen and Mikoshiba, 1978; Kingsbury et al., 1980; Hosli et al., 1980; Palacios et al., 1980; Skerritt and Johnston, 1982; Meier and Schousboe, 1982).

To elucidate this question, experiments were performed at the light as well as the electron microscope level in which primary cultures of cerebellar granule cells were treated with GABA receptor specific agonists or antagonists (Meier et al., 1985). As a GABA receptor agonist, THIP was chosen since it has been shown to bind specifically to GABA receptors (Krogsgaard-Larsen and Johnston, 1978) and not to cross the plasma membrane of neurons (Schousboe et al., 1985a) Bicuculline methobromide was used as the GABA receptor specific antagonist (Curtis et al., 1971).

Experiments were performed on cerebellar granule cells cultured for 4 and 7 days in plain culture media or in the presence of 50 µM GABA, 150 µM THIP or 50 µM GABA and 150 µM bicuculline methobromide. As shown in Table I treatment with THIP for 4 days led to a significant increase in the number of neurite extending cells. Morphometric analyses at the electron microscope level showed that cerebellar granule cells treated with GABA or THIP exhibited a statistically significant increase in the cytoplasmic density of rough endoplasmic reticulum, Golgi apparatus, neurotubules, vesicles and coated vesicles as compared to cultures grown under standard conditions (Meier et al., 1985). No significant effect on the cytoplasmic density of smooth endoplasmic reticulum, mitochondria and ribosomes was observed. This result showed that THIP could completely replace GABA for its

---

Figure 7. Electron micrographs illustrating different types of vesicles in the perikaryon of cerebellar granule cells. Dense core vesicles (dv), coated vesicles (cv) as well as "smooth vesicles" (ve) with varying electron density are observed. Nucleus (nu), nuclear pores (po), ribosomes (ri), rough endoplasmic reticulum (rer), mitochondria (mi) and neurotubules (nt). Bars indicate 200 nm. Unpublished material of G.H. Hansen.

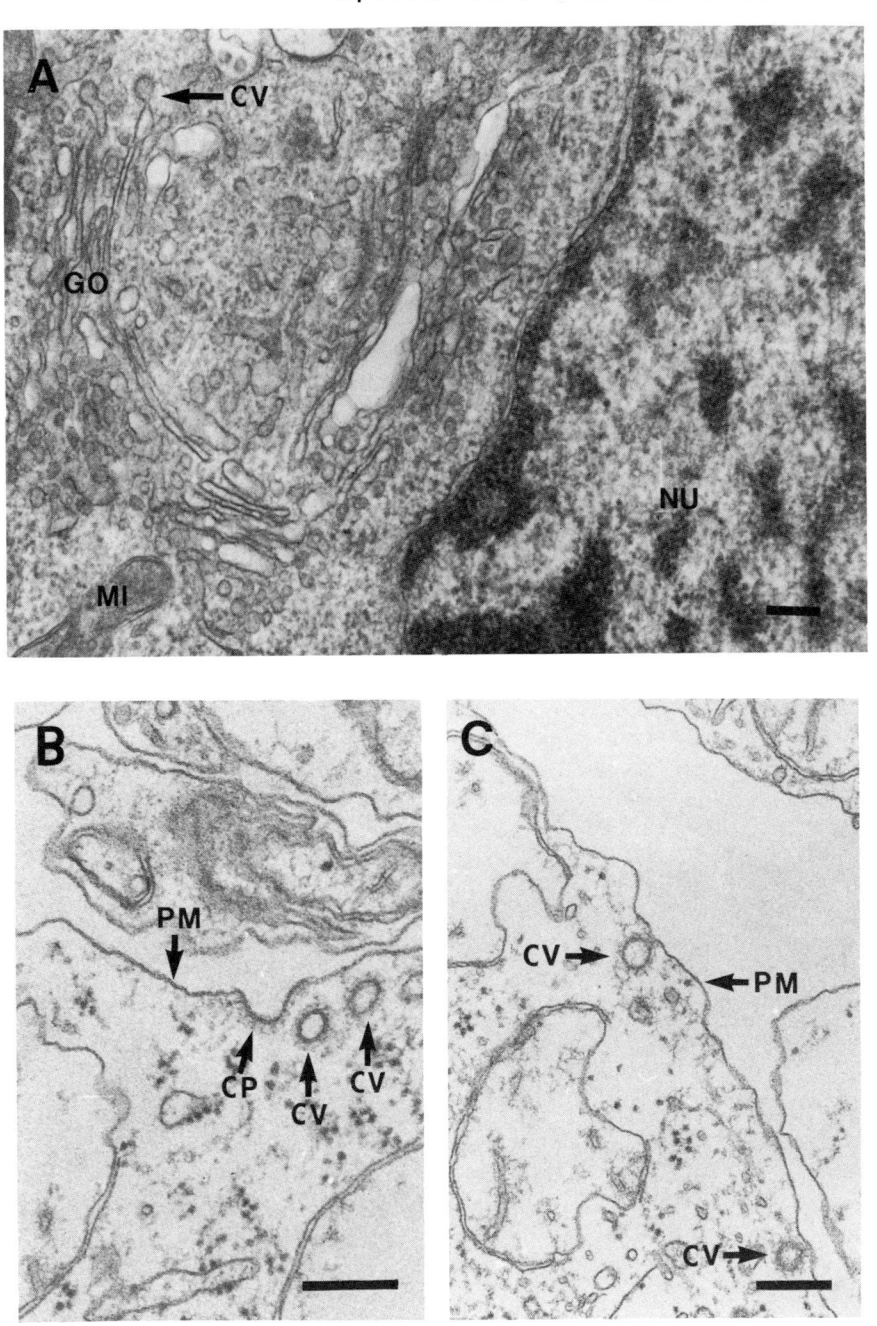

Fig. 8. Legend on next page

neurotrophic action. In cerebellar granule cells cultured for 4 and 7 days in the simultaneous presence of bicuculline methobromide and GABA the neurotrophic action of GABA was completely abolished (Meier et al., 1985).

These findings (cf. Table III) strongly indicate that the neurotrophic effect of GABA is mediated by GABA receptors in the plasma membrane of the cerebellar granule cells. Since it has been shown that cerebellar granule cells cultured in plain culture media, i.e. in the absence of GABA, express only GABA receptors of the high affinity type (Meier and Schousboe, 1982; Meier et al., 1984; Belhage et al., 1986; Meier et al., this volume) it is likely that such GABA receptors are responsible for the mediation of the neurotrophic action of GABA. These GABA receptors are generally believed to be associated with chloride channels (Olsen, 1981). Thus, it is possible that the action of GABA may be coupled to a hyperpolarization of the cells. Such a mechanism would be compatible with the previous demonstration that bromide acts as a neurotrophic agent (Joo et al., 1980; Spoerri and Wolff, 1981; 1982; Toldi et al., 1986). The involvement of ion channels in the neurotrophic action of GABA also seems compatible with the mechanism of action of other neurotrophic factors such as the nerve growth factor which has been shown to affect sodium channels in chick dorsal root ganglionic cells (Skaper and Varon, 1980).

Temporal development of the trophic action

In the study by Hansen et al., (1984) it was shown that the neurotrophic action of GABA could be detected after 1 day of exposure of the cells to GABA with maximal effects after 4 days. No conclusion as to the exact

---

Figure 8. Electron micrographs showing the different location of coated vesicles (cv) in cerebellar granule cells. A. Golgi apparatus (go). Note that a coated vesicle (cv) is either budding from or fusing with the trans cisterna of the Golgi apparatus. Nucleus (nu) and mitochondria (mi). B. A coated pit (cp) in the plasma membrane (pm) and coated vesicles located close to the plasma membrane are observed. C. Coated vesicles are observed close to the plasma membrane. Bars indicate 200 nm. Unpublished material of G.H. Hansen.

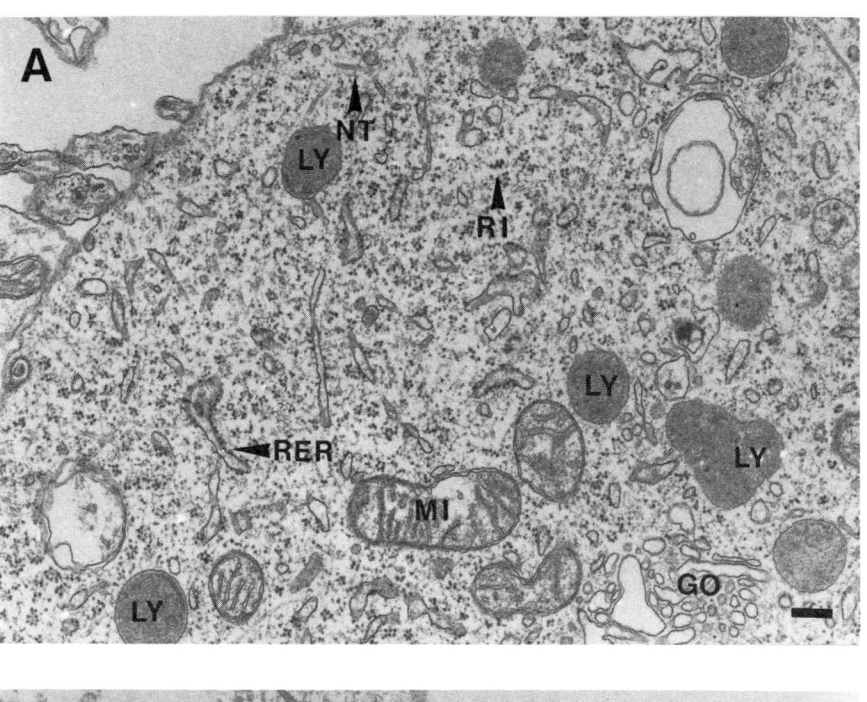

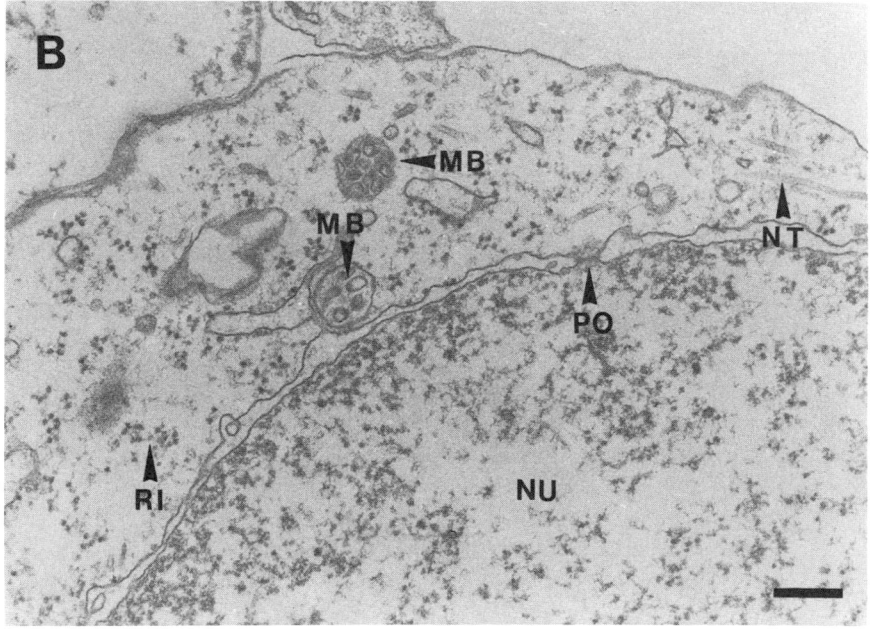

Fig. 9. Legend on next page

temporal development of the trophic action could, however, be reached.

In order to elucidate in more detail the temporal development of the neurotrophic effect of GABA agonists, cerebellar granule cells were cultured in plain media for 4 days, before 150 μM THIP was added to the media. After treatment with THIP for respectively 1, 3, 6 and 24 hours, the cells were prepared for electron microscopy and morphometric analysis. It was found that treatment with THIP for 1 hour led to a significant increase in the cytoplasmic density of rough endoplasmic reticulum, Golgi apparatus, vesicles and coated vesicles concomitant with a significant decrease in the density of smooth endoplasmic reticulum (Hansen et al., 1987). This is further illustrated in Table IV which also contains results for treatment with THIP for 24 hours. It is seen that no further differences were observed between 1 and 24 hours of exposure to THIP.

TABLE III. Summary of effects of GABA agonists and antagonists on morphological development of cerebellar granule cells

Culture condition	Morphological development
Plain culture media	normal
Media + 50 μM GABA	enhanced
Media + 150 μM THIP	enhanced
Media + 50 μM GABA and 150 μM bicuculline	normal

Cerebellar granule cells were cultured for respectively 4 and 7 days in either plain culture media or in the presence or GABA, THIP or GABA + bicuculline. From Hansen et al., (1984); Meier et al. (1985) and unpublished experiments of J. Abraham, G.H. Hansen and A. Schousboe.

Figure 9. Electron micrograph of lysosomes (ly) in a cerebellar granule cell (A). Mitochondria (mi), ribosomes (ri), rough endoplasmic reticulum (rer), Golgi apparatus (go) and neurotubules (nt). B. Electron micrograph illustrating multivesicular bodies (mb) in a cerebellar granule cell. Nucleus (nu), nuclear pores (po), ribosomes and neurotubules. Bars indicates 200 nm.

TABLE IV. Temporal development of the neurotrophic effect of THIP on cerebellar granule cells

Organelle	Cytoplasmic density (%)			
	1 h		24h	
	Control	THIP	Control	THIP
Rough endoplasmic reticulum	3.60±0.44	5.65±0.44*	3.57±0.44	5.93±0.44*
Smooth endoplasmic reticulum	3.36±0.21	2.85±0.21*	3.43±0.21	2.79±0.21*
Golgi apparatus	5.35±0.77	6.75±0.77*	4.97±0.77	6.94±0.77*
Vesicles	9.04±0.74	12.13±0.74*	8.32±0.74	11.73±0.74*
Coated vesicles	1.34±0.18	2.14±0.18*	1.28±0.18	2.28±0.18*

Cerebellar granule cells were cultured for 4 days in plain culture media prior to the addition of 150 μM THIP. The cultures were prepared for morphometric analysis after exposure to THIP for respectively 1 and 24 hours. The results are averages $\pm$ SEM of 27 independent countings calculated on the basis of a two-way analysis of variance. Asterisks indicate statistically significant differences from the controls ($P < 0.002$). From Hansen et al., (1987).

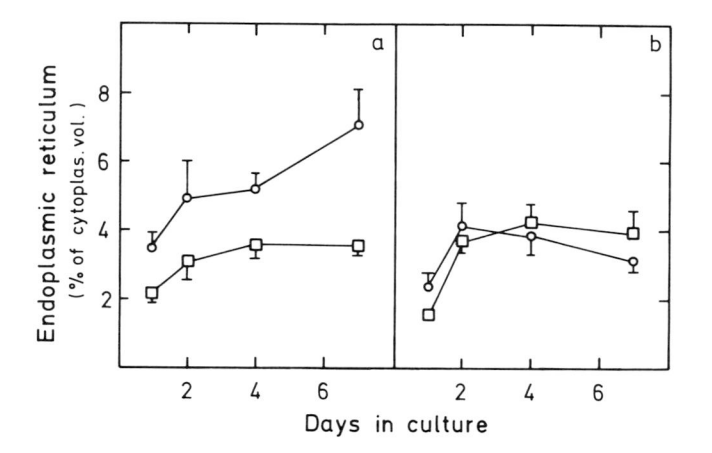

Figure 10. Density of rough endoplasmic reticulum (a) and smooth endoplasmic reticulum (b) expressed as per cent of total cytoplasmic volume in cultured cerebellar granule cells as a function of the culture period. Cells were grown under standard conditions (□) or in the presence of 50 μM GABA (O). Each point represents the average of countings of 25 different electron micrographs, and SEM are indicated by vertical bars if they extend beyond the symbols. (a) GABA-treated cells differed significantly from control cultures (p < 0.025).
From Hansen et al. (1984).

CONCLUSIONS

The results of the light and electron microscopic investigations of primary cultures of cerebellar granule cells grown in the presence of GABA or GABA agonists and antagonists have clearly demonstrated that GABA plays a major role in the development of differentiation of cerebellar granule cells in culture, i.e. GABA has a neurotrophic effect. This conclusion is well in agreement with the original suggestion by Wolff and coworkers (Wolff et al., 1978) that GABA modulates neuronal developmet in vivo. Moreover, using an experimental approach analogous to the one discussed in this review similar results have recently been obtained with cortical neurons (Spoerri, 1986) and tectal neurons (Michler-Stuke and Wolff, 1986) in culture. By the use of specific GABA receptor agonists and antagonists it was furthermore demonstrated that the neurotrophic effect of GABA is mediated by GABA receptors in the plasma membrane (Meier et al., 1985). This is in line with what has been demonstrated with regard to the neurotrophic effect of GABA in retina (Madtes and Redburn, 1983a).

The findings that it is in particular the cytoplasmic density of rough endoplasmic reticulum, Golgi apparatus, vesicles and coated vesicles which is increased after exposure of the cells to GABA agonists, might indicate that protein synthesis at least partly is stimulated by GABA. This suggestion would be in keeping with the early reports stating that GABA enhances brain protein synthesis (Campbell et al., 1966; Tewari and Baxter, 1969; Snodgrass, 1973; Goertz, 1979). Whether the morphological findings indicate a general increase in the synthesis of proteins in cerebellar granule cells or a selective effect on the synthesis of proteins destined for insertion into membranes can not be elucidated at the present time. However, recent studies in our laboratory have indicated that the total amount of proteins as well as of the neuron specific antigens N-CAM (neuronal cell adhesion molecule) and enolase are increased in cerebellar granule cells grown in the presence of GABA or GABA agonists (Meier and Jorgensen, 1986). It has also been demonstrated that exposure of cerebellar granule cells to GABA or GABA agonists induces low affinity GABA receptors (Meier et al., 1983; 1984; Belhage et al., 1986; Meier et al., this volume). As discussed in the adjoining paper (Meier et al., this volume) it has been shown that inhibitors of protein synthesis (actinomycin D and cycloheximide) block the ability of GABA agonists to induce low affinity GABA receptors. This implies that the effect of GABA involves a stimulation of protein synthesis and the result fits well with the observed increase in the cytoplasmic density of organelles involved in synthesis of plasma membrane proteins in cells grown in the presence of GABA. Morphometric analysis of the effects of protein synthesis inhibitors on the ultrastructure of cerebellar granule cells could contribute to the elucidation of the interrelationship of the neurotrophic effect of GABA and the development of the machinery for protein synthesis. In this context it should be kept in mind that the temporal development of the GABA-induced effect on the ultrastructure precedes that of the induction of low affinity receptors (Hansen et al., 1987).

Although the neurotrophic effect of GABA has been documented it still remains unknown whether this effect is general for cerebellar granule cells throughout development or may be restricted to certain stages of cell development and differentiation. That the trophic effect may indeed be restricted to a specific developmental period is indicated by the findings that induction of GABA receptors seems to be restricted to early stages of development (Hansen et al., 1986; Madtes and Bashir-Elahi, 1986).

It has been demonstrated that the neurotrophic effect of GABA is mediated by preexisting high affinity GABA receptors in the plasma membrane of cerebellar granule cells (Meier et al., 1985). However, the actual mechanism by which the GABA receptors mediate the morphological changes in the cells is only speculative at the present time. Several possibilities seem to exist. GABA receptor ligands could be internalized by receptor mediated endocytosis and thereby exert their neurotrophic effect through an intracellular action. Alternatively, the interaction between GABA agonists and the GABA receptors might activate second messengers. By analogy with the proposed mechanism of action for the nerve growth factor (Skaper and Varon, 1980) GABA agonists might via GABA receptors alter the function of ion channels which, in turn, mediate the neurotrophic effect. This latter possibility is favored by the findings that bromide exerts a neurotrophic effect similar to that of GABA (Joo et al., 1980; Spoerri and Wolff, 1981; 1982; Toldi et al., 1986) and that picrotoxin blocks the induction of GABA receptors presumably by its antagonistic action on chloride channels (Meier et al., this volume).

In order to furnish additional information, immunocytochemical studies at the electron microscope level would be of interest. By use of quantitative immunogold staining it could be determined whether the rate of synthesis of specific proteins such as N-CAM and GABA receptors is enhanced in cerebellar granule cells during exposure to GABA agonists. In this context it should be emphasized that it has recently been shown that administration of GABA to rats during early postnatal development enhances the maturation of N-CAM (Meier et al., 1987).

Recent studies of other neurotransmitters such as serotonin, dopamine, and noradrenaline (Narumi et al., 1978; Lauder, 1983; Haydon et al., 1984; Konig et al., 1986) have indicated that these neurotransmitters also exert important regulatory control in the development of the nervous system. It seems accordingly safe to postulate that neurotransmitters in addition to their traditional roles could also be regarded as factors responsible for correct development and differentiation of the central nervous system. Such regulatory actions could also be exerted by neurotoxic agents. Glutamate, one of the most abundant neurotransmitters (Fonnum, 1984), might serve this function since it is known to be a very powerful neurotoxin (Olney, 1978).

ACKNOWLEDGEMENTS

The work has been financially supported by grants from the Danish Medical Research Council (12-389; 12-3334; 12-4599; 12-4492; 12-4767; 12-6340) and the Novo Foundation.

REFERENCES

Belhage B, Meier E, Schousboe A (1986). GABA-agonists induce the formation of low affinity GABA-receptors on cultured cerebellar granule cells via preexisting high affinity GABA-receptors. Neurochem Res 11: 599-606.

Campbell MK, Mahler HR, Moore WJ, Tewari S (1966). Protein synthesis systems from rat brain. Biochemistry 5: 1174-1184.

Curtis DR, Duggan AW, Felix D, Johnston GAR (1971). Bicuculline, an antagonist of GABA and synaptic inhibition in the spinal cord of the cat. Brain Res 32: 69-96.

Eins E, Spoerri PE, Heyder E (1983). GABA or sodium bromide-induced plasticity of neurites of mouse neuroblastoma cells in cultures. A quantitative study. Cell Tiss Res 229: 457-460.

Fonnum F (1984). Glutamate: A neurotransmitter in mammalian brain. J Neurochem 42: 1-11.

Gallo V, Ciotti MT, Coletti A, Aloisi F, Levi G (1982). Selective release of glutamate from cerebellar granule cells differentiating in culture. Proc Natl Acad Sci USA 79: 7919-7923.

Goertz B (1979). Effect of GABA on cell-free protein synthesizing systems from mouse brain. Exp Brain Res 34: 365-372.

Hansen GH, Meier E, Schousboe A (1984). GABA influences the ultrastructure composition of cerebellar granule cells during development in culture. Int J Devl Neurosci 2: 247-257.

Hansen GH, Belhage B, Meier E, Schousboe A (1986). Developmental aspects of the trophic activity of GABA agonists on cerebellar granule cells in culture. Int J. Devl Neurosci 4: Suppl 1: S36.

Hansen GH, Belhage B, Schousboe A, Meier E (1987). Time course of the GABA induced change in ultrastructure composition and GABA receptor expression in cultured cerebellar granule cells. Int J Devl Neurosci Vol 5 In press.

Haydon PG, McCobb DP, Kater SB (1984). Serotonin selectively inhibits growth cone motility and synaptogenesis of specific identified neurons. Science 226: 561-564.

Haydon PG, McCobb DP, Murphy AD, Kater SB (1985). Serotonin and dopamine inhibit neurite outgrowth and growth cone motility. Neurosci Lett Suppl 22: S239.

Hertz L, Juurlink BHJ, Fosmark H, Schousboe A (1982). Astrocytes in primary culture. In Pfeiffer SE (ed): "Neuroscience Approached Through Cell Culture, vol. 1". Boca Raton: CRC Press, pp 175-186.

Hosli E, Mohler H, Richards JG, Hosli L (1980). Autoradiographic localization of binding sites for $[^3H]\gamma$-aminobutyrate,[3H] muscimol, (+) [3H]bicuculline methiodide and [3H]flunitrazepam in cultures of rat cerebellum and spinal cord. Neuroscience 5: 1657-1665.

Joo F, Dames W, Wolff JR (1980). Effect of prolonged sodium bromide administration on the fine structure of dendrites in the superior cervical ganglion of adult rat. Prog Brain Res 51: 109-115.

Kingsbury AE, Wilkin GD, Patel AJ, Balazs R (1980). Distribution of GABA receptors in the rat cerebellum. J Neurochem 35: 739-742.

Konig N, Drian M-J, Privat A, Lamande N, Pares-Herbute N, Schachner M (1986). Dissociated cells of foetal rat pallium grown in culture medium supplemented with noradrenaline: Effects of the expression of neuron-specific enolase and cell adhesion molecule L1. Neurosci Lett 66: 67-72.

Krogsgaard-Larsen P, Johnston GAR (1978). Structure-activity studies on inhibition of GABA binding to rat brain membranes by muscimol and related compounds. J Neurochem 30: 1377-1382.

Lauder JM (1983). Hormonal and humoral influences on brain development. Psychoneuroendocrinology 8: 121-155.

Madtes PC, Bashir-Elahi R (1986). GABA receptor binding site 'induction' in rabbit retina after nipecotic acid treatment. Changes during development. Neurochem Res 11: 55-61.

Madtes PC, Redburn DA (1983a). GABA as a trophic factor during development. Life Sci 33: 979-984.

Madtes PC, Redburn DA (1983b). Synaptic interactions in the GABA system during postnatal development in retina. Brain Res Bull 101: 741-745.

Meier E, Schousboe A (1982). Differences between GABA receptor binding to membranes from cerebellum during postnatal development and from cultured cerebellar granule cells. Dev Neurosci 5: 546-553.

Meier E, Drejer J, Schousboe A (1983). Trophic actions of GABA on the development of physiological active GABA receptors. In Mandel P, De Feudis FV (eds): "CNS-Receptors from Molecular Pharmacology to Behavior". New York: Raven Press, pp 47-58.

Meier E, Drejer J, Schousboe A (1984). GABA induces functionally active low-affinitive GABA receptors on cultured cerebellar granule cells. J Neurochem 43: 1737-1744.

Meier E, Hansen GH, Schousboe A (1985). The trophic effect of GABA on cerebellar granule cells is mediated by

GABA-receptors. Int J Devl Neurosci 3: 401–407.

Meier E, Jorgensen OS (1986). γ-Aminobutyric acid affects the developmental expression of neuron-associated proteins in cerebellar granule cell cultures. J Neurochem 46: 1256–1262.

Meier E, Jorgensen OS, Schousboe A (1987). Effect of repeated treatment with a GABA receptor agonist on postnatal neural development in rats. J Neurochem Submitted.

Messer A (1977). The maintenance and identification of mouse cerebellar granule cells in monolayer cultures. Brain Res 130: 1–12.

Michler-Stuke A, Wolff JR (1986). Modulatory effects of GABA, NGF, and potassium on neurite extension of chick tectal neurons. Int J Devl Neurosci 4: Suppl 1: S71.

Narumi S, Kimmelberg HK, Bourke RS (1978). Effects of norepinephrine on the morphology and some enzyme activities of primary monolayer cultures from rat brain. J Neurochem 31: 1479–1490.

Oertel WH, Schmechel DE, Mugnaini E, Tappaz ML, Kopin IJ (1981). Immunocytochemical localization of glutamate decarboxylase in rat cerebellum with a new antiserum. Neuroscience 6: 2715–2735.

Olney JW (1978). Neurotoxicity of excitatory amino acids. In McGeer EG, Olney JW, McGeer PL (eds): "Kainic Acid as a Tool in Neurobiology". New York: Raven Press, pp 95–121.

Olsen RW (1981). GABA-benzodiazepine-barbiturate receptor interactions. J Neurochem 37: 1–13.

Olsen RA, Mikoshiba K (1978). Localization of gamma-aminobutyric acid receptor binding in the mammalian cerebellum. High levels in granule layer and depletion in agranular cerebella of mutant mice. J Neurochem 30: 1633–1636.

Palacios JM, Young S, Kuhar MJ (1980). Autoradiographic localization of γ-aminobutyric acid (GABA) receptors in the rat cerebellum. Proc Natl Acad Sci USA 77: 670–674.

Palay SL (1982). Current status of neuroanatomical research in the cerebellum. In Palay SL, Chan-Palay V (eds): Exp Brain Res Suppl 6 "The Cerebellum New Vistas". Berlin Heidelberg New York: Springer-Verlag, pp 1–8.

Redburn DA, Madtes PC (1986). Postnatal development of ^{3}H-GABA-accumulating cells in rabbit retina. J Comp Neurol 243: 41–57.

Schousboe A, Larsson OM, Krogsgaard-Larsen P (1985a). Lack

of a high affinity uptake system for the GABA agonists THIP and isoguvacine in neurons and astrocytes cultured from mouse brain. Neurochem Int 7: 505-508.

Schousboe A, Drejer J, Hansen GH, Meier E (1985b). Cultured neurons as model systems for biochemical and pharmacological studies on receptors for neurotransmitter amino acids. Dev Neurosci 7: 252-262.

Schousboe A, Hansen GH, Belhage B, Meier E (1987). Role of the inhibitory neurotransmitter GABA as a signal for neuronal growth and differentiation. In Tucek S (ed): "Metabolism and Development of the Nervous System". N.Y.: John Wiley and Sons, in press.

Seil J (1979): Cerebellum in tissue culture. Rev Neurosci 4: 105-177.

Simantov R, Oster-Granite ML, Herndon RN, Snyder SH (1976). Gamma-aminobutyric acid (GABA) receptor binding selectively depleted by viral-induced granule cell loss in hamster cerebellum. Brain Res 105: 365-371.

Skaper SD, Varon S (1980). Properties of the sodium extrusion mechanism controlled by nerve growth factor in chick embryo dorsal root ganglionic cells. J Neurochem 34: 1654-1660.

Skerritt JH, Johnston GAR (1982). Postnatal development of GABA binding sites and their endogenous inhibitors in rat brain. Dev Neurosci 5: 189-197.

Snodgrass SR (1973). Studies of GABA and protein synthesis. Brain Res 59: 339-348.

Spoerri PE, Wolff JR (1981). Effect of GABA-administration on murine neuroblastoma cells in culture. Cell Tiss Res 218: 567-579.

Spoerri PE, Wolff JR (1982). Morphological changes induced by sodium bromide in murine neuroblastoma cells in vitro. Cell Tiss Res 222: 379-388.

Spoerri PE (1986). GABA induces developmental alterations in cultured neurons. Int J Devl Neurosci 4: Suppl S71.

Tewari S, Baxter CF (1969). Stimulatory effect of GABA upon amino acid incorporation into protein by a ribosomal system from immature rat brain. J Neurochem 16: 171-180.

Toldi J, Farkas Z, Feher O, Dames W, Kasa P, Gyurkovits K, Joo F, Wolff JR (1986). Promotion by sodium bromide of functional synapse formation from foreign nerves in the superior cervical ganglion of adult rat with intact preganglionic nerve supply. Neurosci Lett 69: 19-24.

Wolff JR Foo F, Dames W (1979). Plasticity in dendrites shown by continuous GABA administration in superior cervical ganglion of adult rat. Nature Lond 274: 72–74.

Wolff JR, Rickmann M, Chronwall BM (1979). Axo-glial synapses and GABA-accumulating glial cells in the embryonic neocortex of the rat. Cell Tiss Res 201: 239–248.

Yu ACH, Hertz L (1982). Uptake of glutamate, GABA, and glutamine into a predominantly GABA-ergic and a predominantly glutamatergic nerve cell population in culture. J Neurosci Res 7: 23–35.

Neurotrophic Activity of GABA During Development, pages 139–159
© **1987 Alan R. Liss, Inc.**

THE EXPRESSION OF GABA RECEPTORS ON CULTURED
CEREBELLAR GRANULE CELLS IS INFLUENCED BY GABA

Eddi Meier[1], Bo Belhage, Jorgen Drejer[2] and
Arne Schousboe
Department of Biochemistry A, Pannum Institute,
University of Copenhagen, DK-2200 Copenhagen,
Denmark.

INTRODUCTION

Cultures of cerebellar granule cells have proved to be
a valuable tool in studies of the trophic effects of GABA
since they express high densities of a single class of
GABA-receptors of the high affinity type (Meier and
Schousboe, 1982) and lack the capacity to synthesize and
release GABA in any appreciable amount (Oertel et al.,
1981; Pearce and Dutton, 1982; Gallo et al., 1982). In
this respect cultured cerebellar granule cells are unique
since cultures of neurons derived from other brain areas
express two or more binding sites for GABA and synthesize
and release GABA (Snodgrass et al., 1980). Furthermore,
membranes from cerebellum at different developmental
stages as well as other brain areas express two or more
binding sites for GABA (Wang et al., 1979; Olsen et al.,
1981; Falch and Krogsgaard-Larsen, 1982; Meier and
Schousboe, 1982).

The observation that the two receptor types exhibit
separate developmental patterns in the cerebellum (Fig. 1)
as well as in other brain areas (Madtes and Bashir-Elahi,

[1]Present address
   Department of Pharmacology, H. Lundbeck A/S. DK-2500,
   Copenhagen, Denmark.

[2]Present address
   A/S Ferrosan, Research Division, DK-2860, Copenhagen,
   Denmark.

1985) indicates a differential effect of endogenous regulators on the expression of the two receptor sites. The absence of low affinity GABA receptors in cultures of cerebellar granule cells indicates the lack of an endogenous substance which induces the formation of low affinity GABA receptors. As will be apparent from the following this substance appears to be GABA itself.

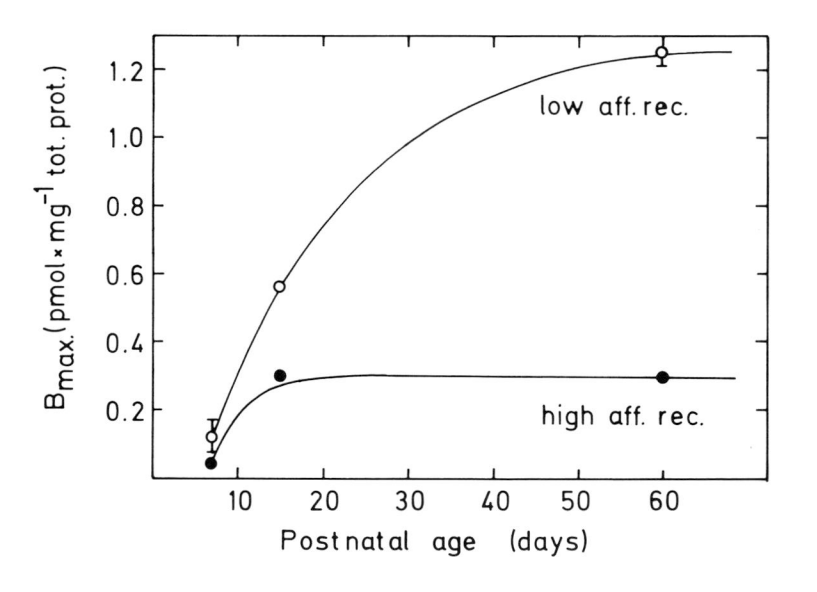

Figure 1. B_{max} for high (K_D 7.1 nM) and low affinity (K_D = 150-750 nM) GABA receptors in cerebellum as a function of the postnatal age of the rats. Values were estimated by computer Scatchard analysis (Munson and Rodbard, 1980; Olsen et al., 1981; McPherson, 1983). Each point represents the average of 3 experiments and the data are expressed on the basis of total protein in the original homogenates from which membranes were prepared. (From Meier et al., 1983).

GABA RECEPTOR EXPRESSION

Cell cultures

Granule cells were cultured from cerebellar of 7-day old rats essentially as described in the preceding chapter (Hansen et al., this volume). The cells were maintained for up to 3 weeks. Such cultures have been shown to consist of 80-90% granule cells and 5-10% astrocytes (Currie, 1980). The glutamatergic nature of the cultured granule cells is illustrated by their ability to release exogenously as well as exogenously supplied glutamate (Fig. 2 and Gallo et al., 1982) in a calcium dependent manner when stimulated either by high concentrations of potassium or L-glutamate (Drejer et al., 1983, 1986).

Effect of GABA-containing culture media

As seen in Fig. 3a granule cells cultured for 8 days in standard culture media exhibit a single class of GABA receptors which are of the high-affinity type with a K_D value of 7 nM. It is, moreover, seen (Fig. 3c) that a prolonged culture period (3 weeks) does not per se alter the characteristics of the GABA binding, i.e., only a single class of receptors with a K_D of 6 nM is seen. If, however, the cells are cultured for 8 days in the presence of 50 µM GABA a curvilinear Scatchard plot of the GABA binding is obtained (Fig. 3b), indicating multiple binding sites with different affinities for GABA. Computer analysis of the data revealed two receptor sites with K_D values of respectively 7 nM and 546 nM (Meier et al., 1984).

It is well documented that GABA recognition sites in different brain areas represent a heterogeneous population of receptor sites with at least two different affinities for GABA (Wang et al., 1979; Olsen et al., 1981; Falch and Krogsgaard-Larsen, 1982; Meier and Schousboe, 1982; Skerritt and Johnston, 1982). Also, cerebral cortex neurons cultured for 3 weeks have been shown to exhibit both a high- and low-affinity binding site for GABA (Ticku et al., 1980). On the other hand, similar neurons cultured for only 3 days exhibit only a high-affinity binding site for GABA (DeFeudis et al. 1979) in analogy with the naive granule cells (Meier and Schousboe, 1982). It is characteristic for cultured neurons originating from

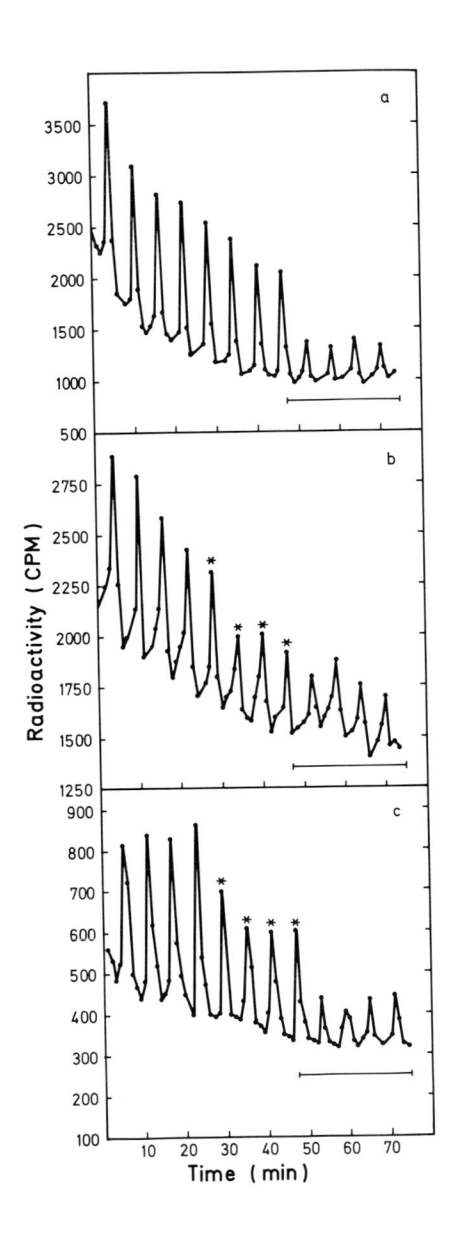

cerebral cortex that the capacity to synthesize and release GABA develops during the second week in culture (Snodgrass et al., 1980; Yu et al., 1984). This means that these neurons exhibit multiple binding sites for GABA at a time when GABA is released into the culture media. This agrees with the observation (Fig. 3) that treatment with GABA of cerebellar granule cells, leads to formation of low-affinity GABA receptors. The number of both high- and low-affinity GABA receptors on the GABA-treated granule cells corresponds to values determined in membranes prepared from cerebella of rats of a corresponding age (Meier and Schousboe, 1982). In this context, it should be kept in mind that treatment of the cultured granule cells with GABA also enhances the morphological development of the cells at the light and electron microcope level (Hansen et al., 1984).

Mechanism of action of GABA

The ability of GABA to promote the expression of low affinity GABA receptors could conceivably involve either an extracellular or an intracellular site of action. In order to elucidate this question cells were grown in the presence of GABA receptor specific agonists such as THIP (4,5,6,7-tetrahydroisoxazolo [5,4-c]pyridin-3-ol) and muscimol (Krogsgaard-Larsen and Johnston, 1978) or the antagonist bicuculline (Curtis et al., 1971). Such an experiment is illustrated in Fig. 4. This shows that membranes prepared from the cells grown in the presence of 150 µM THIP display a curvilinear Scatchard plot with

---

Figure 2. Radioactivies (cpm/sample) in the individual fractions from superfusion experiments performed with 10-20 day old granule cells cultured in the presence of 50 µM GABA. The abscissa shows the time after start of superfusion. Prior to the superfusion, cultures were loaded for 30 min with either D-[^{3}H]-aspartate (a,b) or L-[^{14}C]-glutamine. Superfusion media alternated between low-KCl (5 mM) and high-KCl (100 mM) media, the latter corresponding to the peaks in the graphs. During the last four stimulation periods in each experiment the standard media containing 1.8 mM CaCl$_2$ were substituted with a Ca^{2+}-free mediun containing 1.0 mM CoCl$_2$ (indicated by horizontal bars). Asterisks indicate that the superfusion media contained 50 µM GABA. (From Meier et al., 1984).

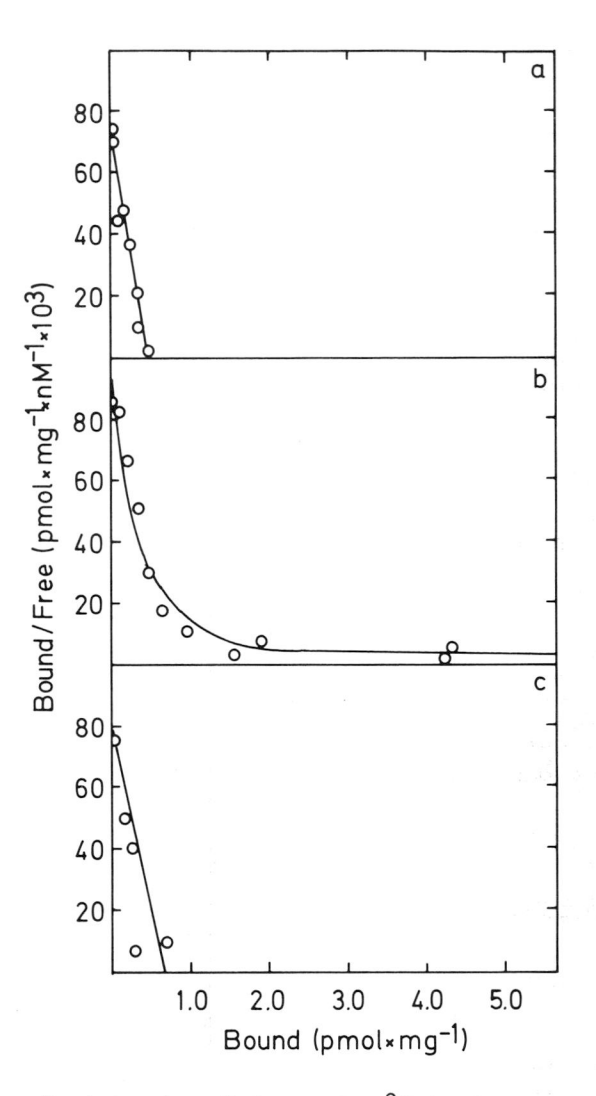

Figure 3. Scatchard plots of ^{3}H–GABA binding to membranes from cerebellar granule cells cultured for 8 days in the absence (a) or presence (b) of 50 μM GABA or for 21 days without GABA (c). Binding data were obtained as in Fig. 1 and kinetic parameters estimated to a) K_D = 7.0 nM, B_{max} 0.466 pmol/mg prot, b) K_{D1} = 7.0 nM, $B_{max}1$ = 0.622; K_{D2} = 550 nM, $B_{max}2$ = 1.0 pmol/mg prot, c) K_D = 5.6 nM, B_{max} = 0.480 pmol/mg prot. (From Meier et al., 1984).

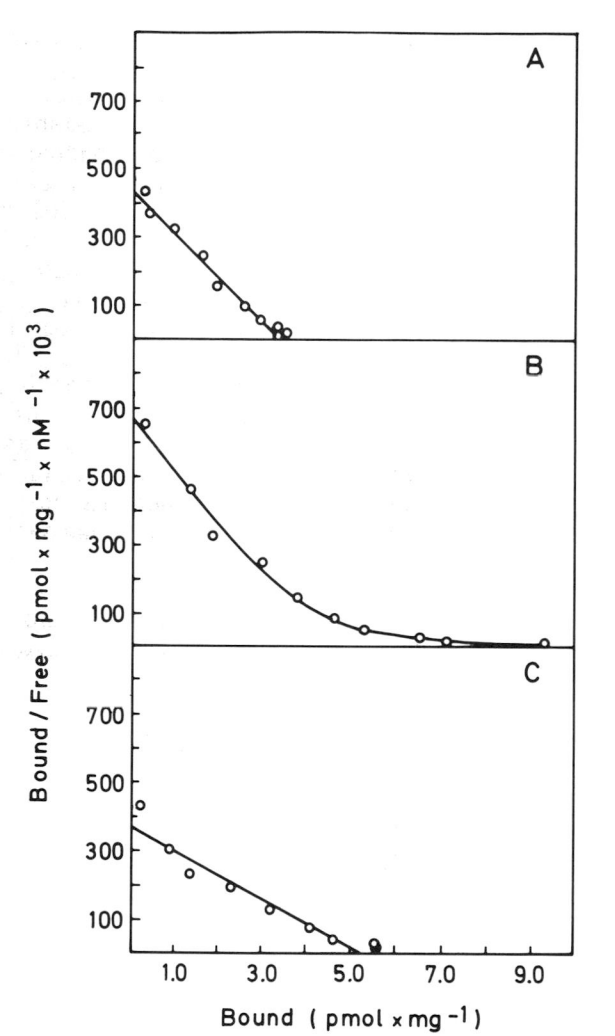

Figure 4. Scatchard plots of ^{3}H-GABA binding to membranes prepared from cerebellar granule cells cultured for 12 days in the absence (A) or presence of 150 μM THIP (B) or the simultaneous presence (C) of THIP and bicuculline methobromide (150 μM of each). Binding data obtained as in Fig. 1.
A) K_D = 7.9 nM, B_{max} = 3.42 pmol/mg prot. B) K_{D1} = 6.8 nM, $B_{max}1$ = 4.41 pmol/mg prot; K_{D2} = 476 nM, $B_{max}2$ = 5.81 pmol/mg prot. C) K_D = 14.3 nM, B_{max} = 5.35 pmol/mg prot. (From Belhage et al., 1986a).

regard to GABA binding whereas cells grown in the presence
of both THIP and bicuculline only display a single high
affinity site for GABA similar to cells grown in the
absence of any GABA analogs (Belhage et al., 1986a). This
strongly suggests that the ability of GABA to induce low
affinity GABA receptors requires the presence of the
preexisting high affinity GABA receptors. This conclusion
is in keeping with the observation by Madtes and Redburn
(1983a) that GABA receptors in retina can be induced by
GABA and GABA receptor agonists. Such a receptor mediated
mechanism of action might suggest the involvement of
chloride channels. That this may indeed be the case is
supported by the observation that picrotoxin which
specifically reacts with GABA-receptor coupled chloride
channels (Olsen, 1981) blocks the ability of GABA or THIP
to induce low affinity GABA receptors (B. Belhage, E.
Meier and A. Schousboe, unpublished results). This
mechanism would probably involve a hyperpolarization of
the cells. This is supported by the finding that Br⁻
exerts a neurotrophic effect similar to that of GABA (Joo
et al., 1980; Spoerri and Wolff, 1981; 1982; Toldi et al.,
1986; Wolff et al., this volume).

Temporal development of GABA receptors

Table 1 shows that kinetic constants (K_D and B_{max})
for GABA binding to membranes prepared from 4-day-old
cultures of cerebellar granule cells exposed to THIP (150
μM) for respectively 1, 3, 6 and 24 hours. It can be seen
that low affinity GABA receptors in addition to high
affinity receptors were observed after exposure of the
cells to THIP for 3 hours. After one hour exposure low
affinity receptors could not be detected. The K_D for
the high affinity receptors was, however, somewhat higher
than the corresponding K_D values calculated for longer
exposure times indicating that low affinity receptors have
started to appear, but their density is too low for the
Scatchard analysis to discriminate between the two binding
sites. After 3 hours no further increase in the formation
of low affinity GABA receptors was observed although
exposure to THIP for respectively 6 and 24 hours increased
the number of high affinity receptors (Hansen et al.,
1987).

In order to study whether a developmental period
exists during which the cells exhibit particularly high

Table I

Kinetic constants (K_D and B_{max}) for GABA binding to membranes prepared from 4-day-old cultures of cerebellar granule cells exposed to THIP for respectively 1, 3, 6 and 24 h

Time of treatment with 150 μM THIP (Hours)	K_D (nM) High	K_D (nM) Low	B_{max} (pmol × mg^{-1}) High	B_{max} Low
1	22.3 ± 5.8	1.00 ± 0.06	0.81 ± 0.02	5.31 ± 0.39
3	6.5 ± 2.4	537 ± 376	1.79 ± 0.09	5.42 ± 0.41
6	5.7 ± 0.9	500 ± 410		
24	7.6 ± 1.8	502 ± 265	1.35 ± 0.18	4.69 ± 0.27

Cells were culture for 4 days in plain culture media and subsequently for 1, 3, 6 and 24 h in the presence of 150 μM THIP. Values for K_D and B_{max} are derived from GABA binding curves by computer analysis (Munson and Rodbard, 1980; McPherson, 1983) and represent the statistically significantly best fits to the curves among either one or two binding sites. Values are given as means ± S.E.M. (From Hansen et al., 1987).

sensitivity to treatment with GABA agonists the following experiments were performed. Cells were cultured for 4, 7, 10 or 14 days prior to treatment with THIP for 6 hours. From Table II it is seen that low-affinity GABA-receptors appear after THIP-treatment in 4- and 7-day-old cultures whereas in 10- and 14-day-old cultures no low affinity GABA receptors could be found in spite of the fact that the number of high affinity receptors was increased compared to 7-day-old cultures (Hansen et al., 1986).

Table II
Kinetic parameters for GABA binding to granule cells cultured in the presence of 150 µM THIP for 6 hours after respectively 4, 7, 10 and 14 days in culture

Developmental age (days in culture)	K_D (nM)		B_{max} (pmol x mg^{-1})	
	High	Low	High	Low
4	5.7	500	1.8	5.4
7	6.6	91	0.7	0.82
10	9.1	–	3.2	–
14	10.3	–	4.7	–

Values for K_D and B_{max} are derived from GABA binding curves by computer analysis as described in Table I. (Unpublished results of B. Belhage, E. Meier and A. Schousboe)

Thus it may be concluded that the cultured granule cells are susceptible to the influence of GABA or GABA agonists only during a restricted developmental period. This conclusion agrees with the observation by Madtes and Bashir-Elahi (1986) that the induction by GABA of GABA receptors in retina is restricted to the early developmental period. Moreover, the induction of the low affinity receptors appears to be extremely rapid. This might suggest that the low affinity receptors are formed by modification of preexisting high affinity receptors. This is, however, incompatible with the finding that the number of high affinity receptors is increased after treatment with THIP (Table I). Alternatively, the induction might require de novo synthesis of low affinity GABA receptors. In this context it should be kept in mind that the effects of THIP on the cytoplasmic densities of organelles involved in protein synthesis precedes the effect on receptor expression by several hours (Hansen et al., 1987 and Hansen et al., this volume).

Role of protein synthesis

Early studies of brain protein synthesis (Campbell et al., 1966; Tewari and Baxter, 1969; Snodgrass, 1973; Goertz, 1979) have indicated that GABA may enhance this process. In order to eludicate whether protein synthesis is involved in the GABA induced receptor formation the effect of protein synthesis inhibitors on this process was investigated. It was found that both actinomycin D (transcription blocker) and cycloheximide (translation blocker) prevented the induction of low affinity GABA receptors by THIP (Belhage et al., 1986b).

PHYSIOLOGICAL FUNCTION OF LOW AFFINITY GABA RECEPTORS

In order to obtain information about a possible function of the inducible low affinity GABA receptors, it was investigated whether GABA could inhibit transmitter release from the granule cells. Since these neurons are glutamatergic (cf. Drejer et al., 1982; 1983; Gallo et al., 1982) the effect of GABA on evoked release of glutamate or D-aspartate was studied (Fig. 2). It can be seen that granule cells cultured for 10-12 days in the presence of 50 µM GABA and subsequently preloaded with D-[^{3}H] aspartate exhibit a pronouned stimulation of D-aspartate release upon repeated stimulations (20 s) with 100 mM KCl. It is also seen that this stimulation is dependent on the presence of Ca^{2+} in the superfusion media. Figure 2b shows a corresponding release experiment performed on an identical culture of cerebellar granule cells, i.e., cultured in the presence of 50 µM GABA. It is seen that GABA significantly inhibits the K^+-induced D-aspartate release (Meier et al., 1984).

The possibility of a correlation between the effect of GABA in the culture media on the receptor expression on the cells and the ability of GABA to inhibit evoked glutamate release was assessed by growing the cells in the presence of different concentrations of GABA as well as

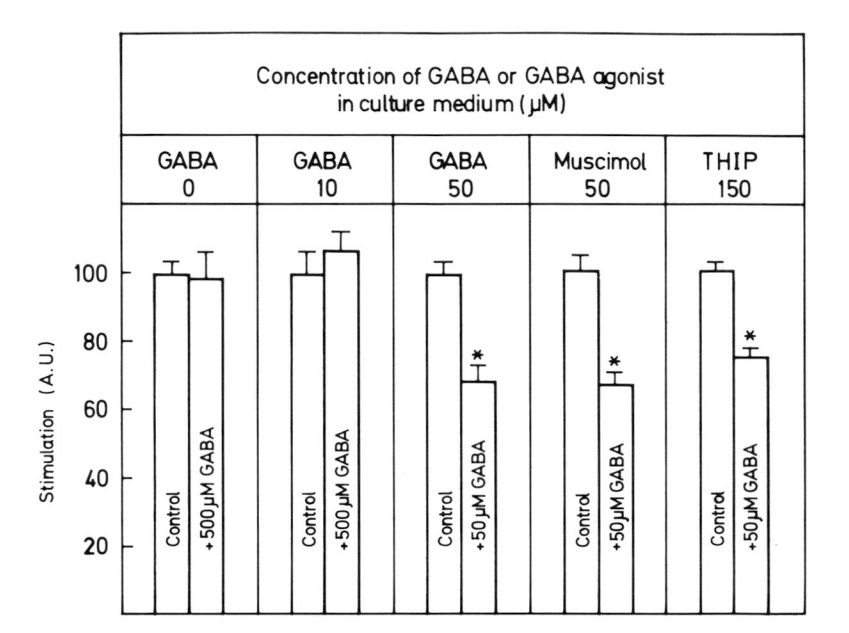

Composition of superfusion medium

Figure 5. Effect of GABA in the superfusion media (cf. Fig. 2) on K^+-stimulated D-$[^3H]$ aspartate release from granule cells cultured in the presence of different concentrations of GABA or its agonists muscimol and THIP (as indicated at the top of the figure) and preloaded with D- $[^3H]$ aspartate. The columns represent the average evoked release (means + SEM) from three successive stimulations (cf. Fig. 2) on three individual cultures. For the sake of comparison the values obtained prior to the addition of GABA to the superfusion media (control columns) have been expressed as 100 arbitrary units (a.u.) in each experiment. The magnitudes of the actual evoked release corresponded to 80–100% of the basal release (cf. Fig. 2) regardless of the culture conditions. Asterisks indicate statistically significant differences from the release in the control experiment (p < 0.01). (From Meier et al., 1984).

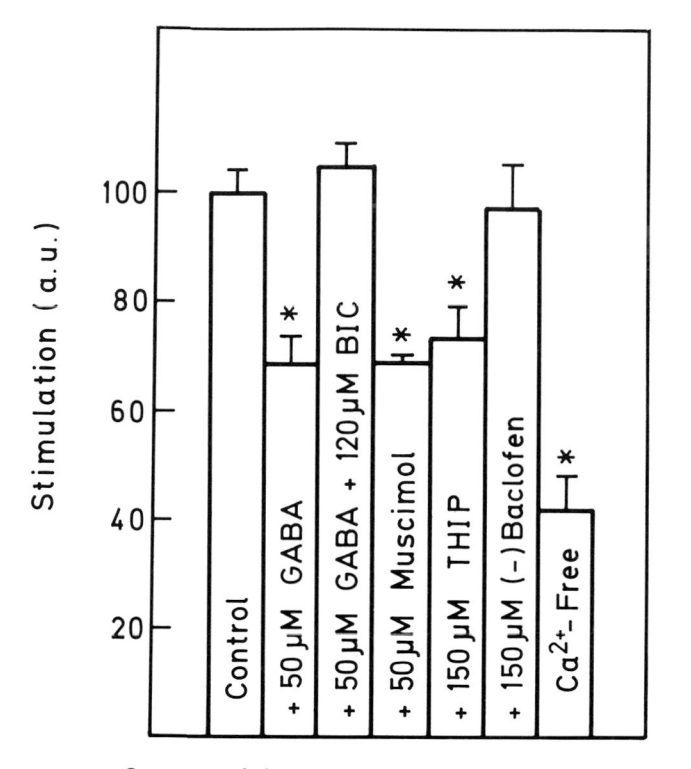

Composition of superfusion medium

Figure 6. Pharmacological characterization of the GABA–mediated inhibition of evoked glutamate release from cerebellar granule cells cultured in the presence of 50 μM GABA and preloaded with D– [³H] aspartate. The composition of the superfusion media during part of the release experiment (cf. Fig. 2) is indicated in the individual columns. The columns represent the average evoked release (mean ± SEM) expressed in arbitrary units (a.u.) from three successive stimulations (cf. Fig. 2) on three individual cultures. The control has been given as 100 a.u., which corresponds to an actual evoked release amounting to 80–100% of the basal release (cf. Fig. 2). Asterisks indicate stastistically significant differences from the release in the control experiment (p < 0.01). (From Meier et al., 1984).

GABA agonists such as muscimol and THIP. Fig. 5 shows that granule cells cultured in the absence of GABA or in the presence of 10 μM GABA did not exhibit a GABA-mediated inhibition of evoked glutamate release. On the other hand, cells cultured in the presence of 50 μM GABA, 50 μM muscimol, or 150 μM THIP, i.e. under conditions where low affinity GABA receptors are induced, exhibited a GABA-mediated inhibition of evoked glutamate release (Meier et al., 1984). It can accordingly be concluded that the ability of GABA to inhibit transmitter release in these neurons requires the presence of low affinity GABA receptors on the cells.

The pharmacological properties of the GABA mediated inhibition of evoked glutamate release are shown in Fig. 6. It is seen that the inhibitory effect of GABA could be blocked completely by the addition to the superfusion media of bicuculline methobromide. Moreover, both muscimol and THIP mimicked the effect of GABA by inhibiting the Ca^{2+}-dependent, K^{+}-induced glutamate release by approximately 50%. In contrast, (-)-baclofen had no effect on the evoked glutamate release. These findings would classify the low affinity GABA receptors as $GABA_A$ receptors (Hill and Bowery, 1981). This also agrees with the autoradiographic demonstration that the cerebellar granule layer is relatively devoid of baclofen binding (Wilkin et al., 1981).

The finding that low affinity GABA receptors mediate the inhibition of a potassium stimulated transmitter release suggests that these receptors are presynaptically localized. That this may indeed be the case is supported by the results shown in Table III. It is seen that the KCl induced depolarization of cerebellar granule cells, as monitored by the intracellular content of TPP^{+} (tetraphenylphosphonium) which reflects the membrane potential (Friedman et al., 1985), cannot be affected by GABA. In agreement with this it has been shown that low affinity GABA receptors do not seem to be coupled to chloride channels (Meier et al., 1985).

CONCLUSIONS

From studies on the effect of GABA on cultured granule cells described in this and the previous chapter (Hansen et al., this volume) it may be concluded that GABA or GABA agonists are able to induce the formation of low affinity GABA receptors and quantitatively alter the ultrastructural composition in cultured granule cells. These effects appear in both cases to be mediated by the preexisting high affinity GABA$_A$ receptors on cultured granule cells via GABA sensitive chloride channels. Furthermore, the processes are extremely rapid and requires, with respect to the formation of low affinity GABA receptors, the functional integrity of protein synthesis in the granule cells. Also the effect appears to be observable only during a restricted early developmental period.

The induced low affinity GABA receptors have the characteristics of a presynaptic GABA$_A$ receptor and appear not to be associated with chloride channels. Furthermore, the fact that their formation requires de novo protein synthesis suggests that high and low affinity receptors differ in their primary protein structures which also agrees with their supposed different cellular localization on the postsynaptic and presynaptic membrane,

Table III
Content of TPP$^+$ in cultured cerebellar granule cells as a function of the external condition

Condition	TPP$^+$ content (cpm x mg^{-1})
Control	571.5 + 1.54 (6)
+ KCl (50 mM)	206.4 ∓ 13.4* (8)
+ KCl (50 mM) + GABA (100 µM)	218.7 ∓ 3.7* (8)

Cells cultured in the presence of 150 µM THIP were preincubated for 30 min at 37°C in the presence of TPP$^+$ (1 µCi/culture). Subsequently, the incubation media were changed to media with the composition given in the Table. After 5 min the cellular amount of TPP$^+$ was determined. Results are averages + SEM with numbers of experiments given in parentheses. Asterisks indicate statistically significant differences from controls (P<0.001). (Unpublished results of A. Schousboe and J. Drejer).

respectively. The association of high affinity GABA receptors with the postsynaptic membrane is supported by the finding that GABA stimulates chloride conductance in granule cell cultures irrespective of the absence or presence of GABA in the culture media i.e. irrespective of the absence or presence of low affinity GABA receptors (Meier et al., 1985). GABA sensitive chloride channels are known to be responsible for the postsynaptic inhibitory spike potentials observed during exposures of nerve cells to GABA (Hosli and Hosli, 1983) and therefore this suggests a postsynaptic localization of the high affinity GABA receptors.

Effects similar to those seen in granule cell cultures of GABA or GABA agonists have been observed in other neuronal systems as previously pointed out with respect to the observations made in the retina system in vitro and in vivo (Madtes and Redburn, 1983a,b; Madtes and Bashir-Elahi, 1986). The effect of GABA on the GABA receptor density appears to be a general phenomenon in neuronal tissues since treatment either with GABA-transaminase inhibitors, which increase cortical GABA levels several fold, or GABA agonists in vivo, increase the GABA receptor density in cerebral cortex (Sykes et al., 1984; Beart et al., 1985).

The effect of GABA on neuronal tissue appears not only to affect the synthesis of GABA receptors, but the synthesis and expression of other nerve cell associated proteins as well. It has recently been demonstrated that GABA treatment increases the total protein content in granule cell cultures and more specifically accelerates the developmental expression of the mature forms of the neural-cell adhesion molecule (N-CAM) and neuron specific enolase (Meier and Jorgensen, 1986). In accordance with these findings in culture, it was found that treatment of rats during rearing with THIP accelerated the developmental expression of N-CAM and glutamate decarboxylase (Meier et al., 1987), which may be regarded as nerve cell markers (Roberts, 1979; Balazs et al., 1980; Bock et al., 1980; Jorgensen and Moller, 1980; Jorgensen et al., 1980; Meier et al., 1982).

The studies of the effect of GABA on biochemical, morphological and functional parameters of nerve cells over the past years (as reviewed in this volume) support the hypothesis that GABA during neuronal development promotes differentiation and maturation of neurons and even may be involved in the reorganization of neuronal fibers in mature tissue during acquisition of new neuronal circuits.

It is striking that GABA appears to have properties which are almost exactly opposite to the other major amino acid neurotransmitter, glutamate. GABA inhibits neuronal firing, whereas glutamate stimulates neuronal firing. Furthermore, GABA promotes neuronal development whereas glutamate hinders or extinguishes neuronal development. These complementary properties of GABA and glutamate may not only be of importance for the correct balance of the immediate firing pattern of the neuronal network but also play a crucial part in the shaping of the complex integrated neuronal network which constitutes the mature brain.

REFERENCES

Balazs R., Reagan C, Meier E, Woodhams GL, Wilkin GP, Patel NJ, Gordon RD (1980). Biochemical properties of neuronal cell types from rat cerebellum. In Giacobini E, Vernadakis A, Shahar A (eds): "Tissue Culture in Neurobiology," New York: Raven Press, pp 155–185.

Beart PM, Scatton B, LLoyd K (1985). Subchronic administration of GABAergic agonists elevates [^{3}H]-GABA binding and produces tolerance in striatal dopamine catabolism. Brain Res 335:169–173.

Belhage B, Meier E, Schousboe A (1986a). GABA-agonists induce the formation of low affinity GABA-receptors on cultured cerebellar granule cells via preexisting high affinity GABA-receptors. Neurochem Res 11:599–606.

Belhage B, Hansen GH, Meier E, Schousboe A (1986b). Effect of inhibitors of protein synthesis and axonal transport on THIP-induced development of GABA receptors in cultured cerebellar granule cells. In Tucek S, Stipek S, Stastny F, Krivanek J (ed): "Molecular Basis of Neural Function," Prague: Eur Soc Neurochem, p 207.

Bock E, Yavin Z, Jorgensen OS, Yavin E (1980). Nervous system-specific protein in developing rat cerebral cells in culture. J Neurochem 35:1297–1302.

Campbell MK, Mahler HR, Moore WJ, Tewari S (1966). Protein synthesis systems from rat brain. Biochemistry 5:1174–1184.

Currie DN (1980). Identification of cell types by immunofluorescence in defined cell cultures of cerebellum. In Giacobini E, Vernadakis A, Shahar A (eds): "Tissue Culture in Neurobiology," New York: Raven Press, pp 75–87.

Curtis DA, Duggan AW, Felix O, Johnston GAR and McLennan H (1971). Antagonism between bicuculline and GABA in the rat brain. Brain Res 33:57–73.

DeFeudis FV, Ossola L, Schmitt G, Mandel P (1979). High-affinity binding of ^{3}H-muscimol to subcellular particles of a neuron-enriched culture of embryonic rat brain. Neurosci Lett 14:195–199.

Drejer J, Larsson OM, Schousboe A (1982). Characterization of L-glutamate uptake into and release from astrocytes and neurons cultured from different brain regions. Exp Brain Res 47:259–269.

Drejer J, Larsson OM, Schousboe A (1983). Characterization of uptake and release processes for D- and L-aspartate in primary cultures of astrocytes and cerebellar granule cells. Neurochem Res 8:231–243.

Drejer J, Honore T, Meier E, Schousboe A (1986). Pharmacologically distinct glutamate receptors on cerebellar granule cells. Life Sci 38:2077–2085.

Falch E., Krogsgaard-Larsen P. (1982). The binding of the GABA agonist ^{3}H-THIP to rat brain synaptic membranes. J Neurochem 38:1123–1129.

Friedman JE, Lelkes PI, Larie E, Rosenheck K, Schneeweiss F, Schneider AA (1985). Membrane potential and catecholamine secretion by bovine adrenal chromaffin cells: Use of tetraphenylphosphonium distribution and carbocyanine dye fluorescence. J Neurochem 44:1391–1402.

Gallo V, Ciotti MT, Coletti A, Aloisi F, Levi G (1982). Selective release of glutamate from cerebellar granule cells differentiating in culture. Proc Natl Acad Sci USA 79:7919–7923.

Goertz B (1979). Effect of GABA on cell-free protein synthesizing systems from mouse brain. Exp Brain Res 34:365–372.

Hansen GH, Meier E, Schousboe A (1984). GABA influences the ultrastructure composition of cerebellar granule cells during development in culture. Int J Devl Neurosci 2:247–257.

Hansen GH, Belhage B, Meier E, Schousboe A (1986). Developmental aspects of the trophic activity of GABA agonists on cerebellar granule cells in culture. Int J Devl Neurosci 4:suppl 1:S36.

Hansen GH, Belhage B, Schousboe A, Meier E (1987). Time course of the GABA induced change in ultrastructure composition and GABA receptor expression in cultured cerebellar granule cells. Int J Devl Neurosci Submitted.

Hill DR, Bowery NG (1981). ^{3}H-baclofen and ^{3}H-GABA bind to bicuculline-insensitive GABA$_B$ sites in rat brain. Nature 290:149–152.

Hosli L, Hosli E (1983). Electrophysiological and autoradiographic studies on GABA and glutamate neurotransmission at the cellular level. In Hertz L, Kvamme E, McGeer EG, Schousboe A (eds): "Glutamine, Glutamate, and GABA in the Central Nervous System," New York: Alan R Liss, pp 441–455.

Joo F, Dames W, Wolff JR (1980). Effect of prolonged sodium bromide administration on the fine structure of dendrites in the superior cervical ganglion of adult rat. Prog Brain Res 51:109–115.

Jorgensen OS, Moller M (1980). Immunocytochemical demonstration of the D2 protein in the presynaptic complex. Brain Res 194:419–429.

Jorgensen OS, Deleuvee A, Thiert J–P, Edelman GM (1980). The nervous system specific protein D2 is involved in adhesion among neurites from cultured rat ganglia. FEBS Lett 111:39–49.

Krogsgaard-Larsen P, Johnston GAR (1978). Structure-activity studies on inhibition of GABA-binding to rat brain membranes by muscimol and related compounds. J Neurochem 30:1377–1382.

Madtes PC, Bashir-Elahi R (1986). GABA receptor binding site 'induction' in rabbit retina after nipecotic acid treatment: Changes during development. Neurochem Res 11:55–61.

Madtes PC, Redburn DA (1983a). GABA as a trophic factor during development. Life Sci 33:979–984.

Madtes PC, Redburn DA (1983b). Synaptic interactions in the GABA system during postnatal development in retina. Brain Res Bull 10:741–745.

McPherson GA (1983). A practical computer-based approach to the analysis of radioligand binding experiments. Comp Prog Biomed 17:107–114.

Meier E, Schousboe A (1982). Differences between GABA receptor binding to membranes from cerebellum during postnatal development and from cultured cerebellar granule cells. Dev Neurosci 5:546–553.

Meier E, Reagan C, Balazs E, Wilkin GP (1982). Specific recognition of the neuronal cell surface by an antiserum against plasma membrane preparations of immature rat cerebellum. Neurochem Res 7:1031–1043.

Meier E, Drejer J, Schousboe A (1983). Trophic actions of GABA on the development of physiologically active GABA receptors: In Mandel P, DeFeudis FV (eds): "CNS-Receptors from Molecular Pharmacology to Behavior," New York: Raven Press, pp 47–58.

Meier E, Drejer J, Schousboe A (1984). GABA induces functionally active low-affinitive GABA receptors on cultured cerebellar granule cells. J Neurochem. 43:1737–1744.

Meier E, Braestrup C, Schousboe A (1985). Direct demonstration of the coupling between high affinity GABA receptors and chloride channels in the neuronal membrane. J Neurochem 44 (suppl):S66.

Meier E, Jorgensen OS (1986). γ-Aminobutyric acid affects the developmental expression of neuron-associated proteins in cerebellar granule cell cultures. J Neurochem 46:1256–1262.

Meier E, Jorgensen OS, Schousboe A (1987). Effect of repeated THIP treatment on postnatal neural development in rats. J Neurochem Submitted.

Munson PI, Rodbard D (1980). A versatile computerized approach for characterization of ligand binding systems. Anal Biochem 107:220–239.

Oertel WH, Schmechel DE, Mugnaini E, Tappaz ML, Kopin IJ (1981). Immunocytochemical localization of glutamate decarboxylase in rat cerebellum with a new antiserum. Neuroscience 6:2715–2735.

Olsen RW (1981). GABA-benzodiazepine-barbiturate receptor interactions. J Neurochem 37:1–13.

Olsen RW, Bergman MO, Van Ness PC, Lummis SC, Watkins AE, Napias C, Greenlee DV (1981). γ-Aminobutyric acid receptor binding in mammalian brain. Heterogeneity of binding sites. Mol Pharmacol 19:217–227.

Pearce BR, Dutton GR (1982). Amino acid neurotransmitter release. In Pfeiffer SE (ed): "Neuroscience Approached Through Cell Culture," Vol. I, Boca Raton, Florida: CRC Press, pp 143–156.

Roberts E (1979). New directions in GABA research I: Immunocytochemical studies of GABA neurons. In Krogsgaard-Larsen P, Scheel-Kruger J, Kofod H (eds): "GABA-Neurotransmitters, Pharmacochemical, Biochemical and Pharmacological Aspects," Munksgaard, Copenhagen, pp 28–45.

Skerritt JH, Johnston GAR (1982). Postnatal development of

GABA binding sites and their endogenous inhibitors in rat brain. Dev Neurosci 5:189-197.

Snodgrass SR (1973). Studies of GABA and protein synthesis. Brain Res 59:339-348.

Snodgrass SR, White WF, Biales B, Dichter M (1980). Biochemical correlates of GABA function in rat cortical neurons in culture. Brain Res 100:123-138.

Spoerri PE, Wolff JR (1981). Effect of GABA-adminstration on murine neuroblastoma cells in culture. Cell Tiss Res 218:567-579.

Spoerri PE, Wolff JR (1982). Morphological changes induced by sodium bromide in murine neuroblastoma cells in vitro. Cell Tiss Res 222:379-388.

Sykes C, Prestwich S, Horton R (1984). Chronic administration of the GABA-transaminase inhibitor ethanol amine O-sulphate leads to up-regulation of GABA binding sites. Biochem Pharmacol 33:387-393.

Tewari S, Baxter CF (1969). Stimulatory effect of GABA upon amino acid incorporation into protein by a ribosomal system from immature rat brain. J Neurochem 16:171-180.

Toldi J, Farkas Z, Feher O, Dames W, Kasa P, Gyurkovits K, Joo F, Wolff JR (1986). Promotion by sodium bromide of functional synapse formation from foreign nerves in the superior cervical ganglion of adult rat with intact preganglionic nerve supply. Neurosci Lett 69:19-24.

Ticku MK, Huang A, Barker JL (1980). Characterization of γ-Aminobutyric acid receptor binding in cultured brain cells. Mol Pharmacol 17:285-289.

Wang Y-J, Salvaterra P, Roberts E (1979). Characterization of ^{3}H-muscimol binding to mouse brain membranes. Biochem Pharmacol 28:1123-1128.

Wilkin GP, Hudson AL, Hill DR, Bowery NG (1981). Autoradiographic localization of GABA$_B$ receptors in rat cerebellum. Nature 294:584-587.

Yu ACH, Hertz E, Hertz L (1984). Alterations in uptake and release rates for GABA, glutamate, and glutamine during biochemical maturation of highly purified cultures of cerebral cortical neurons, a GABAergic preparation. J Neurochem 42:951-960.

Neurotrophic Activity of GABA During Development, pages 161–187
© 1987 Alan R. Liss, Inc.

ONTOGENY OF THE GABA RECEPTOR COMPLEX

Paul Madtes Jr.

Departments of Biology and Chemistry
Point Loma Nazarene College, 3900 Lomaland Drive
San Diego, CA.   92106

INTRODUCTION

Knowledge of the factors which affect the CNS and an understanding of the mechanisms of their actions are vital in both controlling disorders and diseases and improving learning and memory. One particularly crucial aspect of this is the study of how the CNS develops. By determining the mechanism by which the neurons establish their circuits, we may ascertain the principles upon which the contacts are based. In addition, we can test the affects of both endogenous (e.g., hormones) and exogenous (e.g., drugs) stimuli on the developmental mechanism and how they may function in the adult. Thus, insight into the ability of the developing CNS to adjust can be gained. This plasticity is known to occur in many aspects of CNS function, including its morphology, biochemistry and physiology. What remains unknown is how the changes occur.

The importance of these studies lies in their application to 1) repair of damage to the CNS or 2) behavior such as aggressive behavior, learning, and memory. The issue of neuroplasticity generally relates to whether the CNS has a specific recovery mechanism or simply exhibits developmental mechanisms (Finger and Almli, 1985). Knowing how a particular component in the CNS develops may help us answer this question and may lead to procedures to correct damaged areas. Similarly, the influence of environment on both immature (Jans et al., 1985; Kraemer, 1985; Meaney et al., 1985; Skangiel-Kramska and Kossut, 1985; Alleva et al., 1986) and mature CNS tissue (DeFeudis et al., 1976; DeFeudis, 1982; Kraemer, 1985Da; Vanzo et al., 1986) is pronounced. These studies show that by simply changing the environmental stimuli (e.g., social isolation and handling), the biochemistry of the CNS is altered; they also suggest that appropriate input is essential for proper development of mental and social faculties. Thus, our understanding of the factors which influence CNS development may contribute to improving the capability of individuals to learn and interact socially.

While it is interesting that these types of plasticity occur, we know little of the mechanism(s) behind them. Some progress has been made in answering this question, however. It appears as if at least some aspects of these observations involve the appearance of either new synapses or the activation of previously quiescent ones. The presence of synapses is fundamental to the functioning of the CNS. In the process of forming new contacts, a neuron responds to electrical activity (Cohan and Kater, 1986; for review, see Harris, 1981), which results from environmental stimuli. Therefore, cell-to-cell communication is influenced by the environment.

Two types of neuronal communications are possible: direct contact or use of a molecular messenger. The presence of coupling between neuronal cells and between neurons and glial cells during development has been observed both morphologically (Wolff et al., 1981) and biochemically (Conners et al., 1983). Both studies found that transient contacts are established early in the developmental profile of neurons and decline around the time of rapid synaptogenesis. This would suggest that the second type of regulation must come into play.

It has been known for quite some time that Nerve Growth Factor (NGF) is responsible for promoting the growth and development of neurons (Chun and Patterson, 1977a, b). Recently, many other molecules have been found to have similar regulatory, properties (For review, see Varon and Adler, 1981; Adler, 1982).

Several classes of molecules may play a role. Cyclic AMP accelerates the maturation of rat retinal cholinergic neurons (Yeh et al., 1983), suggesting that this second messenger may be involved in the appearance of functional postsynaptic receptors. Cyclic AMP also increases γ-aminobutyric acid (GABA) receptor binding in chick retinal cultures (Madtes and Adler, 1985). If this hypothesis is true, it would suggest that each neurotransmitter may influence the development of its own neurons by using a second messenger system.

A third class of molecules involved in regulation of development is hormones. Glucocorticoids, applied at physiological concentrations, accelerate the developmental sequence of cholinergic neurons, presumably by acting via their receptors at the transcription level of protein synthesis (Puro, 1983). An interesting finding is that stress, which raises glucocorticoid levels (Maickel et al., 1961), mimics the effect of exogenously applied glucocorticoids (Puro, 1983). This is especially interesting in light of the fact that γ-aminobutyric acid (GABA) receptors, which demonstrate a change after stress (Biggio et al., 1980; Skerritt et al., 1981; Yoneda et al., 1983), are also altered by glucocorticoids (Majewska et al., 1985). Thus, glucocorticoid hormones represent a class of molecules capable of markedly influencing neurotransmitter systems.

Another hormone, thyroid hormone, alters the development of neurons. Thyroid hormone is essential for synaptogenesis to occur in the rat cerebellum (Vincent et al., 1982; 1983). Treatment of thyroid-deficient rats with thyroxine reverses the inhibition of synaptogenesis, suggesting that thyroid hormone is essential for normal neuronal development in the cerebellum.

Although these molecules are quite diverse, one other group is of particular interest – neurotransmitters. Classically, neurotransmitters act at synapses to mediate communication between neurons. Recent evidence suggests that they also may serve as trophic factors, determining the synaptogenesis of specific neurons. It is known, for example, that serotonin (5-hydroxytryptamine; 5-HT) inhibits the growth and synaptogenesis of some specific neurons in the snail Helisoma, transiently affects some, does not affect others, and possibly may enhance the growth of some (Haydon et al., 1984). Dopamine inhibits growth cone motility and neurite outgrowth in avian retina neurons (Lankford et al., in press). Another monoamine, noradrenaline (NE), influences the development of adrenergic neurons in the cat (Jonsson and Kasamatsu, 1983) and in the rat (Morris et al., 1983).

Interestingly, the influence of NE in the rat CNS can be countered by the effects of acetylcholine (ACh). Apparently, the composition of NE and ACh, plus environmental influences, determines whether a given neuron population matures into an adrenergic or cholinergic system (For review, see Black and Patterson, 1980). Studies of the regulation of the development of cholinergic neurons have revealed some important details which may aid our understanding of the principle involved. While the initial phenotypic expression is dependent upon noradrenergic characters present in the cells (Levitt et al., 1965; Cochard et al., 1978a, b), it is the presence of a cholinergic factor in the growth conditions, but not NGF, which promotes conversion to a cholinergic neuron (Patterson and Chun, 1977; Chun and Patterson, 1977a, b, c).

GABA can also influence many morphological parameters associated with synaptogenesis in rat superior cervical ganglion (Joo et al., 1979; Wolff et al., 1979a; 1981; Dames et al., 1985), mouse neuroblastoma cells (Wolff et al., 1979b; Spoerri and Wolff, 1982), rat cerebellar cells (Hansen et al., 1984), and rabbit retina (Redburn and Madtes, 1986). In addition, the number of receptors present increases after treatment with GABA analogues (Meier and Schousboe, 1982; Madtes and Redburn, 1983a, b; Meier et al., 1983; 1984a, b, 1985; Madtes and Bashir-Elahi, 1986). Finally, GABA also acts to induce metamorphosis in Haliotis refescens (red abalone) and to direct palate morphogenesis in the mouse (Wee and Zimmerman, 1983; Zimmerman and Wee, 1984). Thus, GABA acts in a variety of developing systems to influence subsequent development.

From these observations, it is clear that the neurotransmitters themselves play an active role in the synaptogenesis of neurons which later may use that neurotransmitter for adult functioning. It is our purpose to look at the mechanism by which this occurs, using the GABA system as our model.

While the evidence supporting the hypothesis that GABA acts as a trophic factor during development is extensive, its mechanism of action is unclear. It appears as if the activity directly involves the postsynaptic receptor (Madtes and Redburn, 1983a, b; Meier et al., 1985; Redburn and Madtes, in press). Therefore, we will concentrate on the role that the GABA receptor complex plays in the development of the CNS. This chapter is not intended to be an extensive review of GABA receptor development, but rather an overview of representative studies which demonstrate the role of GABA in GABAergic development.

The development of the GABA receptor complex has been studied in several areas of the central nervous system. While both the GABA binding site and benzodiazepine binding site have been analyzed in vivo and in vitro, only one study has been reported concerning the development of the barbiturate binding site and the chloride channel, showing an increase in the number of sites with age (Tehrani and Barnes, 1986). In order to understand fully the role of GABA in development, these need to be studied more extensively.

DEVELOPMENT OF GABA BINDING SITES

Brain
     Generally, the profile of the changes observed during the development of the GABA binding site is sigmoidal, i.e., low at early times, increasing linearly with age, and reaching adult levels about the time when rapid synaptogenesis terminates (See Fig. 1). In the rat, two populations of $GABA_A$ binding sites are present, high-affinity and low-affinity receptors. The number of receptors (B_{max}) increases with increasing age, reaching adult levels approximately 3-4 weeks after birth (Coyle and Enna, 1976; Aldinio et al., 1980; Skerritt and Johnston, 1982; Saito et al., 1983; Sykes and Horton, 1986); no change in the apparent affinities (K_D) occurs. A third population of GABA binding sites, the $GABA_B$ sites, also have been described using immature rat cerebral cortex. The B_{max} increases with age; however, only three ages were reported (Sykes and Horton, 1986).

The increase in B_{max} in the rat has been correlated with 1) the high level of GABA early in development (Roberts et al., 1951), 2) the increase in glutamic acid decarboxylase (GAD) (Coyle and Enna, 1976) and 3) synapse formation (Aghajanian and Bloom, 1967). Hence, in the rat brain, the development of the GABA receptor coincides with synaptogenesis. In addition, the development of endogenous inhibitors of the activity of the mature GABA receptor complex has been studied. During ontogenesis, the level of inhibitors to GABA binding has been shown to increase (Palacios et al., 1979; Massotti et al., 1980). In contrast, Skerritt and Johnston claim that the reverse is true (Skerritt and Johnston, 1982). However, these data are not contradictory if one considers that they show

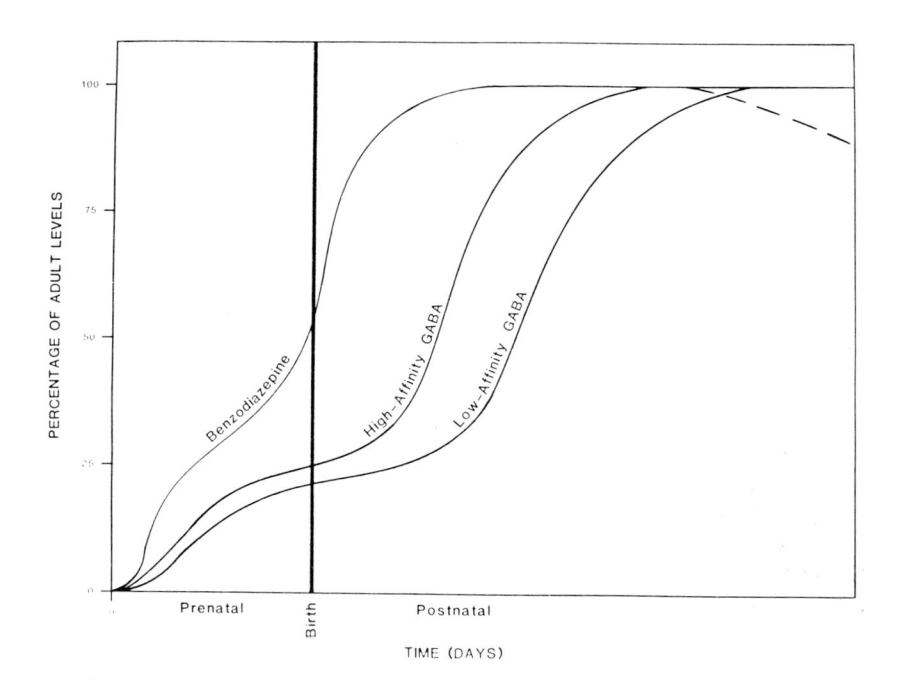

Figure 1: Timecourse of development of benzodiazepine and GABA receptors in the central nervous system. The relative increase in the number of benzodiazepine, high-affinity GABA, and low-affinity GABA receptors is plotted as a function of time, both before and after birth. The relative sequence is benzodiazepine receptors precede high-affinity GABA receptors, which precede low-affinity GABA receptors. The number of benzodiazepine receptors, and maybe both GABA receptor types, decrease after maturation.

that an enhancement of GABA binding in membranes which have been prepared by a single Triton X-100 extraction, decreases with age; this observation suggests that presence of more endogenous inhibitor in older animals. These results indicate that the GABA receptor complex undergoes a type of maturation in biochemistry, if not in function.

In the chick retina, findings similar to those for the rat have been reported. The developmental increase in B_{max} occurs for $GABA_A$ sites, reaching adult levels by hatching (Enna et al., 1976; Fiszer de Plazas, 1982; Jong et al., 1986; Tehrani and Barnes, 1986). This increase parallels synapse formation (Kuriyama et al., 1968) and GAD activity (Enna et al., 1976; Jong et al., 1986), as it did in the rat. Similarly, the level of endogenous inhibitors increases with age (Fiszer de Plazas, 1982). Again, these observations indicate a change in GABA receptor complex biochemistry, and perhaps physiology as well.

An identical developmental profile for GABA binding sites occurs in both feline visual cortex (Shaw et al., 1984) and human cerebral cortex (Lloyd and Dreksler, 1979; Brooksbank et al., 1981), namely low B_{max} early in development, rising to adult levels shortly after birth. In contrast, human cerebellum followed a much slower profile, reaching adult levels at least one year after birth (Brooksbank et al., 1981). It is interesting to note that only in the human cortex does the development of GAD activity not precede receptor development (Brooksbank et al., 1981). It is possible that those areas which have a concentration of GABAergic neurons may mature differently from those that do not. In any case, all these areas apparently have a high correlation between receptor development and synaptogenesis.

Spinal Cord

In the rat spinal cord, the development of GABA binding sites apparently operates differently from the rest of the brain. Quantitatively, the number of receptors decreases, after a transient rise immediately after birth (Saito et al., 1983). The parallel decrease in GABA levels and GAD activity (Saito et al., 1982) suggests that either 1) the spinal cord has essentially

completed its development prior to birth or 2) a
fundamentally different mechanism is involved. Since the
spinal cord tends to mature prior to the brain, the former
is more likely.

Retina

The postnatal development of GABA binding sites in the
retina has been studied primarily in the rabbit. As in
the rest of the CNS, two populations of $GABA_A$ receptors
are present, namely, high- and low-affinity sites. Their
developmental profiles are similar, i.e., both have low
B_{max} values shortly after birth and rise linearly to
adult levels; however, the low-affinity sites lag 2-3 days
behind the high-affinity ones (Madtes and Bashir-Elahi,
1986). The number of high-affinity sites increases during
the time of rapid synaptogenesis, postnatal days (P) 6-12
(McArdle et al., 1977; Madtes and Redburn, 1982; Redburn
and Mitchell, 1982; Madtes and Bashir-Elahi, 1986). The
correlation with other components of the GABA system is
similar to other areas of the CNS, namely, the increase in
GAD activity and GABA levels slightly precede GABA
receptors (Madtes and Redburn, 1983a). Therefore, the
retina makes a good model system for study of the
mechanism of GABAergic development in the CNS.

DEVELOPMENT OF BENZODIAZEPINE RECEPTORS

The second major component of the GABA receptor
complex which has been followed developmentally is the
benzodiazepine binding sites. Study of prenatal rat brain
and spinal cord revealed a caudal-to-rostral progression
of the development of benzodiazepine receptors, a
phenomenon apparently linked to cell differentiation,
though not necessarily with synaptogenesis (Schlumpf et
al., 1983). It is important to determine how the changes
are associated with the development of the GABA binding
sites since, postnatally, the patterns do not appear to be
associated (Palacios and Kuhar, 1982), even though the two
receptors are believed to be part of the same complex.
Possibly, the two only become coupled after maturation.

Postnatally, the development of benzodiazepine sites
in rat brain parallels that for GABA sites, except the
level at birth is much higher than for GABA; neonates have
greater than 50% of the adult benzodiazepine sites levels

compared to 25% greater for GABA sites (Braestrup and Nielsen, 1978; Candy and Martin, 1979; Aldinio et al., 1981) (See Fig. 1). It is of interest to note that studies covering both prenatal and postnatal ages show a dramatic rise in B_{max} after birth, thus revealing a sigmoidal curve which extends from a prenatal age through the postnatal period (Braestrup and Nielsen, 1978; Mallorga et al., 1980). Apparently, the development of the sensitivity of the CNS to benzodiazepines precedes the development of GABA binding sites.

In the spinal cord, similar findings have been reported; benzodiazepine receptor levels are high at birth and decrease as a function of age (Saito et al., 1983), roughly paralleling the results for GABA sites. Again, the development of the spinal cord precedes the other areas of the CNS.

For the chick retina, the level of benzodiazepine binding is low in ovo, rapidly rises around the time of hatching, and reaches adult levels shortly thereafter (Altstein et al., 1981). This exactly parallels the findings for rat brain, if the latter is studied over both prenatal and postnatal age. This lends further support for the use of the retina as a model for general CNS development.

REGULATION OF GABA RECEPTORS

Since the developmental profile of the GABA receptors in the rabbit retina was established, we began to study how their development might be regulated. Our hypothesis is that by blocking uptake in the retina, using nipecotic acid, the extracellular levels of GABA will increase (Madtes and Redburn, 1983a, b), just as it does in the cerebellum (Wood et al., 1980). Our procedure, therefore, is to treat retinal tissue with nipecotic acid (Madtes and Redburn, 1983a). Alteration of GABA uptake was chosen since the mechanism for the uptake of GABA into neurons is nearly mature at birth, suggesting that the transport system may regulate the subsequent development (For a more thorough discussion, see Redburn et al., 1983; Redburn and Madtes, in press).

In vivo treatment with nipecotic acid results in a four-fold increase in the level of GABA binding (Madtes and Redburn, 1983a), which corresponds to an increase in

B_{max} without altering the K_D (Madtes and Bashir-Elahi, 1986). Thus, our model predicts that the higher levels of extracellular GABA "induces" the appearance of postsynaptic receptors. In order to test the mechanism by which this occurs, an in vitro procedure was developed. We found that a 45 min treatment of isolated eyecups results in the same four-fold increase in binding as was found with the in vivo treatment (Madtes and Redburn, 1983b). Therefore, GABA may be acting through a receptor already present. If true, treatment with GABA agonists would also "induce" the appearance of receptors. This, in fact, does occur after treating with GABA, muscimol, or 4,5,6,7-tetrahydroisoxazolo[5,4-c]pyridin-3-ol(THIP), potent GABA agonists. Thus, the induction of postsynaptic receptors must involve interaction with GABA receptors. In addition, the fact that the receptors appear within a short time span (45 min) suggests that they are "unmasked" through exposure of pre-existing receptors. In addition, the B_{max} after treatment never exceeds that found for untreated tissue prepared using Triton X-100, a technique believed to expose all receptors which are present in the membrane (Madtes and Redburn, 1982; Madtes and Bashir-Elahi, 1986). The final answer remains to be fully determined; however, since two additional studies suggest that the mechanism may be more complex. We have been able to see an increase in binding within 25 min after treatment (Madtes and Fuller, unpublished observations), a finding which would support the "unmasking" hypothesis. On the contrary, Belhage et al. have found that, by blocking protein synthesis, the induction of low-affinity GABA receptors in cultured cerebellar granule cells does not occur (Belhage et al., 1986). Blockage of axonal transport did not interfere with induction (Belhage et al., 1986).

The apparent conflict may be resolved by considering the mechanism by which the number of glutamate receptors increases during development or after denervation. An increase in Ca^{2+} activates proteases located in the membrane. These proteases remove the proteins covering the glutamate receptors, resulting in the increase in binding observed. It is possible that a similar mechanism is involved in the induction effect of GABA analogues on the GABA receptor, i.e., activation of proteases. If the protein inhibitors used by Belhage, et al. have an inhibitory action on proteases, their presence would eliminate the unmasking phenomenon. The role of calcium needs to be considered in this action since Ca^{2+} is known to activate proteases. Using mature rat brain membranes, Corda and Guidotti (1983) found that $GABA_B$ binding increases in the presence of Ca^{2+}; however, $GABA_A$ binding decreases. Clearly, Ca^{2+} cannot be responsible for the activation of the proteases involved during development of the GABA system in the same manner as it is in the adult, but this observation does raise the possibility that some specific ion may play a role. This question can be easily tested by treatment with 1) agents known to block proteases to verify the presence of active proteases and 2) ion channel blockers to test the involvement of specific ions.

Alternatively, the unmasking may involve the activity of a phospholipase since this class of enzymes modifies GABA binding (Giambalvo and Rosenberg, 1976; Toffano et al., 1981; Fujimoto and Okabayashi, 1983; Kuriyama et al., 1984; Duman et al., 1986). Through the action of phospholipases, the membrane environment of the GABA receptors can be modified and, hence, result in the appearance of additional sites. This possibility can be tested by treating membranes with inhibitors of phospholipase activity to determine whether GABA receptors can still be induced.

Since repeated exposure of mature tissue to a neurotransmitter classically results in a loss of receptors, and our findings showed an increase with immature retina, apparently a change in sensitivity must occur. We have investigated the time course of this sensitivity to determine when this change occurs. We found that, shortly after birth, the number of high-affinity sites increases after nipecotic acid treatment. This effect is maximal around the time of eye opening (P9-P12). At later ages, the opposite effect is seen, namely, a decrease in receptor number results (See Fig. 2). In contrast, the number of low-affinity sites increased after nipecotic acid treatment only for the first three days after birth, exhibiting classical "desensitization" thereafter (Madtes and Bashir-Elahi, 1986). An interesting observation is that light, the natural stimulus for the retina, apparently is involved in the development mechanism since rearing of the animals in the absence of light eliminates the induction affect in them without altering the normal development profile (Madtes, 1985). Since lower levels of GABA occur when animals are reared without light (Pasantes-Morales et al.,

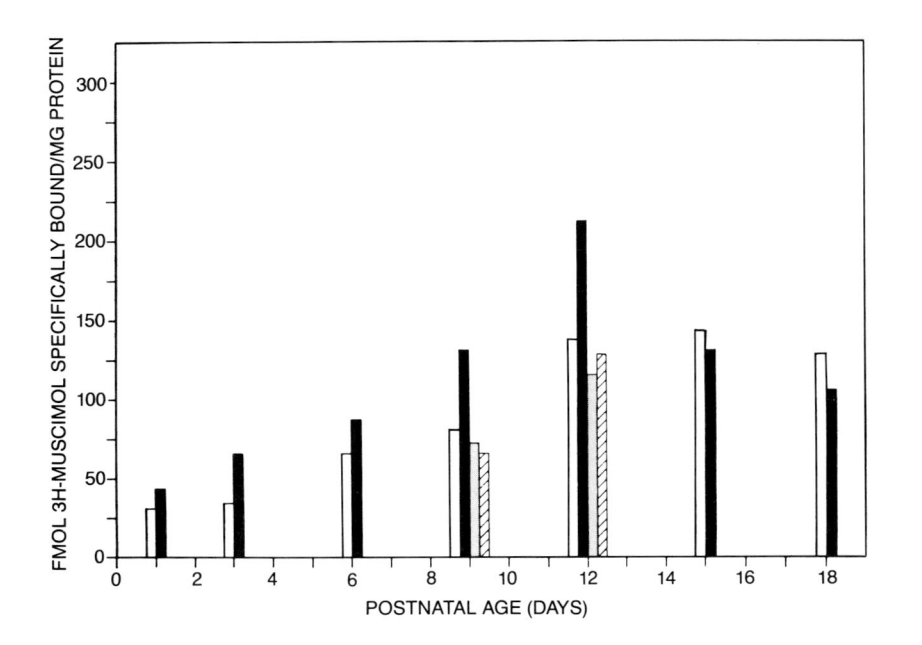

Figure 2: Sensitivity of rabbit retina to treatment with nipecotic acid. Retinas from selected ages were incubated for 45 min in 10 mM nipecotic acid. The presence of high-affinity GABA receptors then was measured using ^{3}H-muscimol. Open bars represent untreated, light-reared controls. Solid bars represent nipecotic acid-treated, light-reared animals. Light gray bars (ages 9 and 12) represent untreated, dark-reared controls. Hashed bars represent nipecotic acid-treated, dark-reared animals. The normal developmental increase occurs in both light-reared and dark-reared animals. Induction after nipecotic acid treatment only occurs in tissue from light-reared animals, being maximally sensitive around the time of eye opening (ages 9-12). Classical desensitization occurs at the mature ages (15-18 days old).

1973), less GABA is available to induce the appearance of receptors. Therefore, the effect should be seen, as would be predicted according to our model. Thus, these findings support our hypothesis that GABA receptors are regulated during development by GABA present in the extracellular space.

MODELS FOR THE MECHANISM OF GABA RECEPTOR INDUCTION BY GABA

It is clear that the GABA receptor itself is involved in the mechanism of action. Our work and that of Meier, Schousboe and co-workers have shown that GABA agonists induce GABA receptors (Madtes and Redburn, 1983a, b; Meier et al., 1983; 1984b; 1985). The question of whether there are multiple mechanisms involved was addressed by incubating eyecups in the presence of both nipecotic acid and THIP. If the GABA receptor is involved in the action of both analogues, the effect of treating with the two together should be equal to treating with each alone. This, in fact, occurs (Madtes and Fuller, unpublished observations). Hence, the induction effect of nipecotic acid treatment acts through the same GABA receptors as THIP acts. In addition, Meier et al. have demonstrated that this induction is sensitive to inhibition by the antagonist bicuculline (Meier et al., 1985), indicating that $GABA_A$ receptors are involved.

Since $GABA_A$ sites are known to play a key role, it is of interest to determine whether $GABA_B$ sites also are involved. A preliminary study using both (-)-baclofen and (+)-baclofen addressed this question. Treatment with (-)-baclofen, the centrally active form, resulted in a slight increase in binding. If co-incubated with THIP, the effects are additive, suggesting that $GABA_B$ sites may play some role in the developmental process. As expected, treatment with (+)-baclofen, the centrally inactive form, was without effect (Madtes and Fuller, unpublished observations). Therefore both $GABA_A$ and $GABA_B$ receptors may be involved in the induction of postsynaptic receptors in immature tissue. One question which is raised by these results in how these effects may occur since $GABA_A$ and $GABA_B$ sites are not thought to exist on the same neurons, although both do exist on Aδ and C primary afferents of rat dorsal root ganglia (Desarmenien et al., 1984). However, further studies are needed to verify these observations and answer this question.

Although the exact mechanism of induction remains to be determined, we can speculate as to how GABA receptors appear. While many explanations are possible, four models are especially worth considering:

Model I: The induction may be a simple pathway. Extracellular GABA levels can be raised by nipecotic acid treatment or by addition of a direct acting agonist. The GABA binds to high-affinity $GABA_A$ sites (and perhaps $GABA_B$ sites as well). These then undergo a change in structure (either by a conformational change or addition of some protein component) to low-affinity sites. This would explain the appearance of functional low-affinity sites and the influence of protein synthesis inhibitors (Meier et al., 1984b; Belhage et al., 1986). However, two shortcomings are present in this model. First, the model does not satisfactorily account for the increase in high-affinity sites (Madtes and Redburn, 1983a, b; Madtes and Bashir-Elahi, 1986). Second, the change from high- to low-affinity has not been found in any tissues. Therefore, the simplest model is unlikely.

Model II: The induction may involve the activation of a critical number of GABA receptors. As the extracellular level of GABA rises, the exposed sites are activated. These receptors are coupled to a "second messenger" which is responsible for turning on general cell metabolism, one aspect of which is protein synthesis. This increase in synthesis provides new receptors for exposure to the cell surface. Although the time course is quite short, the process of synthesis may only involve assembly of subunits, not complete synthesis.

Unfortunately, it does not clarify exactly how the receptors initially present are coupled to the effect of induction, i.e., what is the identity of the "second messenger" in the system. One good candidate is cyclic AMP since cyclic AMP levels have been found to change GABA binding in immature chick retina (Madtes and Adler, 1985). Studies of the relationships between cyclic AMP levels, chloride ion flux, and other candidates for the role of second messenger could help establish the identity.

Model III: This model more directly addresses the

specificity of the induction of GABA receptors. The extracellular GABA again is responsible for binding to the exposed high-affinity sites. Concurrently, the protein synthesis pathway exists in a state of constant activity unless inhibited. This causes a "driving force" (or pressure) to expose new sites. However, in immature tissue, the appearance of new receptors is blocked. When the few sites which are exposed become activated, the conditions preventing exposure are removed and the new receptors are able to appear on the surface of the membrane. When the number of receptors reaches a threshold, the metabolic machinery of the cell turns off. This causes the cell to switch from a "developing" neuron to a "mature" one. This model is superior to both Model I and Model II in that it explains the observation that receptors can be seen within 25 min (Madtes and Fuller, unpublished observations) and can be blocked by treating with protein synthesis inhibitors, but not by axonal transport blockers (Belhage et al., 1986). It also suggests a link between the trophic action of GABA and its neurotransmitter activity. As with Model II, the "second messenger" is unknown. One aspect which could be studied directly is the question of an increase in cell metabolism by measuring changes in other parameters such as glucose consumption, protein synthesis, and DNA synthesis.

Model IV: This model is the most superior in that it encompasses most of the observations to date. Extracellular GABA binds to high-affinity sites, activating a protease, which removes a protein from the surface of the membrane, or a phospholipase, which removes phospholipids. This results in an increase in the number of high-affinity sites. Once a critical number of these sites are activated, the physiology of the cell is stimulated via a second messenger to begin undergoing changes in the general metabolism of the cell. One particular protein which may be produced would be the low-affinity GABA receptors. Thus, the postsynaptic neuron switches to a mature neuron with the classical responses to GABA. Model IV would explain the observed increases in GABA receptors, and their rapid appearance after treatment which can be blocked. However, both a demonstration of the activity of proteases or phospholipases and the identification of the second messenger need to be done to validate this proposal.

Although these models are speculative, they do point

out some areas for future consideration, namely, how the message is conveyed away from the receptor, i.e., what the "second messenger" is. Other questions include: 1) is there a change in the general metabolic activity of the cells; 2) how does this relate to a change in function, i.e., is an activity change related to the change from an immature response to the trophic action of GABA to a mature response to the neurotransmitter action of GABA; and 3) are proteases or phospholipases involved in the increase of GABA receptors.

RELATIONSHIP BETWEEN THE COMPONENTS OF THE GABA SYSTEM DURING DEVELOPMENT AND THOSE AFTER DEVELOPMENT

It is apparent that GABA in particular, and neurotransmitters in general, act during development in a manner quite different from that in an adult. The question then arises as to the relationship(s) between the components of the neurotransmitter system present during development and those present after maturation, i.e., when the neurotransmitter function is operating.

One aspect of the GABA receptor complex which has received little attention is the benzodiazepine receptor. As noted, this component develops prior to either the high- or low-affinity GABA sites. This suggests that either 1) the coupling between the two components occurs after development or 2) the benzodiazepine receptors studied to date are not associated with GABA receptors. This question could be addressed by measuring the effects of a) benzodiazepine on GABA receptor binding and conversely b) GABA on benzodiazepine receptor binding.

The observation that the benzodiazepine receptor matures prior to the GABA sites suggests that this receptor may play a vital role in the developmental mechanism as it relates to synaptogenesis. Possibly, the endogenous ligand for the benzodiazepine receptor may be the initial trophic factor necessary for GABAergic development since benzodiazepines are involved in the regulation of mouse thymoma cell proliferation (Wong et al., 1984). Subsequent to the action of the benzodiazepine ligand, GABA levels may rise to a critical level which allows it to take over the last aspects of connection formation. Once the synapse is formed, GABA serves as a neurotransmitter in the mature CNS. It would be of interest to investigate the changes in the development of the GABA system which occur after manipulation via the benzodiazepine receptor in order to address this possibility.

There is evidence that the components of the GABA system undergo maturation. Morphologically, changes have been studied in both cerebellar cultures (Hansen et al., 1984) and neuroblastoma cultures (Wolff et al., 1979b; Spoerri and Wolff, 1982;). These studies show a characteristic increase in parameters associated with synaptogenesis (For review, see Meier et al., 1983; Redburn and Madtes, in press; Wolff et al., 1984).

Studies on other components of the GABA system indicate that, in addition to morphological changes, biochemical changes also must occur. For example, treatment of both newborn and adult rabbit retinas with nipecotic acid blocks the uptake of GABA; however, the preference appears to be a neuronal block in adults and a glial block in newborns (Madtes and Redburn, unpublished observations). This difference may result from the loss of a high-affinity, low-capacity component of the transport system for GABA during the maturation process (Levi, 1972). In addition, the release mechanism undergoes a maturation, becoming increasingly Ca^{2+}-dependent, i.e., Ca^{2+}-independent in the newborn rat brain growth cones and Ca^{2+}-dependent in mature synaptosomes (Gordon-Weeks et al., personal communication).

Thus, the components of the GABA system goes through a maturation process. It is important to determine whether the second messenger coupled to GABA receptors remains constant during development. This would enable studies to be more directed toward the mechanisms of the action of GABA, both in immature and mature tissues.

It is apparent that GABA acts as a trophic factor in immature tissue and as a neurotransmitter in mature tissue. Therefore, these tissues must undergo a conversion, or maturation, process. Figure 3 is a suggested sequence of events which result in a mature GABAergic synapse. First, the genetic machinery of each neuron controls the growth of neurons and the production of the elements which are required for the initiation of synaptogenesis. One of these elements is the endogenous

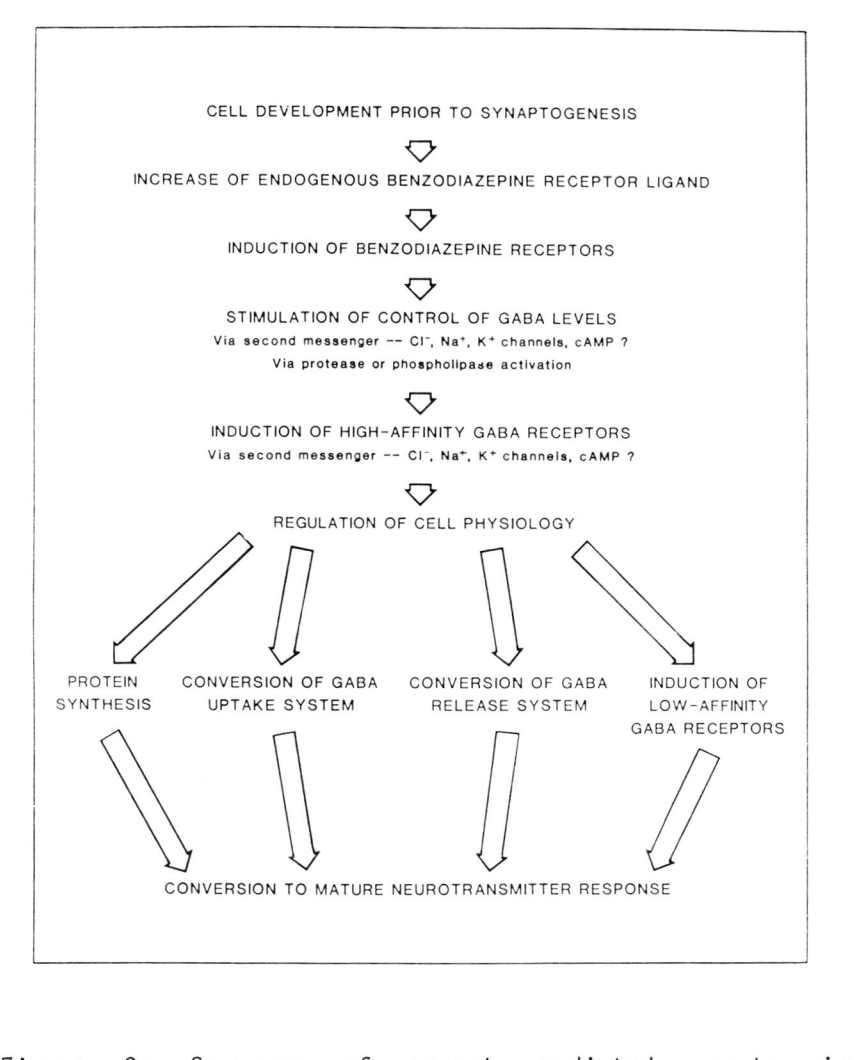

Figure 3: Sequence of receptor—mediated events in GABAergic synaptogenesis. This proposed scheme starts with neurons which are ready to begin synaptogenesis and follows the sequence of events which are the result of actions on benzodiazepine and GABA receptors. Ultimately, a mature, neurotransmitter response is achieved.

ligand for the benzodiazepine receptor. As the incoming neuron grows, the level of this ligand increases. When the target neuron is reached, the ligand binds to the benzodiazepine receptors, inducing their increase. After reaching a critical level of benzodiazepine receptors, the neuronal and glial uptake systems for GABA are stimulated to control the level of GABA in the extracellular space. The GABA then binds to the existing high-affinity receptors which are coupled to a second messenger, possibly Ca^{2+}, Na^+, or K^+ channels, or cyclic AMP, to induce the appearance of more receptors. This exposure may occur by the action of proteases or phospholipases. Once a critical number of high-affinity sites are activated, either the same second messenger, or another one, would regulate the physiology of the cell, such as 1) turning on protein synthesis, 2) altering the specificity of the GABA uptake system and the Ca^{2+}-dependency of the GABA release system, and 3) inducing the appearance of low-affinity receptors. The outcome of these changes is the establishment of the components of the GABA system required for a mature, neurotransmitter response to GABA. Thus, the conversion of the target neuron from a developing cell to a mature one may be mediated via benzodiazepine and GABA receptors.

In conclusion, this suggestion allows some speculation in regard to the development of the GABA system. Since many of the biochemical and morphological components of the GABA system undergo a maturational process, it is possible that two aspects of the transmitter system exist – one used during development and the other used in the adult. The evidence for uptake and release would support this. Similarly, high-affinity GABA receptors may mediate the trophic action of GABA whereas low-affinity sites are involved in the neurotransmitter function. However, high-affinity sites may retain a modulatory function in the adult which is distinct from that of a neurotransmitter since one study has shown that at least one class of GABA receptors (GABA$_B$ sites) can be acted upon without synaptic transmission (Schwartzwelder et al., 1986).

These final suggestions are speculative and need further experimentation for confirmation. However, since several neurotransmitter systems appear to have many characteristics in common with the GABA system during development, these suggestions may allow investigation into the mechanism of CNS development, as it relates to neurotransmitters acting via their receptors. The models give us many areas to investigate and define future experiments that could reveal elements of the trophic action of GABA. Furthermore, from the outline of proposed studies presented here, we may be able to ascertain the role of neurotransmitters in general during synaptogenesis. Ultimately, an understanding of the mechanism of CNS development may be gained.

REFERENCES

Adler R (1982). Regulation of neurite growth in purified retina neuronal cultures: Effects of PNPF, a substratum-bound, neurite-promoting factors. J Neurosci Res 8: 165-177.

Aghajanian GK, Bloom FE (1967). The formation of synaptic junctions in developing rat brains. A quantitative electron microscopic study. Brain Res 6: 710-727.

Aldinio C, Balzano MA, Toffano G (1980). Ontogenic development of GABA recognition sites in different brain areas. Pharmacol Res Commun 12: 495-500.

Aldinio C, Balzano M, Savoini G, Leon A, Toffano G (1981). Ontogeny of ^{3}H-diazepam binding sites in different rat brain areas. Effect of GABA. Devl Neurosci 4: 461-466.

Alleva E, Caprioli A, Laviola G (1986). Postnatal social environment affects morphine analgesia in male mice. Physiol Behav 36: 779-781.

Altstein M, Dudai Y, Vogel Z (1981). Benzodiazepine receptors in chick retina: Development and cellular localization. Brain Res 206: 198-202.

Baudry M, Lynch G (1980). Regulation of hippocampal glutamate receptors: Evidence for the involvement of a calcium-activated protease. Proc Natl Acad Sci USA 77: 2298-2302.

Baudry M, Kramer K, Lynch G (1983). Classification and properties of acidic amino acid receptors in hippocampus. III. Supersensitivity during the postnatal period and following denervation. Mol Pharmacol 24: 229-234.

Belhage B, Hansen GH, Meier E, Schousboe A (1986). Effects of inhibitors of protein synthesis and axonal transport on THIP-induced development of GABA receptors in cultured cerebellar granule cells. Eur Soc Neurochem Abstr.

Biggio G, Corda MG, DeMontis G, Concas A, Gessa GL (1980). Sudden decrease in cerebellar GABA binding induced by stress. Pharmacol Res Commun 12: 489–493.

Black IB, Patterson PH (1980). Developmental regulation of neurotransmitter phenotype. Curr Topics Devl Biol 15: 27–40.

Braestrup C, Nielsen M (1978). Ontogenetic development of benzodiazepine receptors in the rat brain. Brain Res 147: 170–173.

Brooksbank BWL, Atkinson DJ, Balazs R (1981). Biochemical development of the human brain. III. Some parameters of the GABA-ergic system. Devl Neurosci 4: 188–200.

Candy JM, Martin IL (1979). The postnatal development of the benzodiazepine receptor in the cerebral cortex and cerebellum of the rat. J Neurochem 32: 655–658.

Chun LLY, Patterson PH (1977a). Role of nerve growth factor in the development of rat sympathetic neurons in vitro. I. Survival, growth and differentiation of catecholamine production. J Cell Bull 75: 694–704.

Chun LLY, Patterson PH (1977b). Role of nerve growth factor in the development of rat sympathetic neurons in vitro. II. Developmental studies. J Cell Biol 75: 705–711.

Chun LLY, Patterson PH (1977c). Role of nerve growth factor in the development of rat sympathetic neurons in vitro. III. Effect on acetylcholine production. J Cell Biol 75: 712–718.

Cochard P, Goldstein M, Black IB (1978a). Ontogenetic appearance and disappearance of tyrosine hydroxylase and catecholamines in the rat embryo. Proc Natl Acad Sci USA 75: 2986–2990.

Cochard P, Goldstein M, Black IB (1978b). Initial development of the noradrenergic phenotype in autonomic neuroblasts of the rat embryo in vivo. Develop Biol 71: 100–114.

Cohan CS, Kater SB (1986). Suppression of neurite elongation and growth cone motility by electrical activity. Science 232: 1638–1640.

Conners BW, Benardo LS, Prince DA (1983). Coupling between neurons of the developing rat neocortex. J Neurosci 3: 773–782.

Corda MG, Guidotti A (1983). Modulation of GABA receptor binding by Ca^{2+}. J Neurochem 41: 277–280.

Coyle JT, Enna SJ (1976). Neurochemical aspects of the ontogenesis of GABAnergic neurons in the rat brain. Brain Res 111: 119–133.

De Plazas SF (1982). Ontogenesis of GABA receptor sites in chick embryo cerebellum. Devl Brain Res 3: 263-275.

Dames W, Joo F, Feher O, Toldi J, Wolff JR (1985). γ-aminobutyric acid enables synaptogenesis in the intact superior cervical ganglion of the adult rat. Neurosci Lett 54: 159-164.

DaVanzo JP, Chamberlain J, McConnaughey MM (1986). Influence of environment on GABA receptors in muricidal rats. Pharmacol Biochem Behav 25: 95-98.

DeFeudis FV (1982). Time-dependent environmentally-induced changes in cerebral and extra-cerebral morphology and chemistry - the basis of learning, memory and behavior. Gen Pharmac 13: 1-9.

DeFeudis FV, Madtes P, Camacho JG (1976). Binding of glycine and γ-aminobutyric acid to synaptosomal fractions of the brains of differentially-housed mice. Exp Neurol 50: 207-213.

Desarmenian M, Feltz P, Occhipinti G, Santangelo F, Schlichter R (1984). Coexistence of $GABA_A$ and $GABA_B$ receptors on Aδ and C primary afferents. Br J Pharmac 81: 327-333.

Duman RS, Karbon EW, Harrington C, Enna SJ (1986). An examination of the involvement of phospholipase A_2 and C in the β-adrenergic and γ-aminobutyric acid receptor modulation of cyclic AMP accumulation in rat brain slices. J Neurochem 47: 800-810.

Enna SJ, Yamamura HI, Snyder SH (1976). Development of muscarinic cholinergic and GABA receptor binding in chick embryo brain. Brain Res 101: 177-183.

Finger S, Almli CR (1985). Brain damage and neuro-plasticity: Mechanisms of recovery or development. Brain Res Rev 10: 177-186.

Fujimoto M, Okabayashi T (1983). Influence of phospho-lipase treatments on ligand bindings to a benzodiazepine receptor-GABA receptor-chloride ionophore complex. Life Sci 32: 2393-2400.

Giambalvo CT, Rosenberg P (1976). The effect of phospholipases and proteases on the binding of γ-aminobutyric acid to junctional complexes of rat cerebellum. Biochim Biophys Acta 436: 741-756.

Hansen GH, Meier E, Schousboe A (1984). GABA influences the ultrastructure composition of cerebellar granule cells during development in culture. Int J Devl Neurosci 2: 247-257.

Harris WA (1981). Neural activity and development. Ann Rev Physiol 43: 689-710.

Haydon PG, McCobb DP, Kater SB (1984). Serotonin selectively inhibits growth cone motility and synaptogenesis of specific identified neurons. Science 226: 561-564.

Jans JE, deVillers S, Woodside B (1985). The effects of rearing environment on pup development. Devl Psychol 18: 341-347.

Jong Y-J, Thampy KG, Barnes EM Jr (1986). Ontogeny of GABAergic neurons in chick brain: Studies in vivo and in vitro. Devl Brain Res 25: 83-90.

Jonsson G, Kasamatsu T (1983). Maturation of monoamine neurotransmitters and receptors in cat occipital cortex during postnatal critical period. Exp Brain Res 50: 449-458.

Joo F, Dames W, Wolff JR (1979). Effect of prolonged sodium bromide administration on the fine structure of dendrites in the superior cervical ganglion of adult rat. In Cuenao M, Kreutzberg GW, Bloom FE (eds): "Development and Chemical Specificity of Neurons". Prog Brain Res 51: 109-115.

Kraemer G (1985). The primate social environment, brain neurochemical changes and psychopathology. Trends Neurosci 8: 339-340.

Kuriyama K, Sisken B, Haber B, Roberts E (1966). The γ-aminobutyric acid system in the developing chick embryo cerebellum. Brain Res 11: 412-430.

Kuriyama K, Yoneda Y, Taguchi J, Takahashi M, Ohkuma S (1984). Properties of purified γ-aminobutyric acid (GABA) receptors and modulation of GABA receptor binding by membrane phospholipids. Neuropharmacol 23: 839-840.

Lankford K, DeMello FG, Klein WL (in press). A transient embryonic dopamine receptor inhibits growth cone motility and neurite outgrowth in a subset of avian retina neurons. Neurosci Lett.

Levi G (1972). Transport systems for GABA and for other amino acids in incubated chick brain tissue during development. Arch Biochem Biophys 151: 8-21.

Levitt M, Spector S, Sjoerdsma A, Udenfriend S (1965). Elucidation of the rate-limiting step in norepinephrine biosynthesis in the perfused guinea-pig heart. J Pharmacol Exp Ther 148: 1-8.

Lloyd KG, Dreksler S (1979). An analysis of [³H]-gamma-aminobutyric acid (GABA) binding in the human brain. Brain Res 163: 77-87.

Madtes P (1985). Light-dependent regulation of GABA receptors during development. Soc Neurosci Abstr 11:

328.1.

Madtes P Jr, Adler R (1985). Development of muscimol binding sites in chick embryo neural retina in vivo and in vitro: Regulatory effects of cyclic AMP. Int J Devl Neurosci 3: 511-519.

Madtes P Jr, Bashir-Elahi R (1986). GABA receptor binding site "induction" in rabbit retina after nipecotic acid treatment: Changes during postnatal development. Neurochem Res 11: 55-61.

Madtes P, Redburn DA (1982). [^{3}H] GABA binding in developing rabbit retina. Neurochem Res 7: 495-503.

Madtes P Jr, Redburn DA (1983a). Synaptic interactions in the GABA system during postnatal development in retina. Brain Res Bull 10: 741-745.

Madtes P Jr, Redburn DA (1983b). GABA as a trophic factor during development. Life Sci 33: 979-984.

Maickel RP, Westermann EO, Brodie BB (1961). Effects of reserpine and cold-exposure on pituitary-adrenocortical function in rats. J Pharmacol Exp Therap 134: 167-175.

Majewska MA, Bisserbe J-C, Eskay RL (1985). Glucocorticoids are modulators of GABA$_A$ receptors in brain. Brain Res 339: 178-182.

Mallorga P, Hamburg M, Tallman JF, Gallager DW (1980). Ontogenetic changes in GABA modulation of brain benzodiazepine binding. Neuropharmacol 19: 405-408.

Massotti M, Alleva FR, Balazs R, Guidotti A (1980). GABA and benzodiazepine receptors in the offspring of dams receiving diazepam: Ontogenetic studies. Neuropharmacol 19: 951-956.

McArdle CB, Dowling JE, Masland RH (1977). Development of outer segments and synapses in the rabbit retina. J Comp Neurol 175: 253-274.

Meaney MJ, Aitken DH, Bodnoff SR, Iny LJ, Tatarewicz JE, Sapolsky RM (1975). Early postnatal handling alters glucocorticoid receptor concentrations in selected brain regions. Behav Neurosci 99: 765-770.

Meier E, Drejer J, Schousboe A (1983). Trophic action of GABA on the development of physiologically active GABA receptors. In Mandel P, DeFeudis FV (eds): "CNS Receptors - From Molecular Pharmacology to Behavior". New York: Raven Press, pp 47-58.

Meier E, Drejer J, Schousboe A (1984a). GABA as a modulator of glutamatergic neurotransmission. Acta Neurol Scand 69: 334-336.

Meier E, Drejer J, Schousboe A (1984b). GABA induces functionally active low-affinity GABA receptors on cultured cerebellar granule cells. J Neurochem 43: 1737–1744.

Meier E, Hansen GH, Schousboe A (1985). The trophic effect of GABA on cerebellar granule cells is mediated by GABA–receptors. Int J Devl Neurosci 3: 401–407.

Meier E, Schousboe A (1982). Differences between GABA receptor binding to membranes from cerebellum during postnatal development and from cultured cerebellar granule cells. Devl Neurosci 5: 546–553.

Morris G, Seidler FJ, Slotkin TA (1983). Stimulation of ornithine decarboxylase by histamine or norepinephrine in brain regions of the developing rat: Evidence for biogenic amines as trophic agents in neonatal brain development. Life Sci 32: 1565–1571.

Palacios JM, Kuhar M (1982). Ontogeny of high affinity GABA and benzodiazepine receptors in the rat cerebellum: An autoradiographic study. Devl Brain Res 2: 531–539.

Palacios JM, Niehoff DL, Kuhar MJ (1979). Ontogeny of GABA and benzodiazepine receptors: Effects of Triton X–100, bromide and muscimol. Brain Res 179: 390–395.

Patterson P, Chun LLY (1977). The induction of acetylcholine synthesis in primary cultures of dissociated rat sympathetic neurons. I. Effects of conditioned medium. Develop Biol 56: 263–280.

Pasantes–Morales H, Klethi J, Ledig M, Mandel P (1973). Influence of light and dark on the free amino acid pattern of the developing chick retina. Brain Res 57: 59–65.

Puro DG (1983). Glucocorticoid regulation of synaptic development. Devl Brain Res 8: 283–290.

Redburn DA, Madtes P Jr (1986). Postnatal development of ^{3}H–GABA–accumulating cells in rabbit retina. J Comp Neurol 243: 41–57.

Redburn DA, Madtes P Jr (1987). GABA – its role and development in retina. In Chader GJ, Osborne NN (eds): Prog Retinal Res Vol 6: 69–84.

Redburn DA, Massey SC, Madtes P (1983). The GABA uptake system in rabbit retina. In: Hertz L, Kvamme E, McGeer EG, Schousboe A (eds): "Glutamine, Glutamate, and GABA in the Central Nervous System". New York: Alan R Liss, Inc, pp 273–286.

Redburn DA, Mitchell CK (1981). ^{3}H–muscimol binding in synaptosomal fractions from bovine and developing brain retinas. J Neurosci Res 6: 485–487.

Roberts E, Harman PJ, Frankel S (1951). γ–aminobutyric acid content and glutamic decarboxylase activity in developing mouse brain. Proc Soc Exp Biol (NY) 78: 799–803.

Saito K-I, Goto M, Fukuda H (1982). Postnatal development of the GABA system in the rat spinal cord. Japan J Pharmacol 32: 1–7.

Saito K-I, Goto M, Fukuda H (1983). Postnatal development of the benzodiazepine receptors in the rat spinal cord. Japan J Pharmacol 33: 906–909.

Schlumpf M, Richards JG, Lichtensteiger, Mohler H (1983). An autoradiographic study of the prenatal development of benzodiazepine–binding sites in rat brain. J Neurosci 3: 1478–1487.

Shaw C, Needler MC, Cynader M (1984). Ontogenesis of muscimol binding sites in cat visual cortex. Brain Res Bull 13: 331–334.

Skangiel-Kramska J, Kossut M (1985). Monocular deprivation affects GABA receptor in the visual cortex of kittens. Physiol Bohemoslov 34: 145–147.

Skerritt JH, Johnston GAR (1972). Postnatal development of GABA binding sites and their endogenous inhibitors in rat brain. Devl Neurosci 5: 189–197.

Skerritt JH, Trisdikoon P, Johnston GAR (1981). Increased GABA binding in mouse brain following acute swim stress. Brain Res 215: 389–403.

Spoerri PE, Wolff JR (1982). Morphological changes induced by sodium bromide in murine neuroblastoma cells in vitro. Cell Tissue Res 222: 379–388.

Swartzwelder HS, Bragdon AC, Sutch CP, Ault B, Wilson WA (1986). Baclofen suppresses hippocampal epileptiform activity at low concentrations without suppressing synaptic transmission. J Pharmacol Exp Ther 237: 881–887.

Sykes CC, Horton RW (1986). Development of the γ-aminobutyric acid neurotransmitter system in the rat cerebral cortex during repeated administration of the GABA-transaminase inhibitor ethanolamine O-sulphate. J Neurochem 46: 213–217.

Tehrani MHJ, Barnes EM Jr (1986). Ontogeny of the GABA receptor complex in chick brain: Studies in vivo and in vitro. Devl Brain Res 25: 91–98.

Toffano G, Aldinio C, Balzano M, Leon A, Savoini G (1981). Regulation of GABA receptor binding to synaptic plasma membrane of rat cerebral cortex: The role of endogenous phospholipids. Brain Res 222: 95–102.

Varon S, Adler R (1981). Trophic and specifying factors directed to neuronal cells. Adv Cell Neurobiol 2:

115–163.

Vincent J, Legrand C, Rabie, Legrand J (1982–1983). Effects of thyroid hormone on synaptogenesis in the molecular layer of the developing rat cerebellum. J Physiol Paris 78: 729–738.

Wang JKT, Morgan JL, Spector S (1984). Benzodiazepines that bind at peripheral sites inhibit cell proliferation. Proc Natl Acad Sci USA 81: 753–756.

Wee EL, Zimmerman EF (1983). Involvement of GABA in palate morphogenesis and its relation to diazepam teratogenesis in two mouse strains. Teratol 28: 15–22.

Wolff JR, Balcar VJ, Zetzsche T, Bottcher H, Schmechel DE, Chronwall BM (1984). Development of GABA-ergic system in rat visual cortex. In: Lauder JM, Nelson PG (eds): "Gene Expression and Cell-Cell Interactions". New York: Plenum Press, pp 215–239.

Wolff JR, Joo F, Dames W, Feher O (1979a). Induction and maintenance of free postsynaptic membrane thickenings in the adult superior cervical ganglion. J Neurocytol 8: 549–563.

Wolff JR, Rickman M, Chronwall BM (1979b). Axo-glial synapses and GABA-accumulated glial cells in the embryonic neocortex of the rat. Cell Tissue Res 201: 239–248.

Wolff JR, Joo F, Dames W, Feher O (1981). Neuroplasticity in the superior cervical ganglion as a consequence of long-lasting inhibition. In: Feher O, Joo F (eds): "Cellular Analogues of Conditioning and Neural Plasticity". Adv Physiol Sci 36:1–9.

Wood JD, Schousboe A, Krogsgaard-Larsen P (1980). In vitro changes in the GABA content of nerve endings (synaptosomes) induced by inhibitors of GABA uptake. Neuropharmacol. 19: 1149–1152.

Yeh HH, Battelle BA, Puro DG (1983). Maturation of neurotransmission at cholinergic synapses formed in culture by rat retinal neurons: Regulation of cyclic AMP. Devl Brain Res 10: 63–72.

Yoneda Y, Kanmori K, Ida S, Kuriyama K (1983). Stress-induced alterations in metabolism of γ-aminobutyric acid in rat brain. J Neurochem 40: 350–356.

Zimmerman EF, Wee EL (1984). Role of neurotransmitters in palate development. Curr Topics Devl Biol 19: 37–63.

Neurotrophic Activity of GABA During Development, pages 189–220
© **1987 Alan R. Liss, Inc.**

GABA-mediated developmental alterations in a neuronal cell line and in cultures of cerebral and retinal neurons

P.E. Spoerri

Department of Neurosurgery, University of Gottingen, Robert-Koch-Str. 40, D-3400 Gottingen, Federal Republic of Germany

INTRODUCTION

A possible role for GABA as a trophic or regulatory factor in neuronal development in vitro was identified when it was applied to a neuronal cell - line that had previously failed to form synapses or reveal early signs of active synaptogenesis (Spoerri et al., 1980b). Incubation of these cells in the presence of GABA produced several responses. It increased neurite outgrowth, promoted the differentiation of terminal swellings, and induced the proliferation of clear-core, dense-core and coated vesicles. Coated vesicles were actively involved in the formation of specialized contacts by contributing membrane to the bilateral membrane specializations (Spoerri and Wolff, 1981).

Such an effect of GABA on neuronal cell development was not unexpected, as earlier studies revealed that GABA induced in vivo neuroplastic changes relating to the direct or indirect regulation of synaptogenesis (Wolff et al., 1978; Wolff, 1979; Wolff et al., 1979d; Wolff et al., 1979). It was later shown that addition of exogenous GABA to cultures of neonatal rat cerebellum led to enhanced neuritic outgrowth. At the ultrastructural level GABA treatment led to an increased density of neurotubules, rough endoplasmic reticulum (RER), Golgi apparatus, coated vesicles and other vesicles (Hansen et al., 1984). Additionally, GABA induced the formation of low affinity GABA receptors in contrast to the high affinity receptors which were present (Meier et al., 1984). The effects of

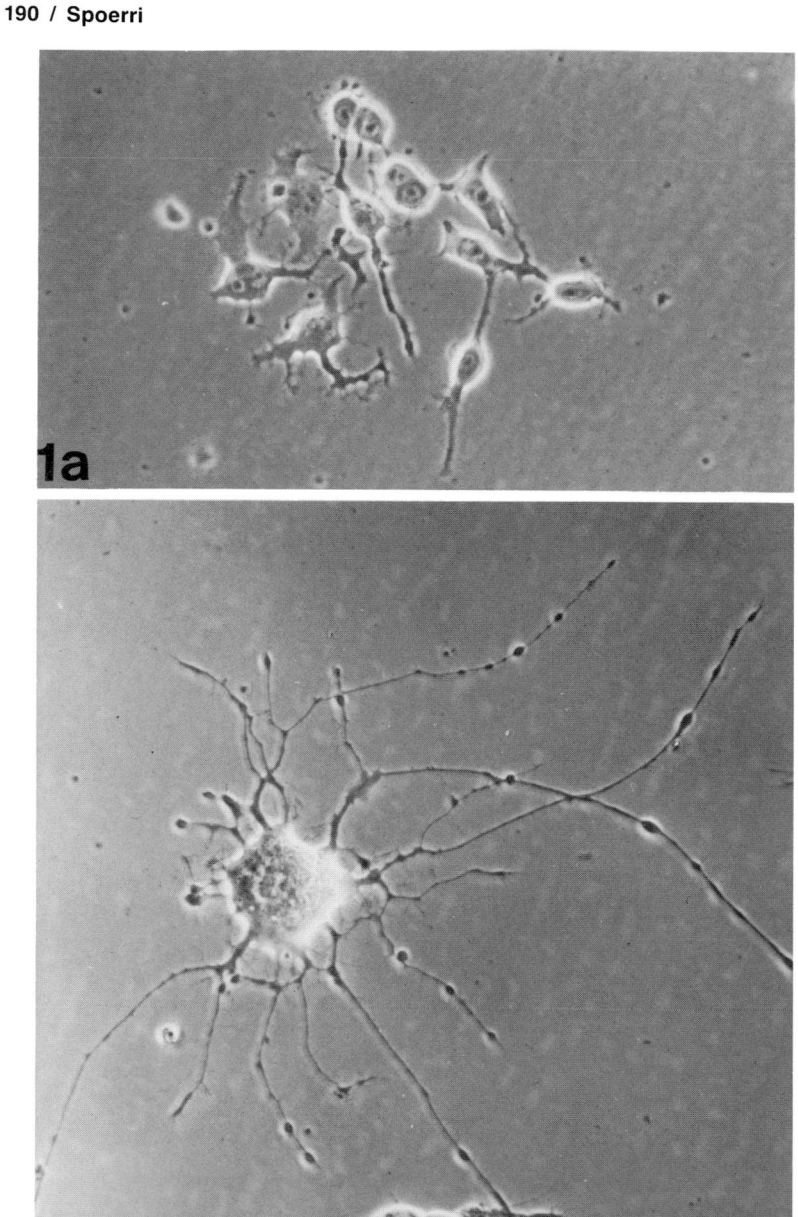

GABA could be completely blocked by the simultaneous presence of the antagonist bicuculline methobromide (150 µM) in the culture media (Meier et al., 1985). In the rabbit retina, treatments which blocked high affinity GABA uptake, led to a significant increase in binding to high affinity GABA receptor, suggesting a relationship between GABA availability in the extracellular spaces and the development of binding sites (Madtes and Redburn, 1983a, b; Redburn et al., 1983). These data were indicative that the formation of GABA receptor sites was influenced by the activity of the GABA uptake system supporting the hypothesis that GABA may function as a trophic factor in the development of at least certain neuron types.

The mechanism of action of GABA particularly at the morphological level is still not clearly understood. In the following report earlier studies on responses to GABA in neuronal cultures will be reviewed. Some additional recent investigations using mainly primary cultures from embryonic chick brain and retina will be described in an attempt to give further insights on the mode of action of this substance.

THE EXPERIMENTAL APPROACH

Preparation of Neuronal Cell Cultures

Stock cultures of C1300 mouse neuroblastoma, clone N-2A, purchased from the American Type Culture Collection (Rockville, MD), were maintained at 37°C in a humidified atmosphere of 5% CO_2 and 95% air. The cultures were grown in plastic Petri-dishes (35 mm, Nunc) or in plastic flasks (Corning) and were fed twice to three times a week with Eagle's minimum essential medium or Ham F-10 medium supplemented with 10% fetal calf serum (FCS) and 1% of 200 mM L-glutamine.

After 5 days in culture the cells were fed with normal medium or with the same medium containing 1-2% FCS instead

---

Figure 1. (a) N-2A cells, living preparation, 48h in medium containing 1% FCS. (b) Same cells after 48h in the same medium supplemented with 10^{-5} M GABA. Note the extensively long, branching neurites with numerous, small, fine projections. Phase; (a) x 480 (b) x 600.

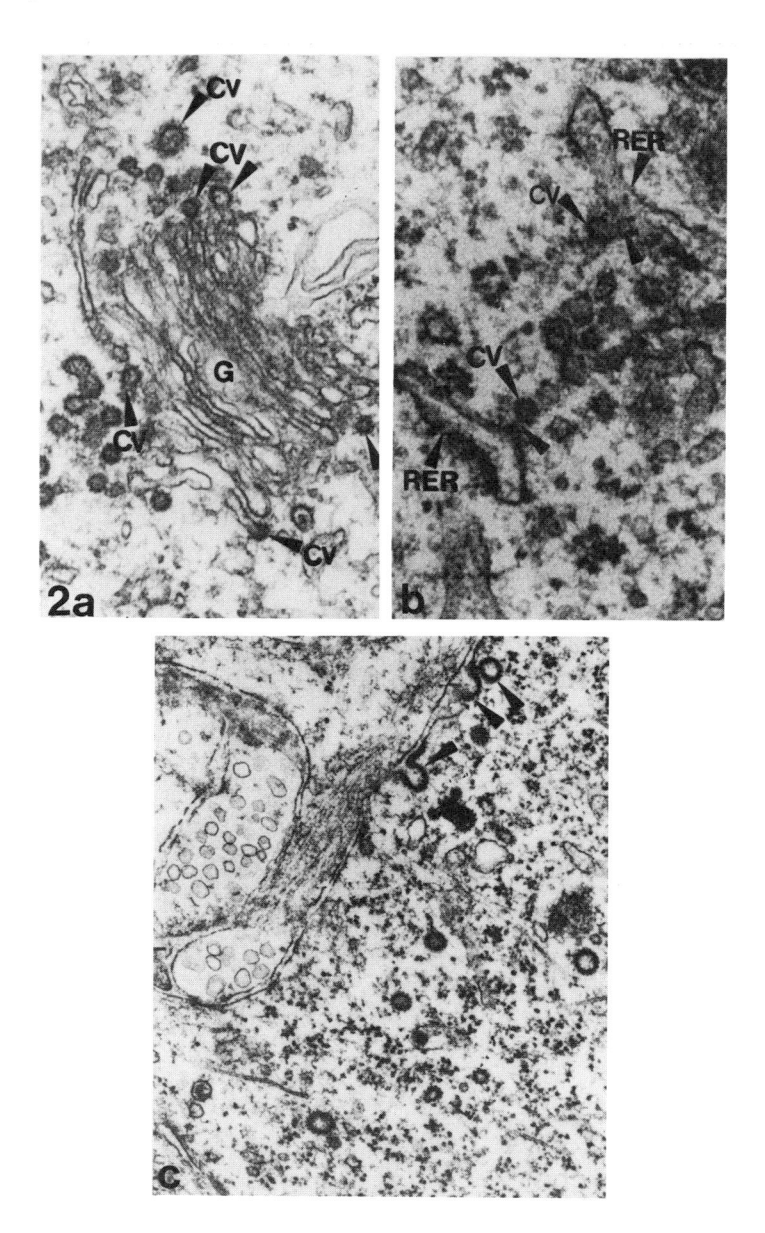

of 10% to which GABA was added (Spoerri and Wolff, 1981; Eins et al., 1983). This substance was dissolved in double distilled water and added to the normal medium producing concentrations of 10^{-4} to 10^{-5} M. GABA was applied to the cultures for a maximum of 2 days.

Primary Cultures

Cerebral Hemisperes. Cultures were prepared from the cerebra of 6-day-old chick embryos as previous described (Pettmann et al., 1979). The cerebral hemispheres were dissected out and the meningeal membranes removed. The brain tissue was then placed in a pool of Hank's balanced salt solution and pieces approximately 1-2 mm, were cut out. The tissue was then gently dissociated by passage through a 22-gauge needle into and out of a 5 ml syringe (five times). After mechanical dissociation, 1.8 ml of Eagle's basal medium (BME), containing 26.4 mM $NaHCO_3$, 33.3 mM D-glucose, 2 mM L-glutamine and 10% FCS, was added to poly-D-lysine treated Petri dishes (35 mm, Nunc), containing 0.2 ml of cell suspension (5 x 10^4 cell density). The cultures were incubated at $37^\circ C$ in a humidified atmosphere consisting of 5% CO_2 and 95% air. The cells were grown either in the absence or presence of 10^{-5} M GABA. After 24h in culture, 40 μM cytosine arabinoside was added and following 2 days in culture the medium was changed to an analogous medium without the mitotic inhibitor. After 3 days the cultures were fed and the respective supply of GABA renewed in the treated cultures.

Figure 2. (a) Coated vesicles located within the Golgi apparatus (G) of N-2A cells and are confluent with membranes of the Golgi cisternae. (b) Coated vesicles associated with RER and apparently budding off from the cisternae (arrowheads). 5 and 10 day-old cultures treated with 10^{-4} M GABA. (c) Coated vesicles (CV) displaying clear centers (80-120 nm in diameter), a filamentous dense substance and thin cytoplasmic protrusions extending radially from the outer surface of the limiting membrane. Such vesicles are seen within the cytoplasm and at the periphery of cells (arrowheads). 7-day-old cultures treated with 10^{-4} M GABA (a) x 40,500; (b) 60,000; (c) 32,500.

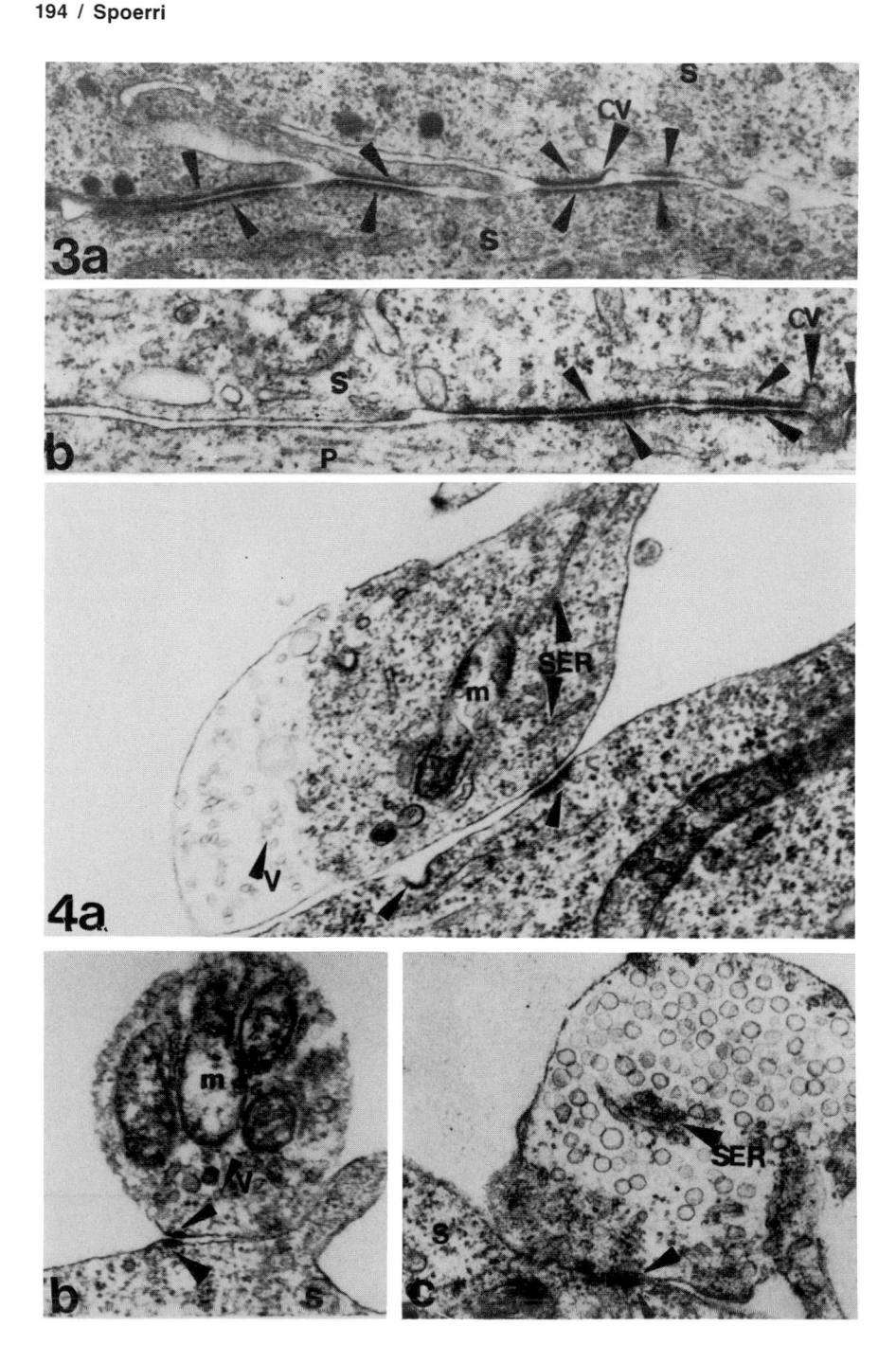

Retina. Glial-free, purified neuronal cultures were prepared as previously described (Adler, 1982; Adler et al., 1982). Neural retina of 8-day chick embryos was dissected free from other ocular tissues. The tissue was mechanically dissociated in 3 ml of serum-free Eagle's basal medium (BME), rinsed with Ca^{+2} and Mg^{+2} free Hank's and the cells incubated at 37ºC for 15 min in 5 ml of 0.1% trypsin in phosphate buffered saline (PBS). The cells were centrifuged, the trypsin supernatant removed and washed 2 x with basic medium BME. The cells were further dispersed by several passes through the tip of a Pasteur pipette and the single cell suspension diluted several fold with culture medium. The culture medium consisted of BME containing 2.2 mg/ml bicarbonate supplemented with 5.0 g/l D-glucose, 2 mM glutamine and 10% FCS. 2 ml aliquots containing 2×10^5 cells/ml were seeded into individual 35 mm dishes (Corning) some containing thermanox (Lux) coverslips. The Petri dishes and coverslips were precoated with rat tail collagen (Sigma) or 0.1 mg/ml of poly-L-ornithine (M.W. 400,000; Sigma). The cultures were incubated at 37ºC in an atmosphere of 5% CO_2 and 95% air for up to 8 days. The cells were grown either in the absence or presence of

---

Figures 3a, b. Bilateral membrane specializations or specialized contacts (arrowheads). Note the dense membrane invaginations (arrowheads), which may form coated vesicles (CV), in continuity with the dense membrane condensation. P = Process, S = Soma, 18 day-old cultures treated with 10^{-4} M GABA for 2 days. X 32,500.

Figures 4a-c. Varicosities displaying vesicles, mitochondria and cisternae of SER. (a) Vesicles, 40-60 nm in diameter, single cisternae of the SER and mitochondria (M), see arrowheads. Opposite to the terminal swelling at the periphery of the neuronal soma (S), a membrane thickening (arrowhead) and a dense membrane invagination are present, both remote from the vesicles (V). (b) Symmetrical densities (membrane thickenings), one on the bouton and the other on the opposed soma (arrowheads). (c) Within the terminal swelling, numerous, large, empty appearing, smooth, round vesicles of varying diameter (up to 200 nm). Note the presence of SER and opposed membrane thickenings. From 10, 18 and 15 day-old cultures treated with 10^{-5} M GABA for 2 days. x 34,000.

10^{-5} M GABA in medium supplemented with 50% of pigment epithelium conditioned medium (PECM; Spoerri et al., in preparation). After 3 days the cultures were fed and the respective supply of GABA renewed in the treated cultures. All cultures were examined daily utilizing a Zeiss IM 35 or a Nikon Diaphot inverted phase contrast microscope.

Transmission and Scanning Electron Microcopy

The culture medium was drained off the cells grown on plastic Petri dishes coverslips or flasks. The neuronal cells were fixed in situ at 36^0 C for 30 min. using 2.5% glutaraldehyhde in 0.08 M phosphate buffer (pH 7.2). The cells were postfixed in 1% osmium tetroxide containing 0.2 M saccharose in 0.08 M phosphate buffer for 1h. After dehydration in ethanol the cultures grown on plastic and half of those grown on coverslips were embedded in Epon 812. The other half of the coverslip cultures were

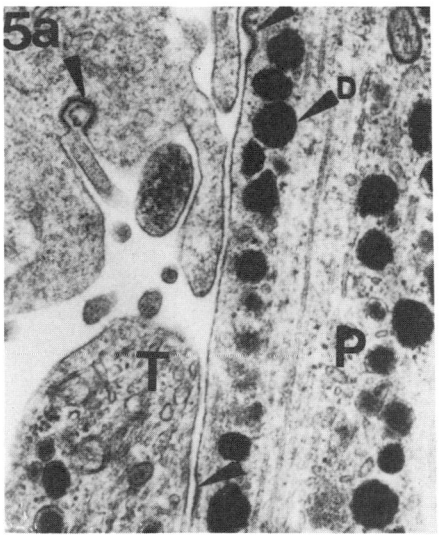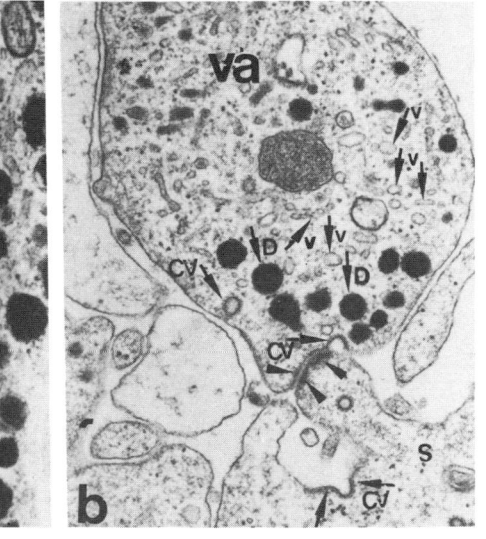

Figures 5a, b. Regions of N-2A cells displaying large amounts of dense-core vesicles (D) within the periphery of a process (P) or within a varicosity (V) or terminal swelling (T) in GABA treated cultures. Note the dense membrane invaginations (arrowheads), vesicles (V) and coated vesicles (CV), S = soma. (a) x 34,000; (b) 25,500.

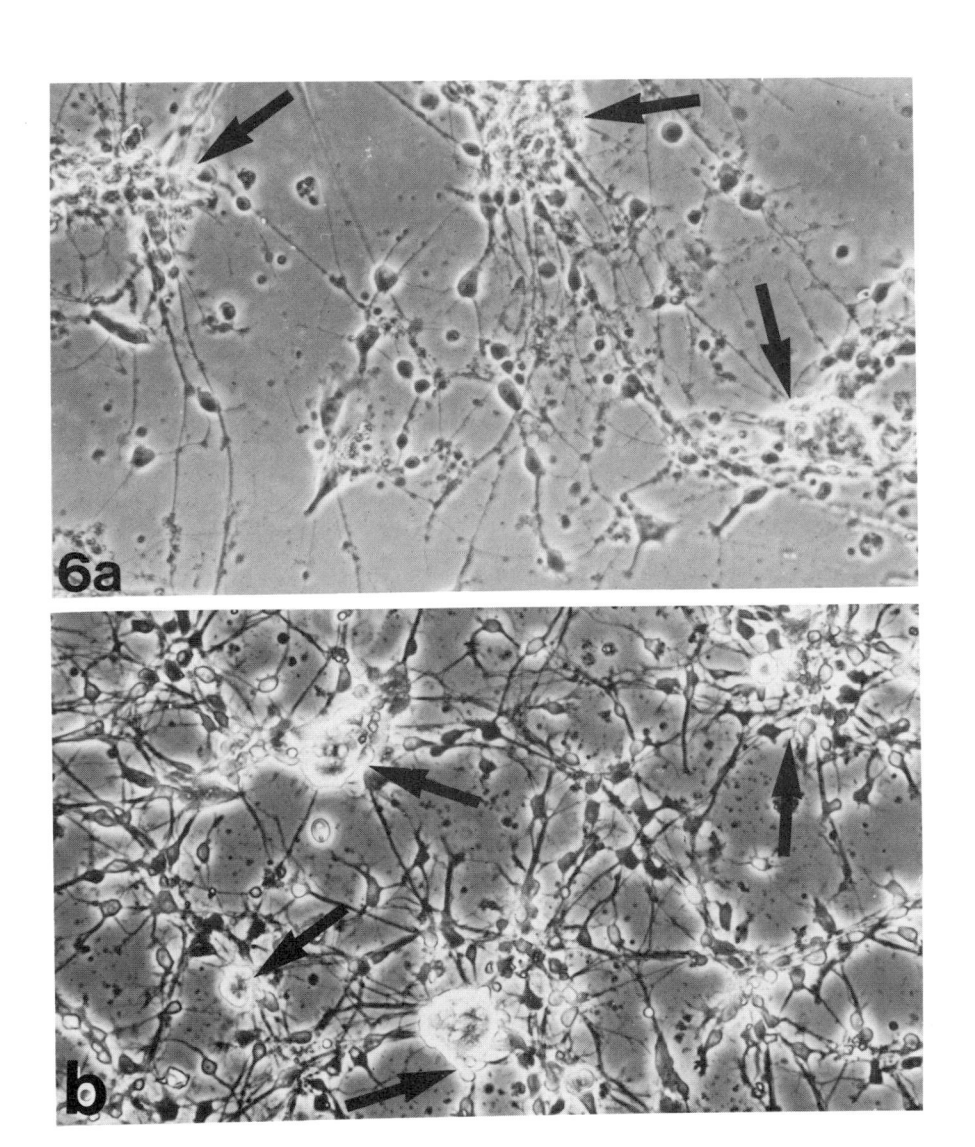

Fig. 6. Legend on next page

processed for scanning electron microscopy (SEM). Cultures embedded in Epon 812 for transmission electron microscopy (TEM) were thin sectioned as described (Spoerri et al., 1980a), stained in uranyl acetate and Reynold's lead citrate and photographed in a Zeiss 95 or 10 CR or Philips 301 transmission electron microscope. For SEM, specimens were critically point dried (Balzers BU 101) mounted on stubs and sputter coated (Technics Hummer X) prior to viewing on a Hitashi 450 S scanning electron microscope.

Morphometric Analysis

Light Microscopy. The following parameters were measured: (1) the number of cells or colonies of neuronal cell bodies, and (2) the number and length of the primary and secondary processes per neuron. The numerically coded cultures were randomly mixed and evaluated microscopically as described (Roisen et al., 1972). Observations were made in representative microscopic field. All rating was accomplished at a magnification of 150x using phase contrast optics. After evaluation the cultures were decoded. At least five Petri dishes of treated and untreated cultures were evaluated for each of three independent experiments. The data were analyzed statistically using Student's t test.

Electron Microscope-Synapse Counts. Quantification was done on primary cultures fixed on day 7, 9 and 11. Each fixed embedded culture was sawed into 4 quarters and from each quarter a reaggregate was sectioned. The sections were collected on nickel grids with hole diameters of 50 x 50 μm. Subsequently, 4 thin sections were selected, each derived from a different quarter. Only sections covered with 90% healthy neuropil were used. Thus 16 tissue samples per culture dish could be

---

Figures 6,a b. Light micrographs taken 2 days after plating cerebral cortical neurons, from 8 day-old chick embryos, in medium supplemented with serum. (a) Note the early aggregation of clusters of neurons (arrows) and the emission of a few single or bundles of neurites. (b) Similar culture supplemented with 10^{-5} M GABA showing in increase in the number of cell aggregates (arrows) and interconnecting neurites. Phase x 350.

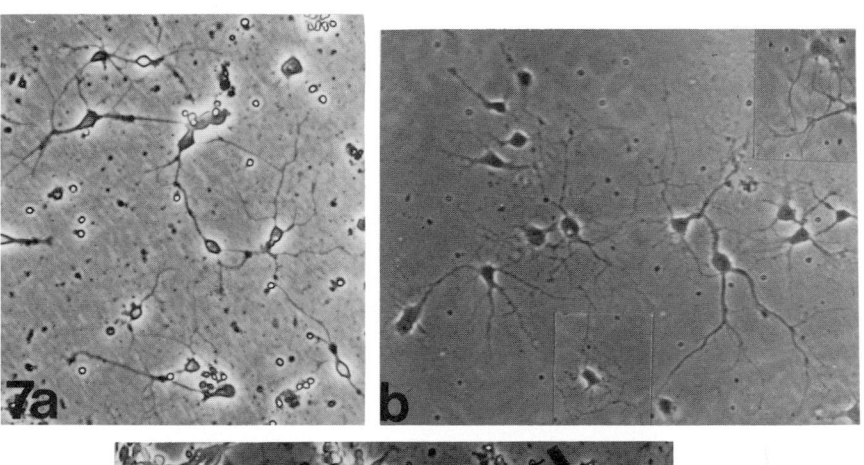

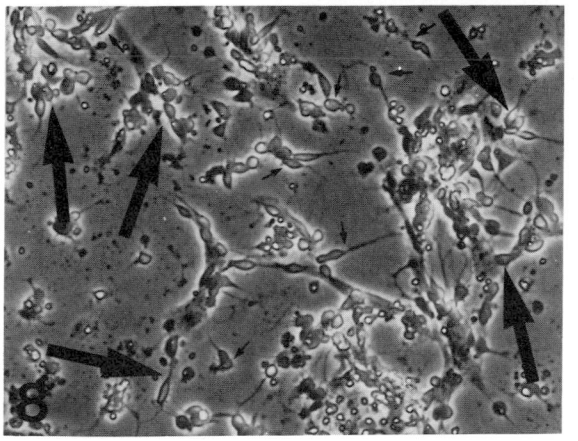

Figures 7a, b. Light micrographs of isolated retinal neurons depicting the sprouting effect of 10^{-5} M GABA, increasing the number of primary and secondary processes of neurons. (a) Untreated, (b) treated culture. Phase; x 350.

Figure 8. Differentiating photoreceptor cells with refractile oil droplets (arrows) from embryonic chick retina 7 days in culture. Phase; x 350.

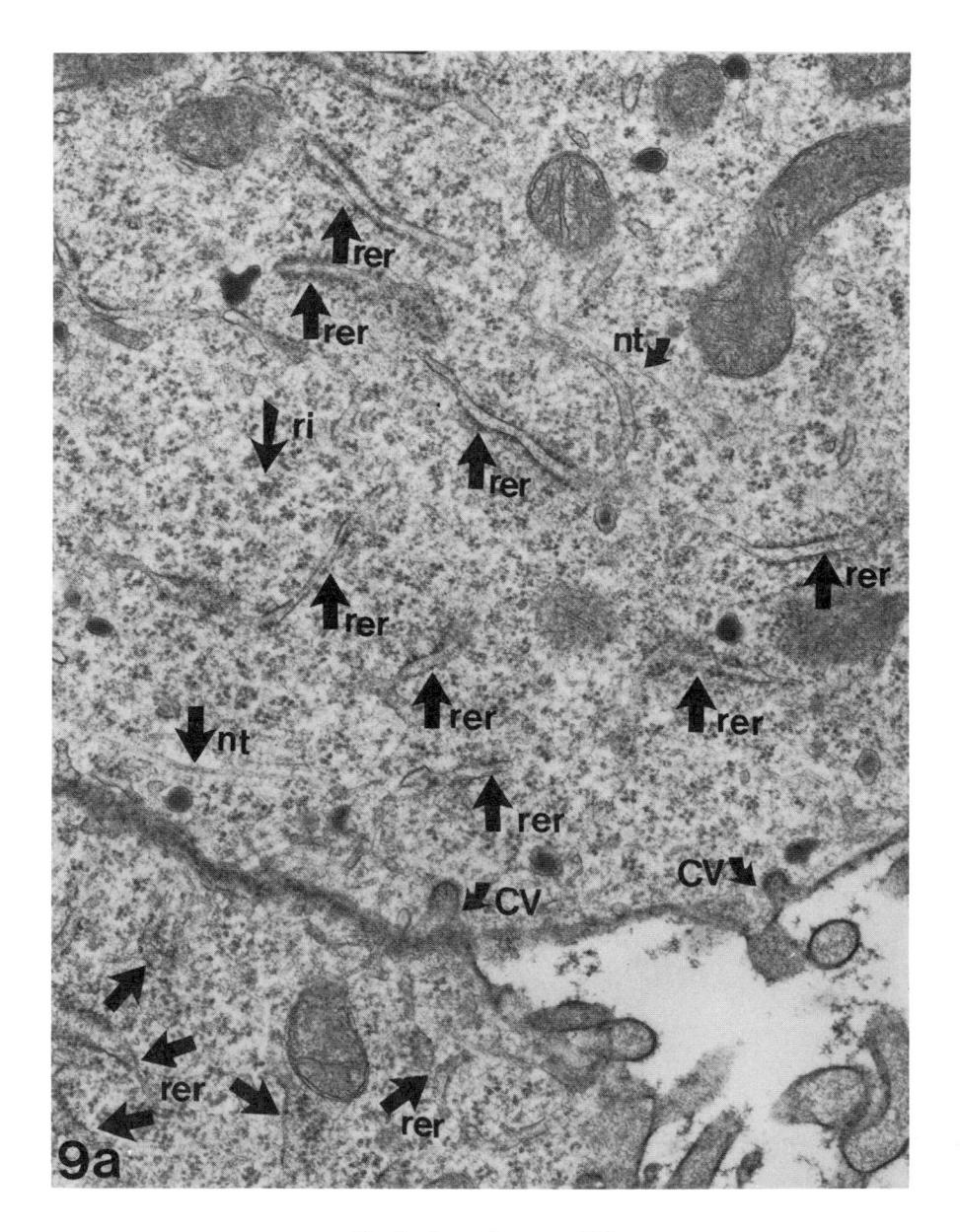

Fig. 9a. Legend on page 202

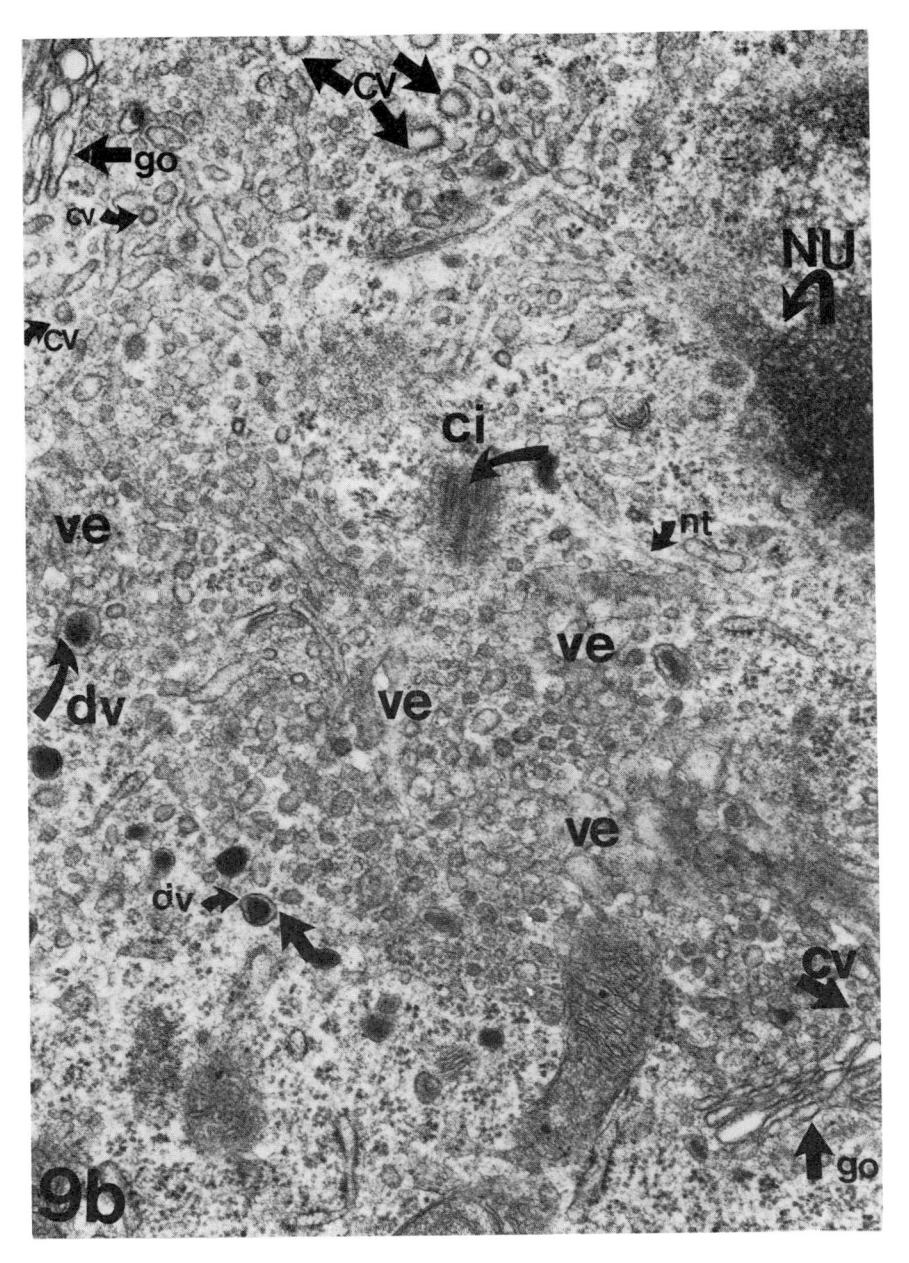

Fig. 9b. Legend on next page

screened as previously described (Romijn et al., 1984).

OBSERVATIONS

Effects of GABA on N-2a cells

N-2A cells grown in monolayer culture in the presence of serum possess few neurites and display a phenotype characterized by slow differentiation and rapid proliferation. This is in contrast to the type of growth observed when serum is deleted and low concentrations are being used. Upon addition of GABA to the non-synchronous cell population, extensive neurite formation with elaborate contacts is observed within 20 - 24h (Figs. 1a, b). This effect has been extensively described elsewhere (Spoerri et al, 1980b; Spoerri and Wolff, 1981; Eins et al., 1983; Spoerri, 1984; 1987b).

Electron microscopy revealed that the effect of a two-day application of 10^{-4} to 10^{-5} M GABA to the cultures advanced the stage of neuronal maturation. There was a proliferation of the exocytotic, 100 nm diameter coated vesicles. These vesicles appeared to originate from the Golgi cisternae and the RER (Figs. 2a-c). Coated vesicles were found in continuity with uni- and bilateral membrane specializations contributing undercoating to the postsynaptic density (Figs. 3a, b).

Following the appearance of the postsynaptic density, a small number of synaptic vesicles were seen in the growth cone cytoplasm, in some stage of its reorganization into a synaptic bouton. However, the synaptic vesicles did not cluster at the active zone. The growth cone cytoplasm still contained a few mound areas and primitive contacts or symmetrical densities (Figs. 4a-c). As clear synaptic vesicles accumulated at the forming presynaptic site, large dense-core vesicles gathered at the periphery of somata or neurites, suggesting that they may play a role in the process of synapse formation (Figs. 5a, b).

Figure 9. Electron micrographs of GABA treated (a) cultured cerebral cortical and (b) retinal neurons, depicting an increase in the density of RER (rer), Golgi apparatus (go) and neurotubules (nt). ri = ribosomes, cv = coated vesicles budding off the Golgi, dv = dense core vesicles, ve - vesicles, ci = cilium. x 10,500.

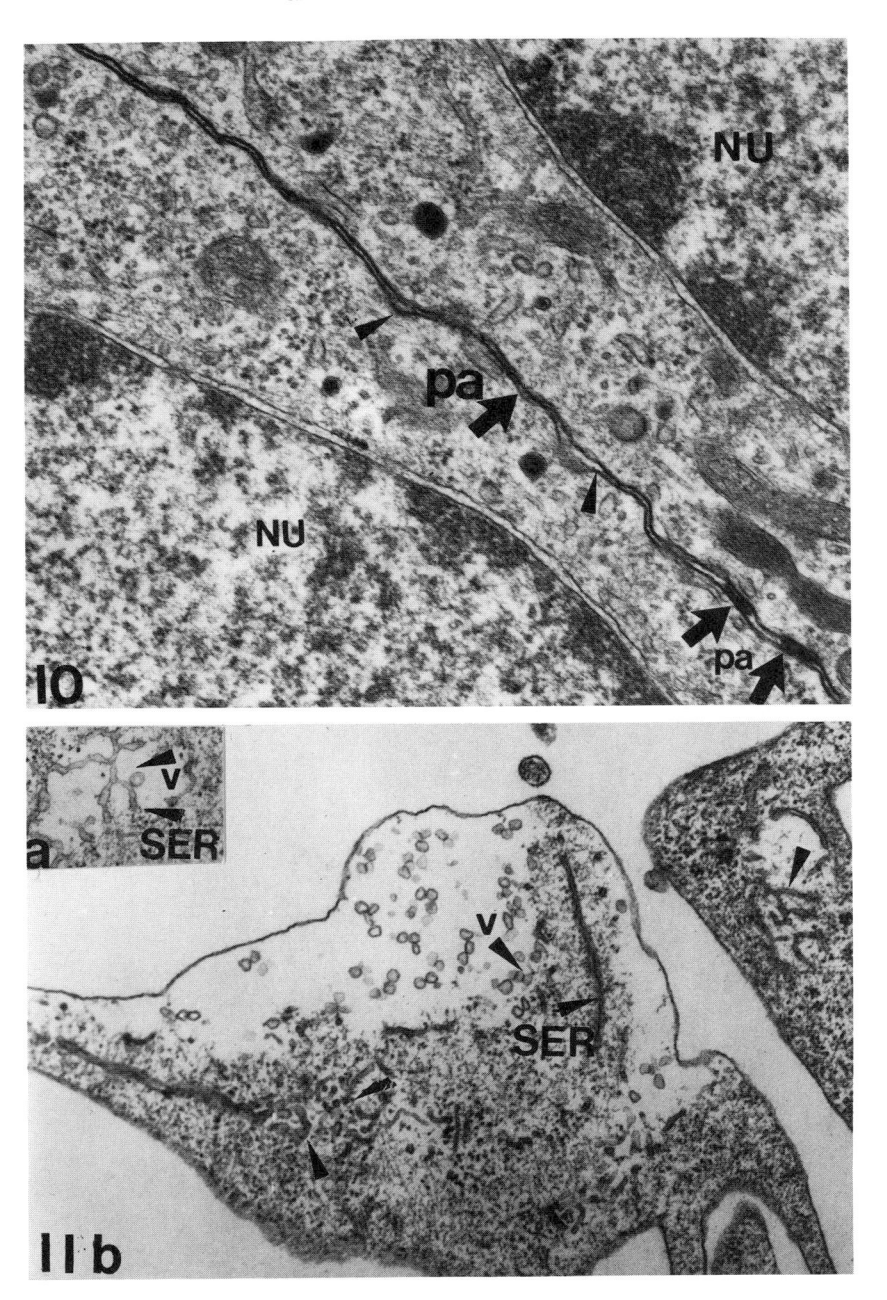

Figs. 10 and 11. Legends on next page

These results have been described in detail elsewhere (Spoerri and Wolff, 1981; Spoerri, 1987b).

Effects of GABA on Primary Cultures

Cerebrum. The development of primary neuronal cell cultures from embryonic chick cerebrum was characterized by aggregation of cells into clusters and by the consequent emission of bundles of neurites interconnecting these clusters. This occurred 3-4 days after cell seeding. As we have previously described (Spoerri, 1986; Spoerri, 1987c), addition of 10^{-5} M GABA to the culture medium caused an earlier formation of clusters and as a consequence an earlier outgrowth of neurites. In cultures supplemented with GABA the network formation due to the extensive branching of the processes was already evident 1 1/2 - 2 days after cell seeding, while in the control the less pronounced growth became obvious only later (Figs. 6a, b). The morphological aspect of the cultures after 4 days in vitro is shown in Table I. There was a considerable increase in the number of cells extending neurites in GABA treated cultures. The number of colonies or reaggregates was also enhanced.

Retina. Neural retina cells treated with GABA had more processes and their number per microscopic field increased. The morphological aspect of the neural retina cultures after 4 days in vitro is shown (Figs. 7a,b; Table II). The light micrographs reveal the sprouting effect of GABA increasing the number of primary and secondary processes. The elongated cells with their refractile vacuoles and the relative short neurites at the distal end, identified as photoreceptor cells (cones; Fig. 8) will be referred to later on.

Figure 10. Profiles of cerebral cortical neurons displaying desmosome-like structures or puncta adhaerentia (pa). Note the dense membrane invaginations (arrowheads). Nu = nucleus. x 32,500.

Figures 11a, b. Clear-core vesicles (V) seen budding from the SER, within a soma or varicosity (arrowheads). x 25,500.

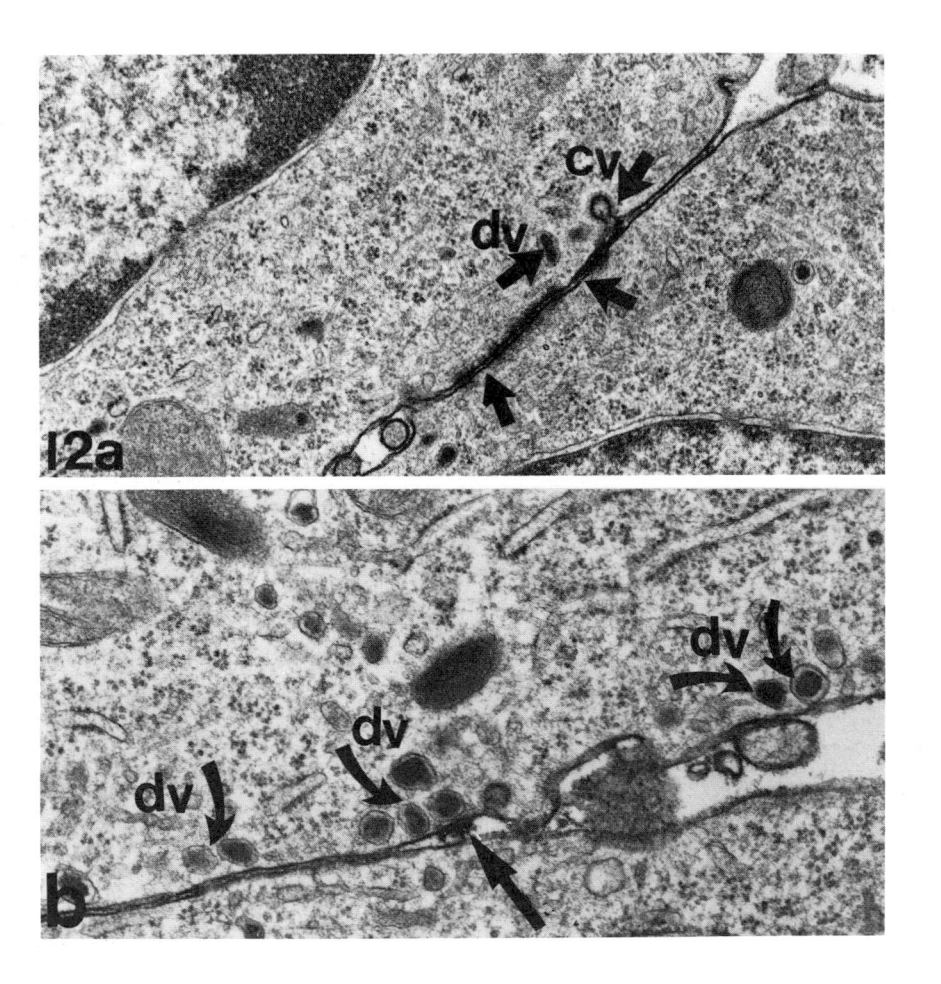

Figure 12. (a) Dense-core (dv) and coated vesicles commonly seen in the vicinity of a bilateral membrane specialization. (b) Dense-core (dv) vesicles gather near the plasmalemma and appear associated with an amorphous electron-dense substance (arrow). (a) x 25,500; (b) x 40,500.

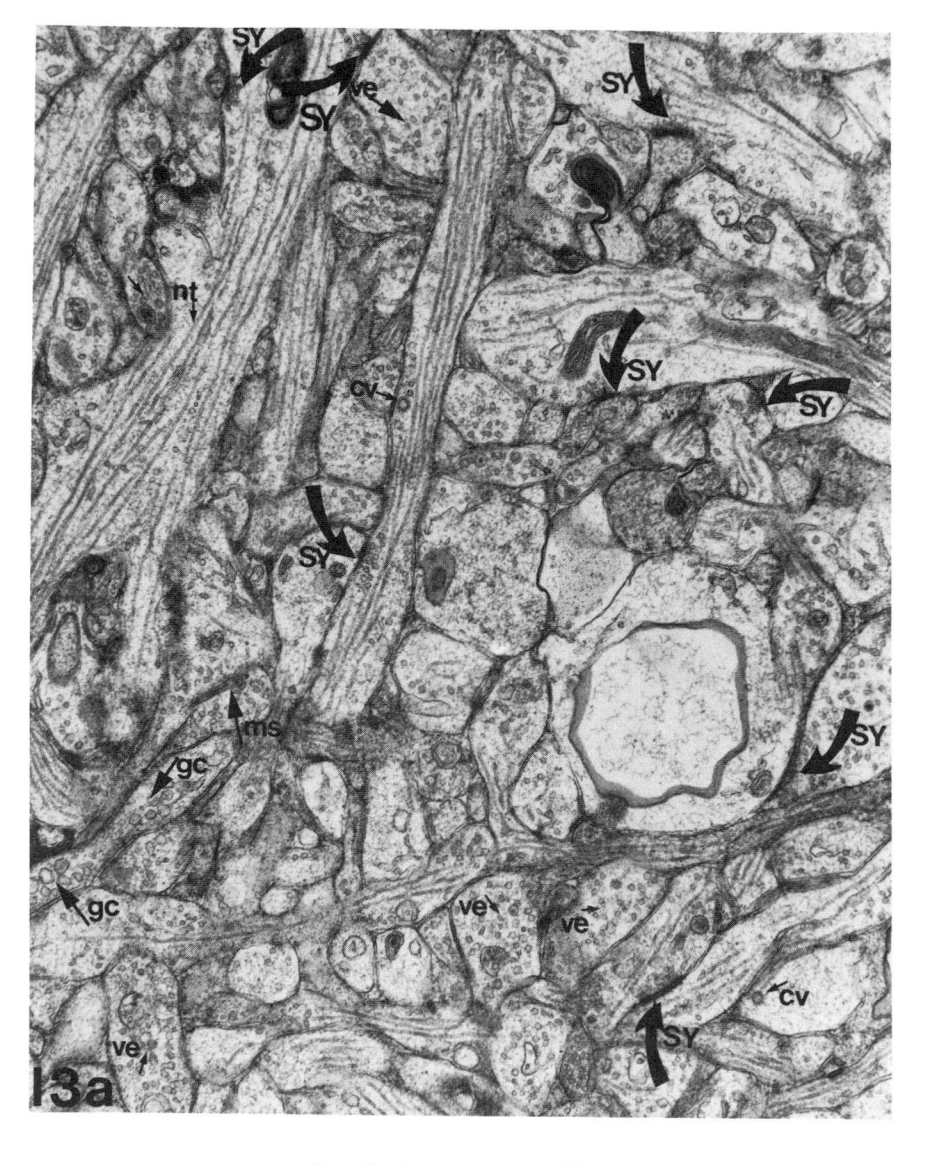

Fig. 13a. Legend on page 210

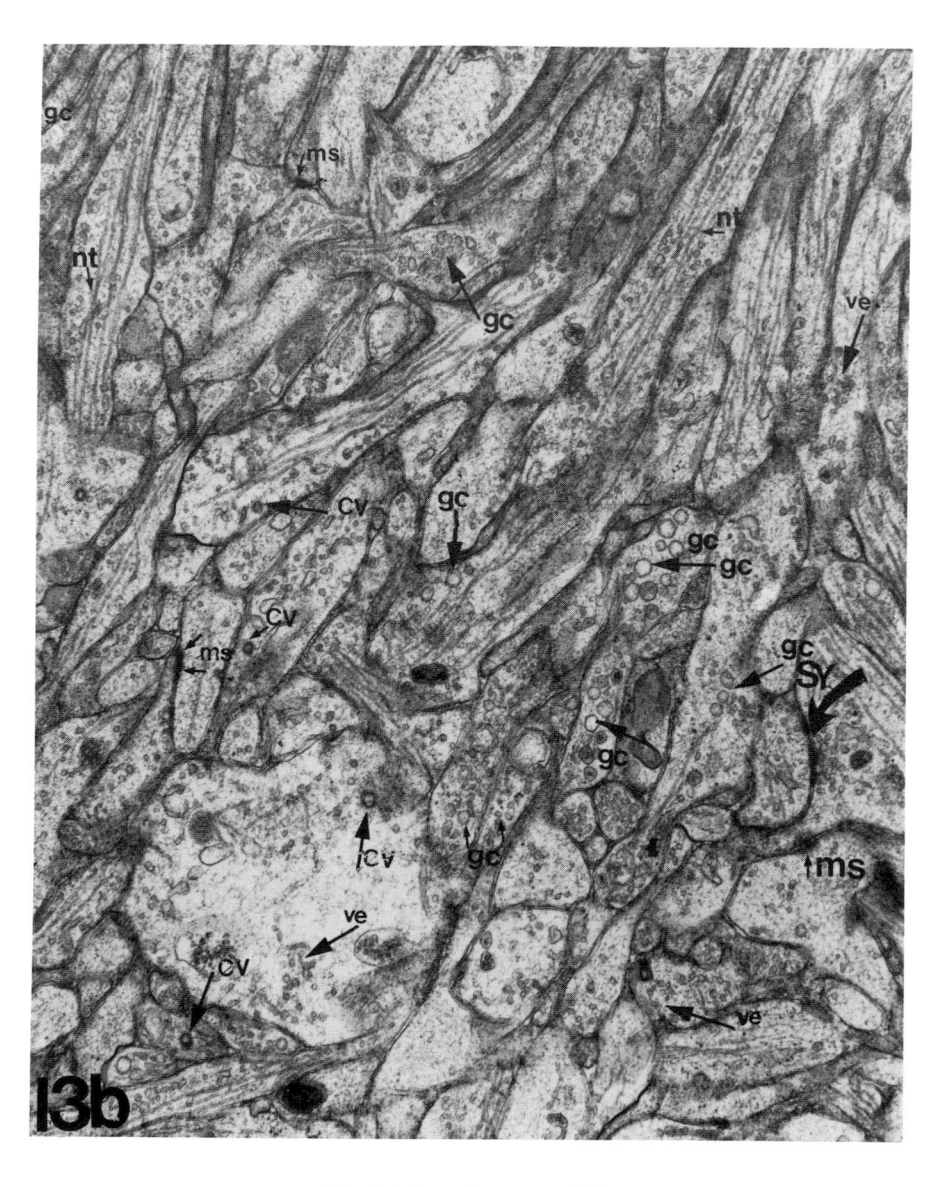

Fig. 13b. Legend on page 210

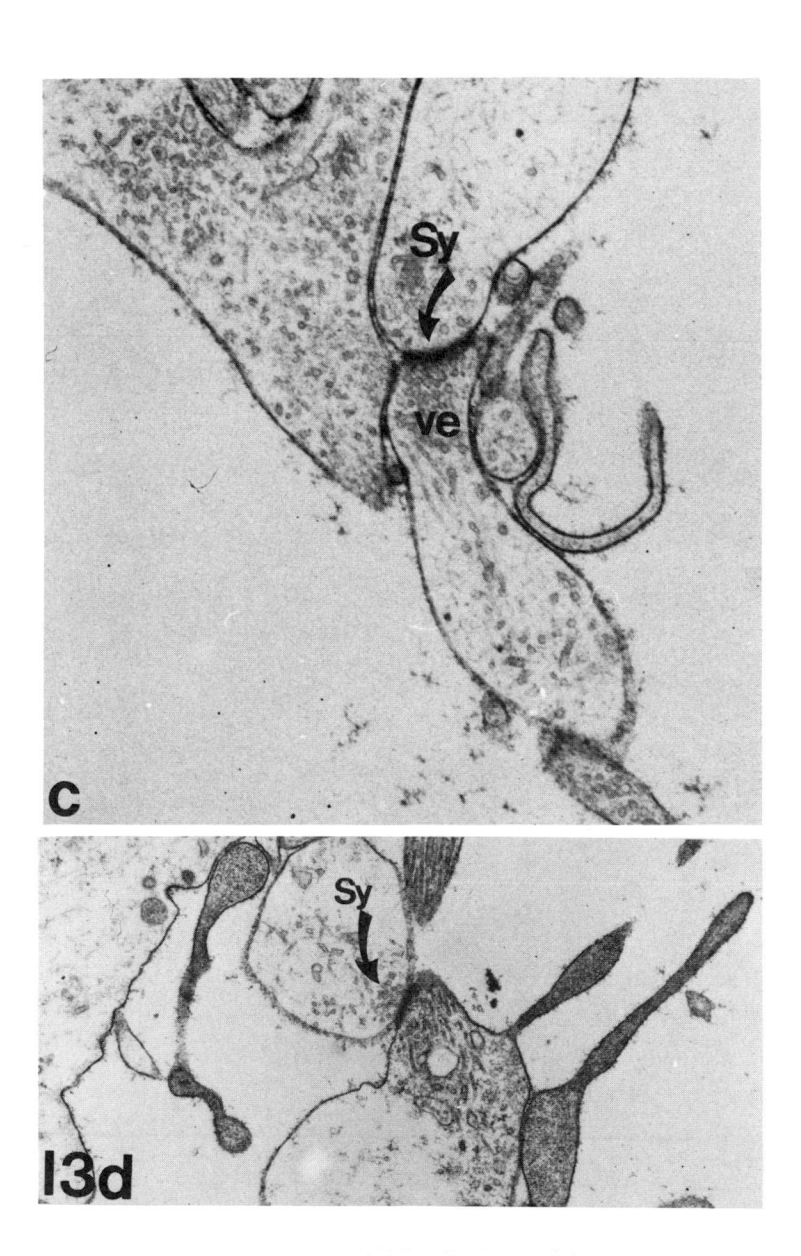

Figs. 13c and 13d. Legends on page 210

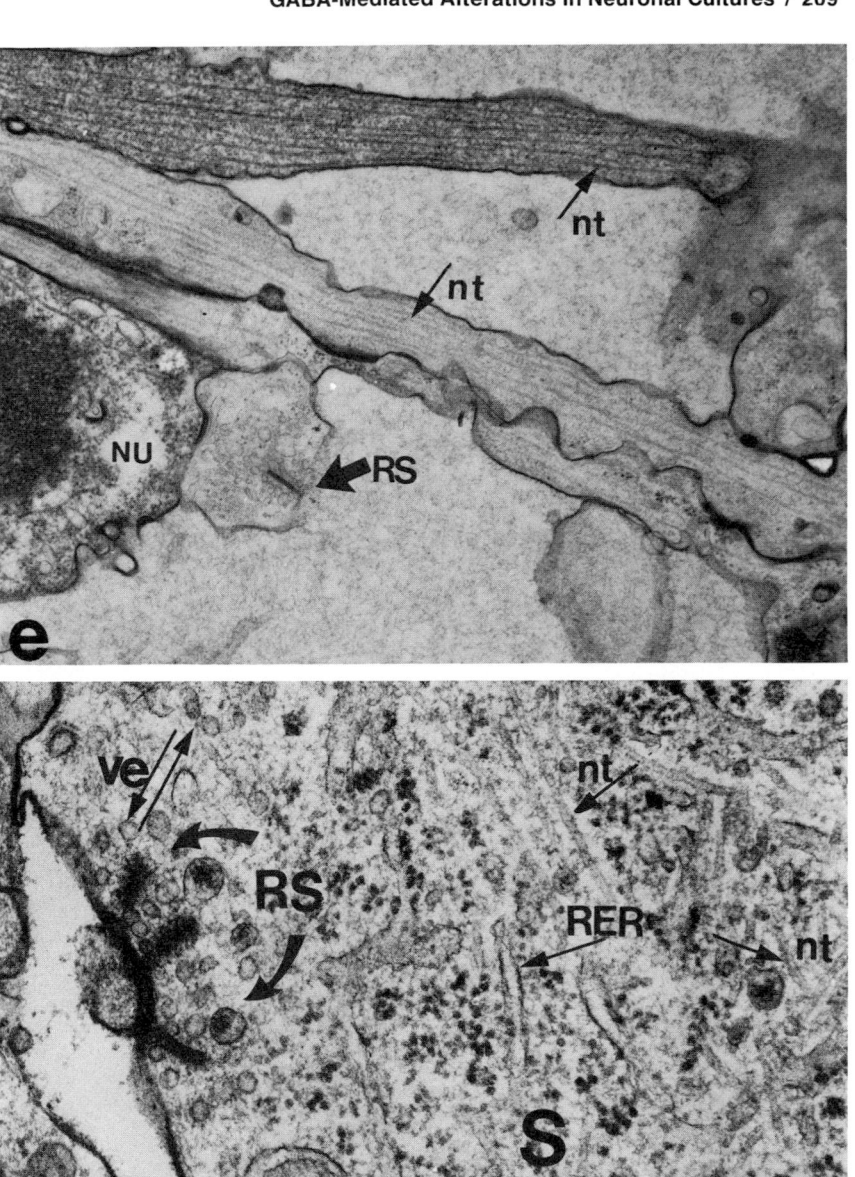

Figs. 13e and 13f. Legends on next page

Ultrastructural examination of the GABA treated neurons in culture revealed an increase in the density of RER, Golgi apparatus and neurotubules (Figs. 9a,b). The most striking phenomenon was the considerable increase in the number of vesicles including clear-core, dense-core and coated vesicle types. As described above, the latter appeared to bud from RER or Golgi. There was also an increase in desmosome-like structures or puncta adhaerentia which apparently precede the appearance of synapses (Fig. 10). Coated vesicles were seen in continuity with electron-dense membrane specializations. Clear-core vesicles were seen budding from the SER within the soma or in varicosities (Fig. 11a, b). There was also a proliferation of dense-core vesicles which was commonly seen near desmosome-like structures (Fig. 12a, b). This type of vesicle may play a role in synaptogenesis.

Quantitative electron microscopic counts of synapses performed on aggregate cultures fixed on day 7, 9 and 11 (Table III), revealed that GABA treated cultures produced a significantly greater number of synapses, including ribbon synapses in the retina (Figs. 13a-f). Noticeable were the great number of clear-core vesicles present in the boutons and the numerous neurotubules seen in the neurites. Coated vesicles, growth cones and dense-core vesicles were still present in small number at this stage of development. Many synapses resembled Gray's type 1 which had a wider cleft and a more pronounced synaptic density compared with those of type 2. There was usually one presynaptic dense projection per presynaptic element

---

Figure 13. (a) Numerous mature synapses (Sy) are present in GABA treated cerebral cortical neurons. Note the increased number of neurotubules present (nt). (b) Less numerous mature synapses (Sy). Note the presence of a large number of vesicles (ve), coated vesicles (CV), growth cones (gc) and membrane specializations (ms). (c,d) Additional single mature synapses (Sy) and numerous vesicles (ve) in GABA treated cortical neurons. (e) Ribbon synapse (RS) in retina cultures; note the large number of neurotubules (nt). Nu = Nucleus. (f) Another ribbon synapse (RS) at the periphery of a soma (S). Note the increased number of RER, and neurotubules (nt) and vesicles (ve). (a,b) x 25,500, (c) 46,750, (d) 25,500, (e) 27,500, (f) 40,500.

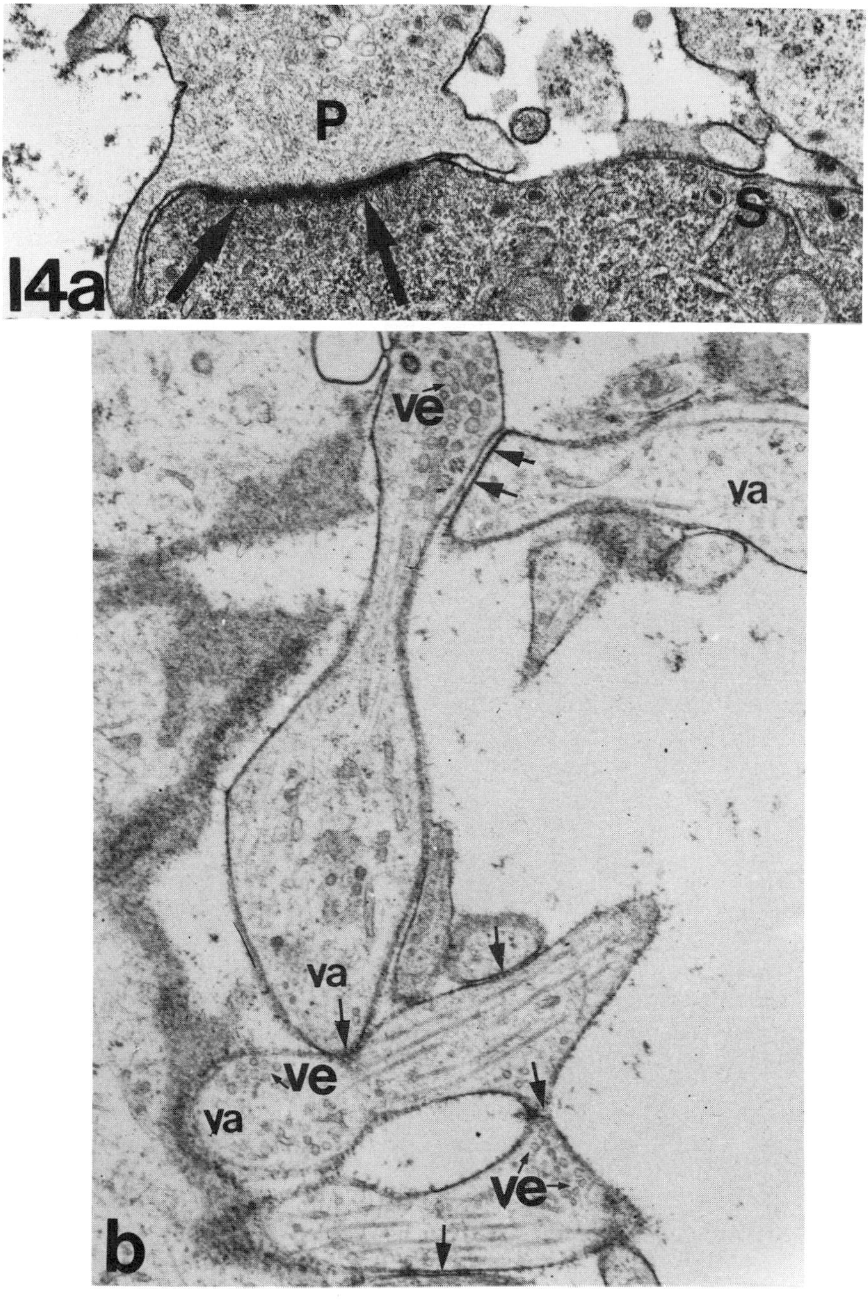

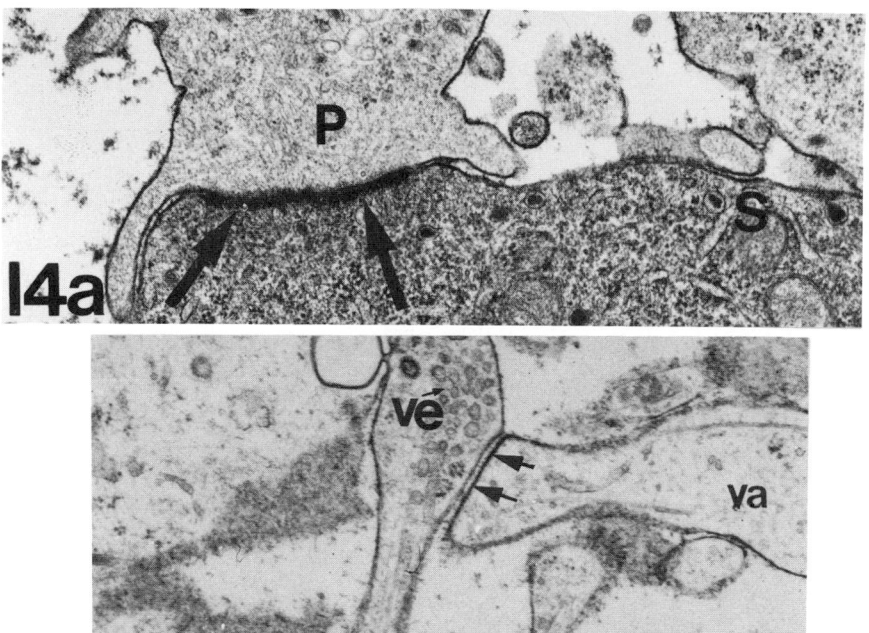

Figs. 14a and 14b. Legends on next page

and it was short and narrow, typical of a young synapse (Burry and Lasher, 1978). Bilateral membrane specializations which may represent early synapses (Fig. 14a, b) were numerous in the untreated control cultures. The results have been described elsewhere (Spoerri, 1987c).

Retina cultures supplemented with 10^{-5} M GABA after 8 days in in vitro showed additionally that the degree of maturation of the photoreceptor outersegment in particular, was affected (Figs. 15, 16). A membranous bulbous structure was been attached to the inner segment as revealed by SEM. At the TEM level, the GABA treated photoreceptor cells had rudimentary outersegments with a large number of membranous inclusions which were absent in controls or were present to a much lesser extend (Spoerri, 1987c).

DISCUSSION

The morphological changes observed in N-2A cells and primary cultures from embryonic chick cerebrum and retina revealed structural changes in the plasma membrane, possible increases in substratum adhesions and enhancement of neurite extension with branching. Ultrastructurally, GABA promoted synaptogenesis and appeared to regulate a wide variety of synaptic mechanisms as shown by the presence of a large number of vesicles other than the coated vesicle. The latter seemed consistently to be closely associated with bilateral membrane specializations or postsynaptic densities.

As presently and previously shown, GABA increased the density of RER (Hansen et al., 1984; Meier et al., 1985), suggestive of an increase in protein synthesis destined for insertion into membranes. The development of the Golgi apparatus was also promoted as was that of coated vesicles, structures apparently involved in the transfer of newly synthesized protein. The coated vesicle may be involved in the insertion of membranous receptor protein

Figures 14a, b. Bilateral membrane specializations or immature synapses are numerous in the untreated control cultures of retina and cerebral cortex (arrows). Ve = Vesicles, P = Process, S = Soma, Va = varicosities. (a) 29,750, (b) 35,700.

into the plasma membrane and thus account for the presence of low affinity receptors in cultured cerebellar granule cells (Meier et al., 1984) and the development of GABA high affinity binding sites in the rabbit retina (Madtes and Redburn, 1983a, b; Redburn et al., 1983). The neurotrophic effect of GABA may have contributed to the maturation of a variety of synaptic mechanisms, thus accounting for the large number of synapses present in GABA treated cultures as revealed morphometrically. In response to an analogous situation one may account for the enhanced maturation of the embryonic chick retina photoreceptor rudimentary outersegment and may reflect similar mechanisms.

In this context, recent studies involving the development of binding sites for (^{3}H) muscimol, a potent agonist of GABA receptors, in chick embryo retina in vivo and in vitro were very striking (Madtes and Adler, 1985). These binding sites were increased by 100% after 24h treatment with dibutyryl cyclic AMP, 8-bromo cyclic AMP or the phosphodiesterase inhibitor IBMX. The results raised the possibility that cylic AMP may be involved in the regulation of the components of the GABA system and may account for the responses observed. Other studies have shown that cyclic nucleotide derivatives stimulate the appearance of cholinergic receptors (Betz, 1983) and other cholinergic properties (Yeh et al., 1983).

TABLE I: Effect of GABA on embryonic chick cerebral neurons grown for 4 days in the presence of GABA

Treatment	Number of colonies per microscopic field	Number of cells extending neurites
NM (control)	53.00 + 5.00	734.00 + 28.00
NM + GABA	78.00 $\mp$ 6.00*	1033.00 $\mp$ 43.00*

NM = Nutrient Medium.
GABA (10^{-5} M) was renewed after 48h.
* Values represent the mean of + S.E.M. of 3 independent experiments of 5 Petri dishes each.
Statistically significant (p< 0.02).

TABLE II: Morphometric analysis of embryonic chick retina neurons grown for 4 days in the presence of GABA

Treatment	Number of cells per microscopic field	Number of primary processes per neuron	Length of primary processes (μm)	Number of secondary processes per neuron	Length of secondary processes (μm)
NM (control)	22.60 ± 0.80	2.53 ± 0.15	40.35 ± 2.36	5.21 ± 0.36	17.15 ± 0.86
NM + GABA	29.79 ± 0.72*	6.29 ± 0.37	77.40 ± 5.69*	12.23 ± 0.54*	31.15 ± 1.16*

NM = Nutrient Medium.
GABA (10^{-5}M) was renewed after 48h.
Values represent the mean of ± S.E.M. of 3 independent experiments of 5 Petri dishes each.
* Statistically significant ($p < 0.02$).

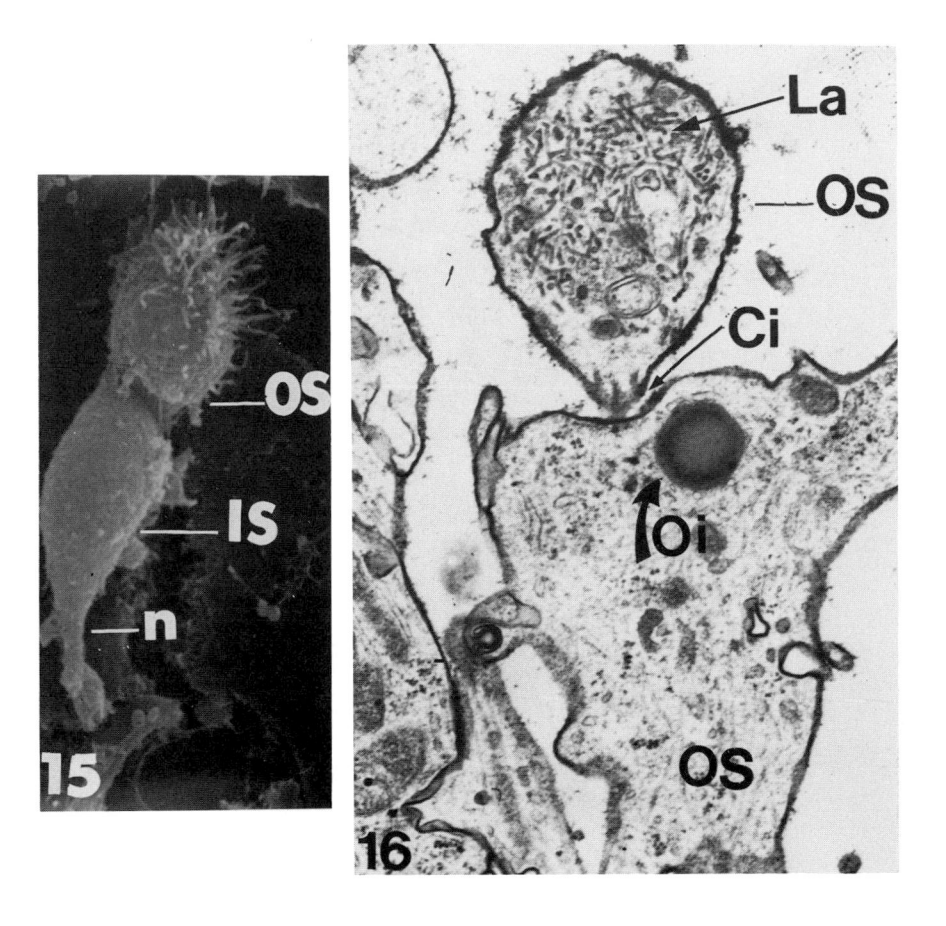

Figure 15. Scanning electron micrograph showing an advanced stage of differentiation of photoreceptor cells. The rudimentary OS is attached to the inner segment (IS). Note the short neurite (n) at the distal end. x 2000.

Figure 16. A differentiating cone cell has an elaborate rudimentary outer segment (OS). The membranous sac is continuous with the plasma membrane surrounding the connecting cilium (Ci) and contains numerous lamellar (La) inclusions (arrow), which were present to a much lesser extend in non-GABA treated cultures. Prominent is the oil droplet (Oi) in the proximal end of the rudimentary outer segment (OS). x 32,500.

The molecular mechanism underlying the trophic effect of GABA is not known. The ionic mechanism may be analogous to that proposed for the neurotrophic effect of NGF involving the control of Na^+, K^+ and other ionic pumps (Skaper and Varon, 1980). NGF also increases the intracellular cAMP which in turn regulates the mobilization of Ca^{+2} ions. These events are correlated with structural changes in the plasma membrane, increases in substratum adhesions and neurite extension (Schubert et al., 1971; Delman et al., 1979). cAMP by acting as a second messenger, may activate enzymes and/or protein synthesis and consequently induce developmental changes including maturation of synapses. A similarity in the mode of action of these trophic agents may exist since earlier findings have suggested that GABA may stimulate the protein synthetic pathway at the level of aminoacyl-t-RNA synthetase, implying GABA in the role of an indirect regulator of protein metabolism (Baxter, 1976). More evidence supporting this view is the observation that gangliosides, (sialic containing glycosphingolipids) produce additive neuritogenic effects when exogenously applied to primary neuronal cultures or cell-lines (Spoerri, 1983; Matta et al., 1986; Roisen et al., 1987). The ganglioside-induced changes in neuronal surface activity were also mediated in part by cAMP dependent processes (Spero and Roisen, 1985).

In summary, the increase in the number and surface area of neurons (length and branching of the neurites) caused by GABA may be correlated with alterations in the

TABLE III. Number of synapses per 2500 μm^2 $\pm$ S.E.M. in neuronal cultures grown in the presence or absence of GABA

Treatment	7 DIV	9 DIV	11 DIV
NM (control)	45.1 $\pm$ 4.3	50.8 $\pm$ 7.6	59.5 $\pm$ 4.5
NM + GABA	72.4 $\pm$ 6.5*	82.7 $\pm$ 5.8*	92.3 $\pm$ 11.4*

NM = Nutrient Medium.
Values given represent average countings of 16 electron micrographs. *GABA - treated cells differed significantly from the controls ($p < 0.05$).

flux of ions favouring the exchanges of solutes and metabolites needed for cell growth and development. The enhancement of the neuronal processes, facilitate the establishment of cell to cell contacts, promoting synaptogenesis and the appearance of structures involved in presynaptic transmission. These events may be mediated by the direct or indirect regulation of protein synthesis which may account for most of the developmental changes induced by this substance in neuronal cell-lines and primary neurons in culture.

ACKNOWLEDGEMENTS

This work was supported by the German Science Foundation, the Universitatsbund Gottingen and NIH grant RO1EYO4590. The authors thanks Wolfgang Bauer and Thomas Gunther for excellent technical assistance.

REFERENCES

Adler R (1982). Regulation of neurite growth in purified retina cultures: Effects of PNPF, a substratum - bound neurite - promoting factor. J Neurosci Res 8:165-177.

Adler R, Magistretti PJ, Hyndman AG, Schoemaker WJ (1982). Purification and cytochemical identification of neuronal and nonneuronal cells in chick embryo retina cultures. Devl Neurosci 5:27-39.

Baxter CF (1976). Effect of GABA on protein metabolism in the nervous system. In Roberts E, Chase TN, Tower DB (eds) "GABA in Nervous System Function". New York: Raven Press, pp 89-102.

Betz H (1983). Regulation of bungarotoxin receptor accumulation in chick retina cultures: effects of membrane depolarization, cyclic nucleotide derivatives, and Ca^{2+}. J Neurosci 3:1333-1341.

Burry RW, Lasher SR (1978). A quantitative electron microscopic study of synapse formation in dispersed cell cultures of rat cerebellum stained by OS-UL or by E-PTA. Brain Res 147:1-15.

Eins E, Spoerri PE, Heyder E (1983). GABA or sodium bromide induced plasticity of neurites of mouse neuroblastoma cells. A quantitative study. Cell Tissue Res 229:457-460.

Delman JR, Brinkley RR, Means AR (1979). Regulation of microfilaments and microtubules by calcium and cyclic AMP. In Greengard P, Robinson GA (eds) "Advances in

Cyclic Nucleotide Research". New York: Raven Press, pp 119-134.

Hansen HG, Meier E, Schousboe A (1984). GABA influences the ultrastructure composition of cerebellar granule cells during development in culture. Int J Devl Neuroscience 2:247-257.

Madtes PC JR, Redburn DA (1983a). Synaptic interactions in the GABA system during postnatal development in the retina. Brain Res Bull 10:741-745.

Madtes P, Redburn DA (1983b). GABA as a trophic factor during development. Life Sci 33:979-984.

Matta SG, Yorke G, Roisen FJ (1986). Neuritogenic and metabolic effects of individual gangliosides and their interaction with nerve growth factor in cultures of neuroblastoma and pheochromocytoma. Dev Brain Res 27:243-252.

Meier E, Drejer J, Schousboe A (1984). GABA induces functionally active low-affinity GABA receptors on cultured cerebellar granule cells. J Neurochem 43:1737-1744.

Meier E, Hansen GH, Schousboe A (1985): The trophic effect of GABA on cerebellar granule cells is mediated by GABA-receptors. Int J Devl Neurosci 3:401-407.

Pettmann B, Louis JC, Sensenbrenner M (1979). Morphological and biochemical maturation of neurones cultured in the absence of glial cells. Nature 281:378-380.

Redburn DA, Massey SC, Madtes P (1983). The GABA uptake system in rabbit retina. In Hertz L, Kvamme E, McGeer EG and Schousboe A (eds) "Glutamine, Glutamate and GABA", New York: Alan R Liss pp 273-286.

Roisen FJ, Murphy RA, Braden WG (1972). Neurite development in vitro I. The effect of adenosine 3',5' cyclic monophosphate (cyclic AMP). J Neurobiol 4:347-368.

Roisen FJ, Matta SG, Yorke G, Rapport MM (1987). The role of gangliosides in neurotrophic interaction in vitro. In Tettamanti G, Ledeen RW, Sandhoff K, Nagai Y, Toffano G (eds) "Neuronal Plasticity and Gangliosides". Padova: Liviana Press (in press).

Romijn HJ, van Huizen F, Wolters PS (1984). Towards an improved serum-free, chemically defined medium for long-term culturing of cerebral cortex tissue. Neurosci Biobehav Rev 8:301-334.

Schubert D, Humphreys S, De Vitry F, Jacob J (1971). Induced differentiation of a neuroblastoma. Devl Biol 25:514-546.

Skaper SD, Varon S (1980): Properties of the sodium extrusion mechanism controlled by nerve growth factor in chick embryo dorsal root ganglionic cells. J Neurochem 34:1654-1660.

Spero DA, Roisen FJ (1984): Gangliosides induce microfilament-dependent changes in membrane surface activity of neuro-2a neuroblastoma cells. Int J Devl Neuroscience 2:247-257.

Spoerri PE (1983). Effects of gangliosides on the in vitro development of neuroblastoma cells: An ultrastructural study. Int J Devl Neuroscience 6:383-391.

Spoerri PE (1984). Mouse neuroblastoma cells in vitro. Substances regulating synapse-like formations. Film B1544, Sektion Medizin, Serie 6, Nummer 15, Institut fur den Wissenschaftlichen Film Gottingen, Federal Rep Germany.

Spoerri PE (1987a). Facilitated establishment of contacts and synapses in neuronal cultures: Ganglioside-mediated neurite sprouting and outgrowth. In Tettamanti G, Ledeen RW, Sandhoff K, Nagai Y, Toffano G (eds) "Neuronal Plasticity and Gangliosides". Padova: Liviana Press, (in press).

Spoerri PE (1987b): Current findings on the morphological induction of synaptogenesis in vitro. In Vernadakis A (ed) "Model Systems of Development and Aging of the Nervous System". Boston: Martinus Nijhoff Publishing (in press).

Spoerri PE (1987c). Neurotrophic effects of GABA in cultures of embryonic chick brain and retina. Synapse (submitted).

Spoerri PE, Wolff JR (1981). Effect of GABA-administration on murine neuroblastoma cells in culture I. Increased membrane dynamics and formation of specialized contacts. Cell Tissue Res 218:567-579.

Spoerri PE, Wolff JR (1982). Morphological changes induced by sodium bromide in murine neuroblastoma cells in vitro. Cell Tissue Res 222:379-388.

Spoerri PE, Dresp W, Heyder E (1980a): A simple embedding technique for monolayer neuronal cultures grown in plastic flasks. Acta Anat 107:221-223.

Spoerri PE, Glees P, Dresp W (1980b). The time course of a synapse formation of mouse neuroblastoma cells in monolayer cultures. Cell Tissue Res 205:411-421.

Spoerri PE, Kelley KC, Allen CB, Ulshafer RJ (1987). Photoreceptor differentiation in cultures of embryonic (rd) retinal degenerate chickens: Influence of optic lobe conditioned media. Cell Tissue Res (submitted).

Spoerri PE, Ulshafer RJ, Allen CB, Kellen KC. Photorecep- tor outersegment differentiation in cultures of embryonic chick retina (in preparation).

Wolff JR (1979). Hinweise auf eine Doppelrolle von GABA als synaptischer Transmitter. In Verh Dtsch Zool Ges. Stuttgart: Gustav Fischer Verlag, pp 194-200.

Wolff JR, Joo F, Dames W (1978): Plasticity in dendrites shown by continuous GABA administration in superior cervical ganglion of adult rat. Nature 274:72-74.

Wolff JR, Richmann M, Chronwall BM (1979a): Axo-glial synapses and GABA-accumulating glial cells in the embryonic neocortex of the rat. Cell Tissue Res 201:239-248.

Wolff JR, Joo F, Dames W, Feher O (1979b): Induction and maintenance of free postsynaptic thickenings in the adult superior cervical ganglion. J Neurocytol 8:849-863.

Yeh HH, Batelle BA, Puro DG (1983): Maturation of neurotransmission at cholinergic synapses formed in culture by rat retinal neurons: regulation by cyclic AMP. Devl Brain Res 63-72.

Neurotrophic Activity of GABA During Development, pages 221–252
© **1987 Alan R. Liss, Inc.**

SYNAPTIC, METABOLIC AND MORPHOGENETIC EFFECTS OF GABA IN
THE SUPERIOR CERVICAL GANGLION OF RATS

Joachim R Wolff, Ferenc Joo[1] and Peter Kasa[2]

Developmental Neurobiology Unit, Department of
Anatomy, University of Gottingen, Kreuzbergring
36, D- 3400 Gottingen, F.R.G.

INTRODUCTION

According to current topics of neuronal communication,
excitatory and inhibitory synaptic transmissions play a
key role in the transient modulation of bioelectric
activity in neurons. During the last decade, evidence
accumulated indicating that long term changes in
bioelectrical activity may influence the synaptogenesis,
not only during ontogenesis (for reference see, van
Huizen, 1986) but also during synaptic reorganization
after de-afferentation (e.g., Rutledge, 1978). In most
experiments designed to gain better understanding of the
cellular and molecular mechanisms of such "trophic" or
neuroplastic effects, the excitatory afferent input to
neuronal populations is manipulated (e.g., sensory
deprivation, action potential blockade, deafferentation).
This review will collect evidence indicating that,
similarly to decreased excitatory input, increased and/or
prolonged inhibition by GABA can also induce neuroplastic
responses in the superior cervical ganglion.

For the respective studies, this ganglion has several
advantages over central nervous tissue: Its neuronal
organizations are relatively simple, the neuroplastic

1 Laboratory of Molecular Neurobiology, Institute of
   Biophysics, Biological Research Center, Szeged, Hungary

2 Central Research Laboratory, University Medical
   School, Szeged, Hungary

responses to partial de-afferentation have been
extensively studied, and GABA being a physiological
component of the SCG suppresses ganglionic transmission
like a typical inhibitory transmitter or modulator.

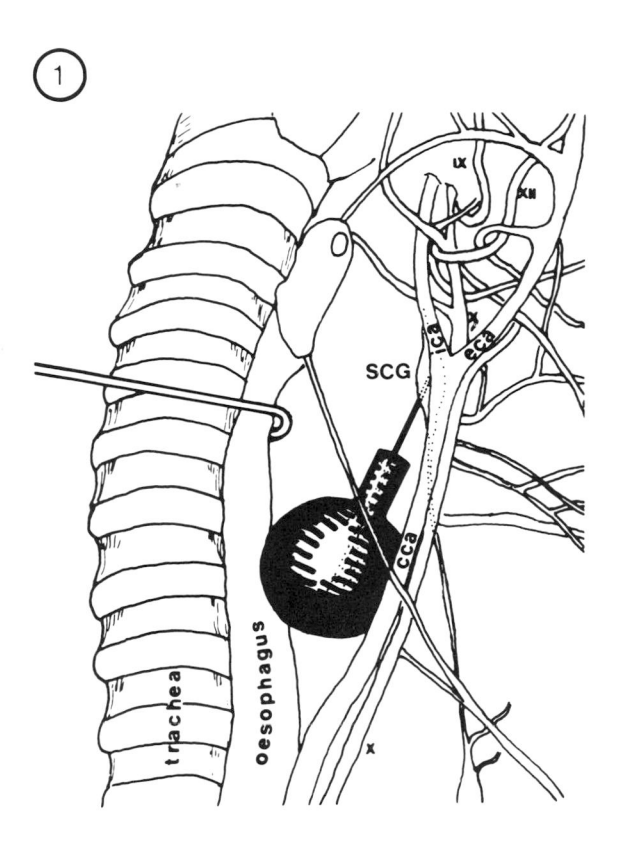

Figure 1. Ventromedial view of the rat's cervical
ganglion showing the position of implanted glass bulb.
SCG, superior cervical ganglion; IX, X and XII, cranial
nerves; cca, common carotid artery; ica, internal carotid
artery; eca, external carotid artery. The longus colli
muscle, to which the glass bulb was glued, is beneath the
bulb. (From Wolff et al., 1979).

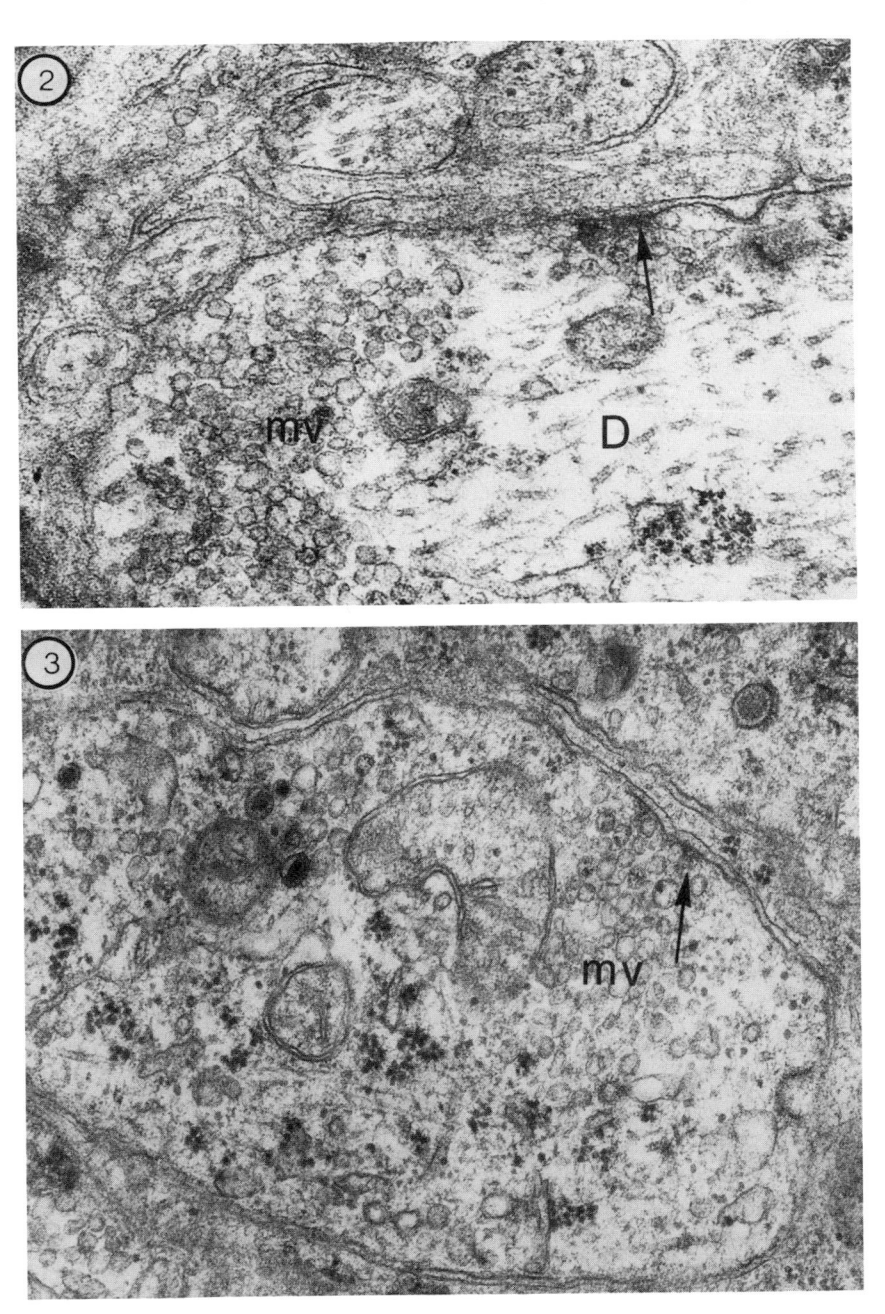

Figs. 2 and 3. Legends on next page

NEURONAL ORGANIZATION OF THE ADULT SCG

The principle ganglion cells are innervated by cholinergic axons which originate from different (C8 – Th7) segments of the spinal cord (Bowers and Zigmond, 1979). Afferent synapses form asymmetric contacts which are mainly located on dendrites while axosomatic contacts are scarce (Joo et al., 1971). The postganglionic axons provide the noradrenergic innervation of various muscular and glandular tissues of the head. Recently, immunohistochemical studies (Olschowska and Jacobowitz, 1983; Jarvi et al., 1986) revealed that, besides containing dopamine-β-hydroxylase, a subpopulation (30-50%) of ganglion cells show positivity for bovine pancreatic polypeptide-like substance. This indicates that not only noradrenaline but also some peptides may be released from the nerve endings innervating the target organs. Ganglionic neurons are concerned as well, because postganglionic axons give off recurrent collaterals which innervate principle ganglion cells (Joo et al., 1971).

The SCG contains several sets of interneurons which are innervated by preganglionic afferents: The SIF cells produce and release, although non-synaptically, various monoamines (noradrenaline, dopamine and histamine, serotonin (Verhofstadt et al., 1981). There is at least one other set of neurons which contains GABA (Fig. 1, Wolff et al., 1986) and probably glutamate decarboxylase (GAD) the GABA synthesizing enzyme (Kanazawa et al., 1976; Kenny and Ariano, 1986). In addition to the neuronal GABA-system, satellite glial cells can accumulate GABA by a high affinity uptake mechanism (Iversen and Kelly, 1975; Wolff et al., 1979) and may contribute to the relatively high GABA content in the SCG of rats (297 pmol/mg protein tissue (Bertilsson et al., 1976). Since depolarizing agents induce the release of GABA in the ganglion (Bowery and Brown, 1972), GABA apparently plays the role of an inhibitory transmitter (see below) in the SCG of rats (Fig. 2).

Figures 2-3. Microvesiculation and presynaptic-like vesicle aggregations in dendrites. mv = micro-vesicles, D = dendrite. Arrow points at a membrane thickening. Fig. 2 : x 65,000; Fig. 3 : x 65,000.

The ACh system

The presence of an acetylcholine system in the SCG is well documented (Hebb and Waites, 1956; Birks and Mac Intosh, 1961; Thoenen et al., 1972; Burt, 1978; Dahlstrom et al., 1980; Fumagalli and De Renzis, 1980; George and Dolivo, 1982; Kwok and Collier, 1982; Taniguchi et al., 1983; Kasa et al., 1985).

The activity of the ACh synthesizing enzyme, choline-0-acetyltransferase (ChAT), drops after preganglionic denervation (Burt, 1978). On the other hand, Fonnum et al., (1984) demonstrated that partial de-afferentation of the SCG, leading to axonal sprouting and formation of new synaptic contacts by the remaining cholinergic fibers, resulted in a small decrease of ChAT activity in the newly developed axon terminals. Since cholinergic interneurons have not been revealed in the SCG, ChAT activity is apparently restricted to the preganglionic cholinergic fibers.

Electron microscopic histochemistry (Kasa and Csernovszky, 1967) revealed that the transmitter hydrolyzing enzyme, acetylcholine esterase (AChE), is present in the cytoplasm and at the surface of principal ganglionic cells. The mAChR and nAChR are localized on pre- and postsynaptic elements, respectively (Dombrowski et al., 1983; Toldi et al., 1983; Chiappinelli and Dryer, 1984).

Stimulation of preganglionic cholinergic axons induces release of ACh (Paton and Thompson, 1953; Birks and MacIntosh, 1961; Kobayashi and Libet, 1970; Dawes and Vizi, 1973; Vizi, 1979; Farkas et al., 1986; Araujo and Collier, 1986), which exerts an excitatory effect on the ganglionic neurons. This effect can be modulated by adrenaline (Bulbring, 1944; De Groat and Volle, 1966; Capuzzo et al., 1983; Paton and Thompson, 1953; Christ and Nishi, 197a, b), noradrenaline (Reinert, 1963; Noon et al., 1975; Dun and Karczmar, 1977), and among other putative transmitters, also by GABA (De Groat et al., 1971; Bowery and Brown, 1974; Farkas et al., 1984; 1986). It has been shown that adrenoreceptors, responsible for the postsynaptic effect of catecholamines, are of an α type (Starke, 1977; Vizi, 1979; 1983). Studies with antagonists suggest that the effect of noradrenaline to depress the ACh release is mediated by a presynaptic α_2-adrenoreceptor, although Araujo and Collier (1986) revealed a mixed population of receptors, which may have different effects on the ACh release. Two types of GABA receptors, $GABA_A$ and $GABA_B$, have been described, which are present on the presynaptic cholinergic axon terminals and inhibit the transmitter release (Farkas et al., 1984, 1986). Thus, monoaminergic and GABAergic interneurons may modulate the release of ACh, apart from their postsynaptic effects.

Summary

The neuronal organization of the SCG is characterized by cholinergic preganglionic afferents which innervate the noradrenergic (and peptidergic) principle ganglion cells as well as interneurons. The latter comprise several sets of neurons which produce various transmitters (e.g., various monoamines, GABA), and probably modulate the ganglionic transmission via various presynaptic and postsynaptic receptors. Thus, GABAergic interneurons play a physiological role in the SCG.

ACUTE EFFECTS OF GABA ON SYNAPTIC TRANSMISSION

Although the role of GABA as a major inhibitory synaptic transmitter in the CNS is universelly accepted, its functions in the PNS are not so well understood. In the SCG, the presence of GABA (Bertilsson et al., 1976) and $GABA_A$ and $GABA_B$ receptors (Farkas et al., 1984; 1986) indicates that this substance may affect synaptic transmission in the ganglion on presynaptic and/or postsynaptic sites. Indeed De Groat et al. (1971) demonstrated that with the application of bicuculline the inhibitory effect of GABA on the synaptic transmission could be reduced.

Depression of ganglionic action potentials

The effects of GABA upon ganglionic transmission have been extensively studied in various preparations and species (De Groat, 1970; Adams and Brown, 1975; Kimura et al., 1977; Brown and Constantini, 1978; Kato et al., 1978). It was unequivocally established that GABA depresses ganglionic action potentials in proportion to the dose given. Adams and Brown (1975) suggested that

GABA induces an increase in Cl⁻ conductance of the postsynaptic membrane and diminishes action potentials by depolarization and by shunting the inward current. Meanwhile, the membrane potential is shifted towards the Cl⁻ equilibrium potential which may then result in a de- or hyperpolarization depending on the actual relation of the two potential values. In addition to these direct effects on ganglion cells, presynaptic indirect effects have to be taken into account.

Inhibition of ACh release

Presynaptic effects of GABA were primarily observed by Kato et al. (1978) in bullfrog sympathetic ganglia. In rat SCG, Brown and Higgins (1979) described an inhibitory effect of GABA on the release of ACh, which can be mediated by GABA$_A$ and GABA$_B$ receptors (Farkas et al., 1984, 1986). It has been shown that, at the GABA$_A$ receptor site, bicuculline (a GABA$_A$ receptor antagonist) is able to reduce the inhibitory effect of GABA while baclofen (a GABA$_B$ receptor agonist) will potentiate the GABA induced inhibition further. These results and those presented by De Groat et al. (1971) suggest that in SCG at least two types of GABA receptors are present. Receptor binding studies support the suggestion of more receptor types, since the combination of bicuculline and baclofen, both applied in large excess, produced less than 100% inhibition of the specific binding of GABA. Until recently, the source of GABA in the SCG was unclear. Radioactive GABA was mainly accumulated by glial cells (e.g., Wolff et al. 1979). Therefore, it has been suggested that the GABA-ergic system may physiologically act as a negative feed-back mechanism which induces glial cells responding to extracellular K⁺ released by depolarized neurons (Wolff et al., 1986). However, immunohistochemistry using anti-GABA antibodies revealed in the SCG a subpopulation of GABAergic neurons which make axon-like processes and axon varicosities containing vesicles and being apposed to ganglionic cells (Wolff, 1986). Thus, the inhibitory transmitter can be released from GABA-ergic interneurons. Since axo-axonic synapses have not been found, the question, whether neuronal or glial release of GABA decreases the ACh release in the CGS, is open for further studies.

Summary

Externally applied GABA suppresses the ganglionic transmission. This may be mediated through $GABA_A$ and $GABA_B$ receptors which are found on pre- and postsynaptic sites. While synapse-like contacts of GABAergic axon terminals have been found on dendrites of principle ganglion cells, axo-axonic synapses have not been observed. Thus, it is still unclear, whether GABA released from synapses inhibits ACh release under physiological conditions and/or which is the role of GABA accumulating glial cells.

NEURONAL PLASTICITY EVOKED BY LONG LASTING GABA TREATMENT

In the beginning of our morphological studies, a micromethod was developed (Dames et al., 1979), by which almost constant amounts of GABA could be continuously released into the SCG from a localized source for long periods of time (hours to months). In short, small glass bulbs connected with 50 µm wide glass tube were filled either with GABA (10 µl of 48 mM solution) or with control solvent and were then inserted ventromedially into the SCG under aseptic conditions (Fig. 1). The microinfusion was carried out from 1 to 30 days, thereafter the ganglia were processed for routine electron microscopy.

Morphological changes in dendrites

Appearance of microvesicles. Three days after implantation of the GABA-containing glass bulbs, one of the most apparent structural changes was the increase in the number of clear microvesicles of varying (40-100 nm) diameter in the dendrites of principal ganglion cells (Fig. 2.).

Occasionally, these vesicles accumulated in clusters at dense projections, which resembled those in presynaptic elements but were not connected to postsynaptic densities (Fig. 3). Similar morphological transformations of dendrites have been observed in the central nervous system after X-ray irradiation (Sotelo, 1977) or after de-afferentation (Hamori and Somogyi, 1982). It is tempting to speculate that these presynaptic-like features represent sites of dendritic release of transmitter substances.

Interestingly enough, microvesiculation of a similar

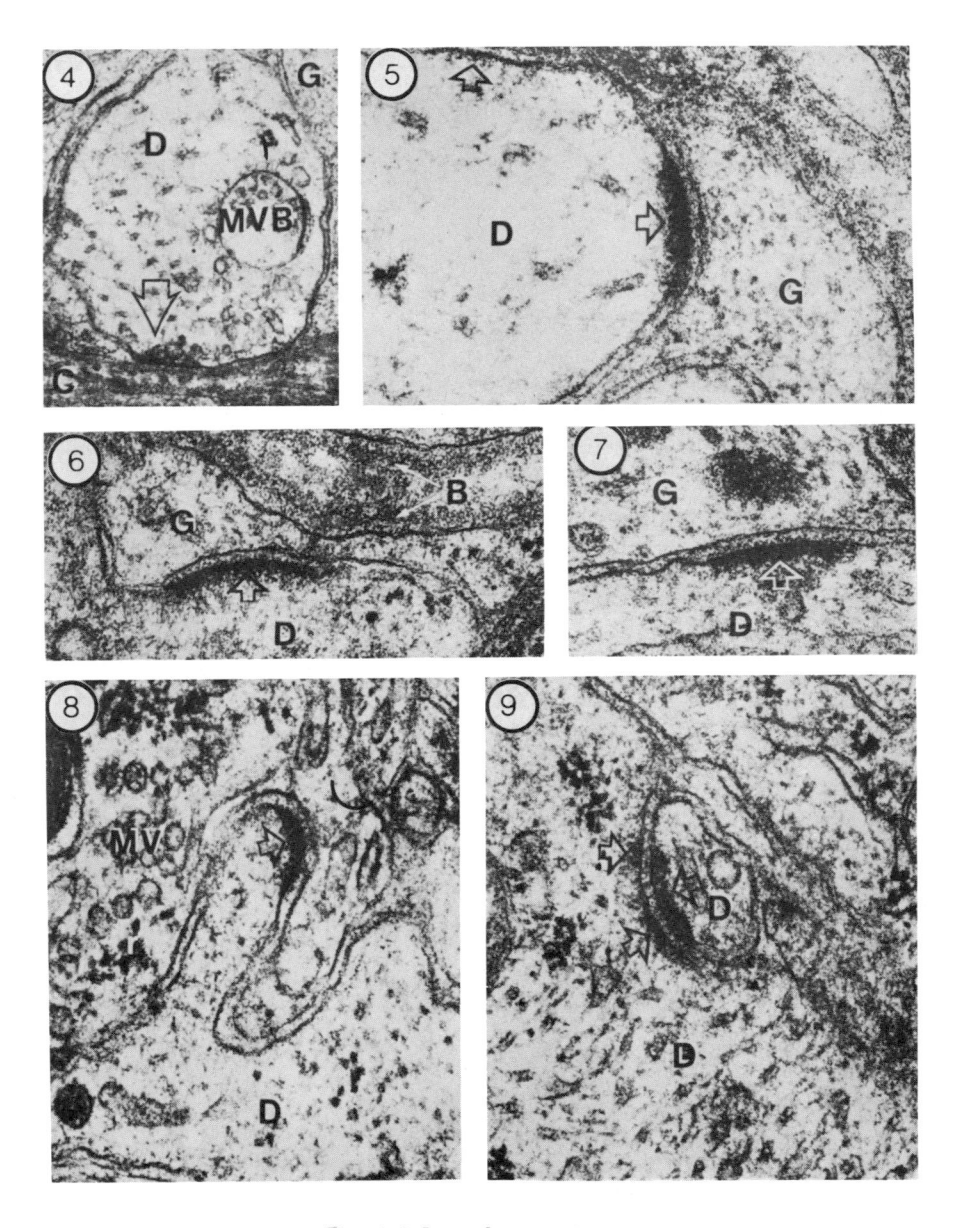

Figs. 4–9. Legends on next page

character was found by Hansen et al. (1984), who studied the influence of GABA on cerebellar granule cells in culture. The mechanism of this plastic change is unknown.

Changes in the shape of dendrites. After GABA application, many dendrites developed spine-like protrusions (Figs. 6 and 8) which probably caused a significant increase of their surface-to-volume ratio. These results are in line with observations indicating that the normal branching pattern of dendrites can change in neurons of the adult SCG, as revealed by repeated imaging in situ (Purves and Hadley, 1985).

Appearance of vacant paramembranous densities. In GABA treated ganglia, localized aggregations of a filamentous material appeared along the inner aspect of dendritic plasma membranes (Figs. 4-8). These structural complexes resemble the postsynaptic membrane thickenings of Gray's type I synapses. Analysis of serial sections (Figs. 10-12) showed that these membrane thickenings, however, were not attached to axon terminals or any other form of presynaptic element. These features were termed, therefore, "free or vacant postsynaptic membrane thickenings" (Wolff et al., 1978; 1979). Symmetrical, desmosome-like structures between dendrites were also found more often in the SCG treated with GABA than in controls (Fig. 9).

Morphological effects on axon terminals and synapses

A detailed morphometric analysis was undertaken, mainly on serial sections, to establish if GABA induces any detectable change in the structure of axon terminals (Joo et al., 1987). This analysis revealed that synapses undergo significant changes consisting of (i) a reduction in size of presynaptic axon terminals, (ii) a decrease in the number of synaptic vesicles per axon terminal and (iii) a diminuition in the size of the postsynaptic

---

Figures 4-9. Non-innervated and postsynaptic-like membrane thickenings (arrows) at dendritic membranes after long-term GABA treatment. D = dendrites, G = glial processes, MVB = multivesicular bodies, B = basal laminae, MV = microvesicles. Fig. 4 = x 30,000; Figs. 5-8 = 80,000; Fig. 9 = 65,000 (From Wolff et al., 1979).

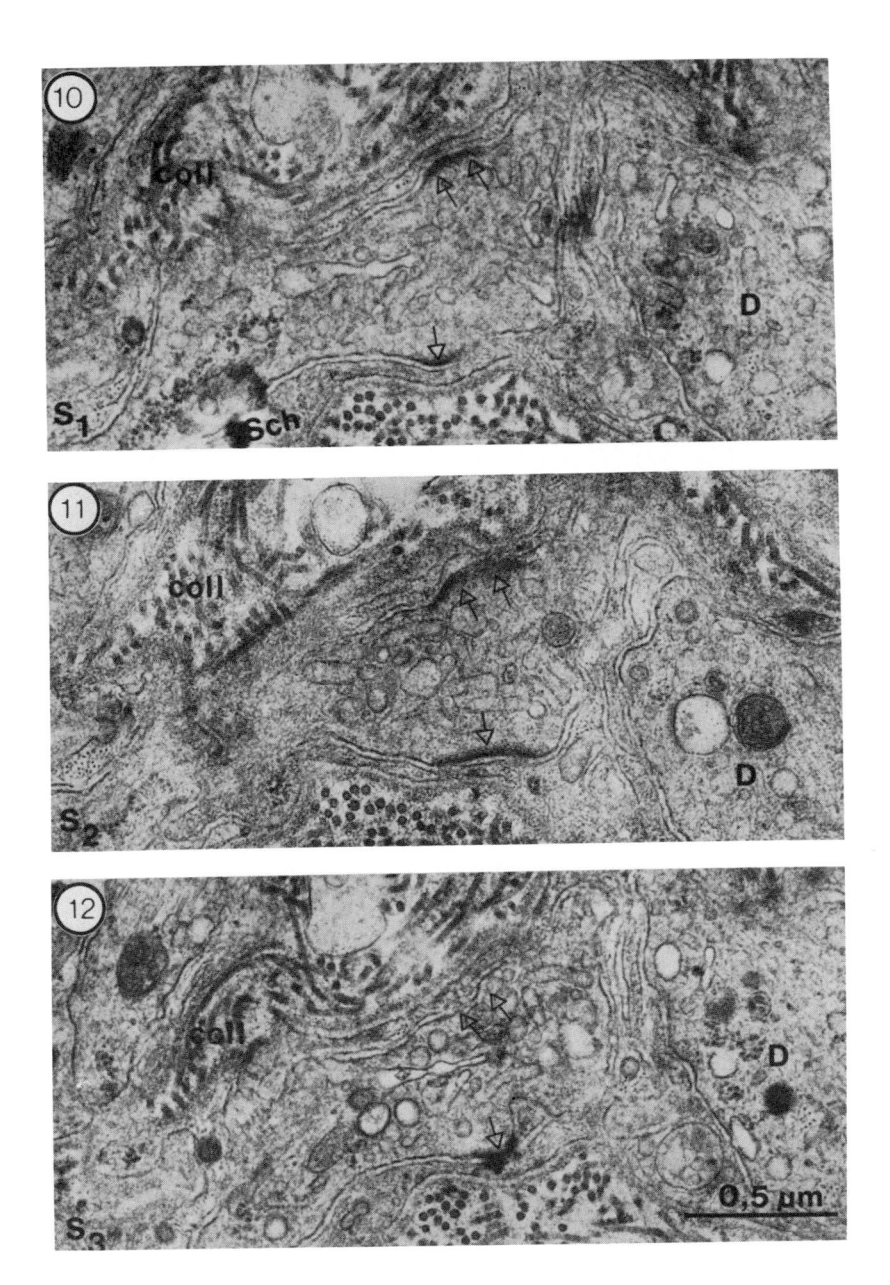

Figs. 10, 11, and 12. Legends on next page

membrane thickenings at the dendritic side (Figs. 13-18).

These results provide morphological evidence that long-term application of GABA to the SCG exerts an effect not only on the dendrites but also on the presynaptic elements made by preganglionic nerve fibers.

Changes in the ACh system

In the SCG, some components of the ACh system can be modulated by various experimental interventions including the long lasting application of GABA. Changes in ChAT activity and the number of nAChR + mAChR have been reported after preganglionic denervation (Dun et al., 1976; Taniguchi et al., 1983; but see Burt 1978), postganglionic axotomy (Fumagalli and De Renzis, 1980), and implantation of the hypoglossal nerve (see below).

Long lasting GABA application induced a transient increase of nicotinic, (+ 87% after 12 h) but not muscarinic, AChR and a drop in AChE activity. ChAT activity and ACh concentration, although showing a tendency for smaller values, did not change significantly (Kasa et al., 1985). These results may be interpreted as a sensitization of the ganglion cells for cholinergic transmission (AChE↓, nAChR↑), which may be an adaption to the suppression of ACh release by GABA. It is not yet clear whether newly formed vacant postsynaptic densities correspond to sites where the extra population of nAChR is accumulated. However, we have tried to determine if both changes may be related to an increased capacity . for forming cholinergic synapses.

Promotion by GABA of synaptogenesis

Since long-term GABA treatment of the SCG resulted in changes of the dendritic morphology and the ACh-system, the question was raised, whether GABA could change the synaptogenetic capacity of the ganglion cells. In order to address this question experimentally, foreign nerves are implanted into the ganglion. Together with the

---

Figures 10-12. Free postsynaptic thickenings (arrows) in serial sections (S1-3). D = dendrite, Sch = Schwann cell process, Coll = collagen fibrils, x 40,000.

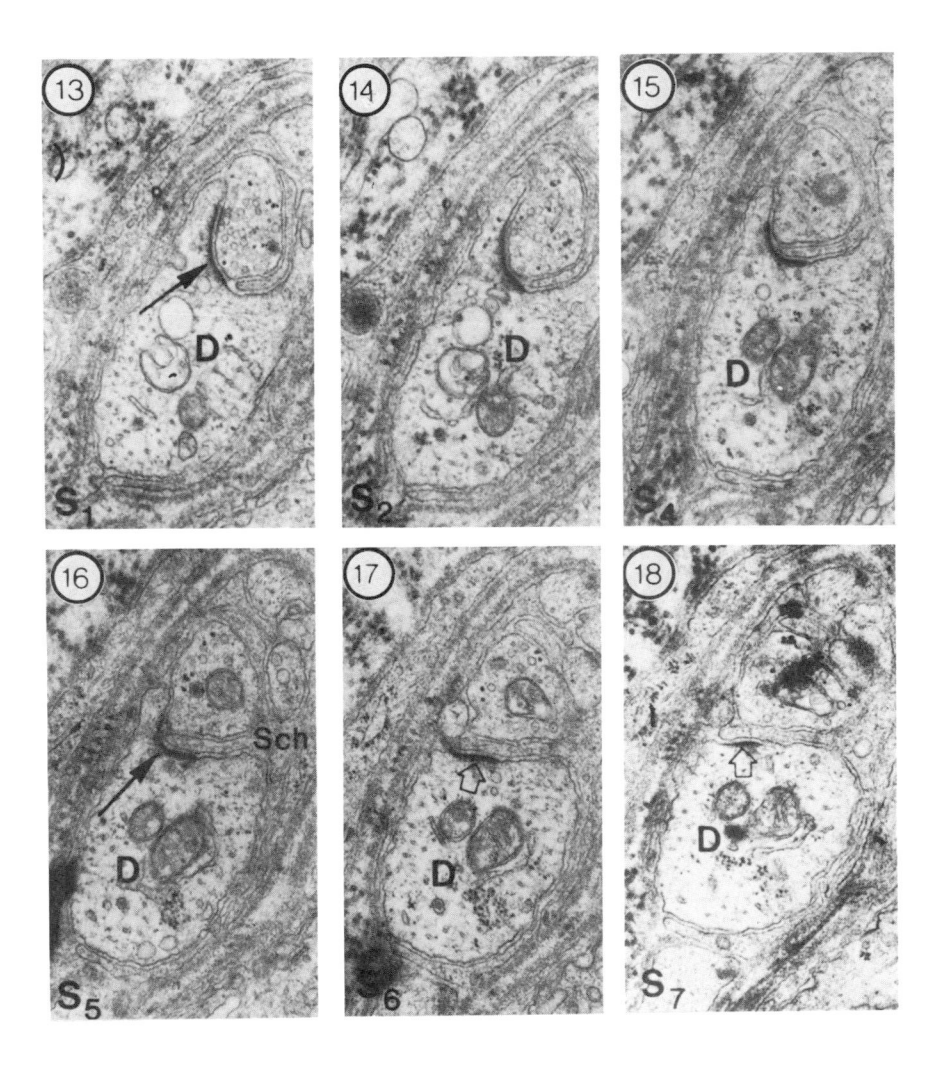

Figures 13-18. Serial sections of a synapse from GABA-(3-day) treated SCG. Arrows point at the postsynaptic membrane thickenings. Note the dissociation of postsynaptic thickenings and presynaptic elements. D = dendrites. x 30,000.

insertion of GABA—containing glass bulbs into the SCG, the hypoglossal nerve (N.XII) was gently positioned to a window cut into the capsule at the ventromedial surface of the ganglion. The animals were kept alive for 2–4 months, then morphological, electrophysiological and neurochemical studies were carried out to check if synapse formation had taken place.

Morphological evidence

In experiments in which the implanted N.XII was cut 24 and 48 hours before electron microscopic processing, we were able to detect degenerating nerve fibers and terminals in the SCG, if GABA had been applied as well (Joo et al., 1983; Figs. 19–20). These results suggested that the effect of GABA on double innervation in the SCG could be obtained in the presence of an intact preganglionic nerve.

Electrophysiological evidence

In control animals, which were implanted with glass bulbs containing artificial CSF and hypoglossal nerve, action potentials were recorded from the SCG only after the stimulation of the preganglionic trunk. In contrast, when the hypoglossal nerve was implanted into the GABA—treated SCG, stimulation of both the preganglionic nerve trunk and N.XII induced action potentials indicating that both types of axon had functional synaptic contacts with principal ganglion cells (Fig. 21). Synaptic transmission from both nerves could be blocked by hexamethonium indicating the involvement of cholinergic transmission in both types of synapses (Dames et al., 1985).

Biochemical evidence

Implantation of the hypoglossal nerve during in vivo application of GABA has a pronounced effect on the AChE activity (Kasa et al., 1985). The AChE activity in the untreated SCG is 7.32 ± 1.26 µmol ACh hydrolysed/h/ganglion (100%). In ganglia treated with GABA and implanted with the hypoglossal nerve, the enzyme activity gradually increased to 140% (10.44 ± 1.54 µmol). In contrast to the decrease of AChE in GABA treated ganglia, an analysis of the molecular forms of AChE (4S, 10S, and 16S; Gisiger et al., 1978; Verdiere and Rieger, 1982) revealed that the 16S form increased selectively (+100%, p≤0.01) after nerve implantation.

Summary

Long-term application of GABA to the SCG results in structural, biochemical and electrophysiological changes which indicate that GABA increases the sensitivity for ACh in ganglion cells. By implantation of a foreign cholinergic nerve, double innervated SCG can be produced only in the presence of GABA. This suggests that GABA increases the synaptogenetic capacity of the sympathetic neurons.

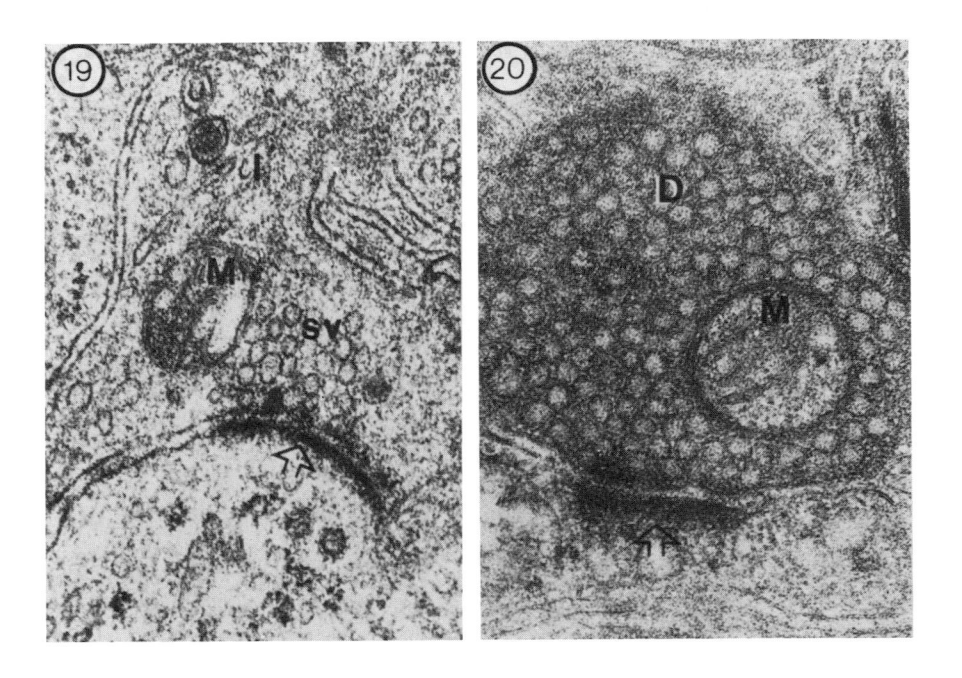

Figures 19-20. Fine structural appearance of synapses from double-innervated SCG, in which the N.XII was cut 24 hours prior to investigation. Fig. 19 = a synapse with normal structure, Fig. 20 = degenerating terminal (D). sv = synaptic vesicles, M = mitochondria, arrows point at the postsynaptic membrane. x 70,000.

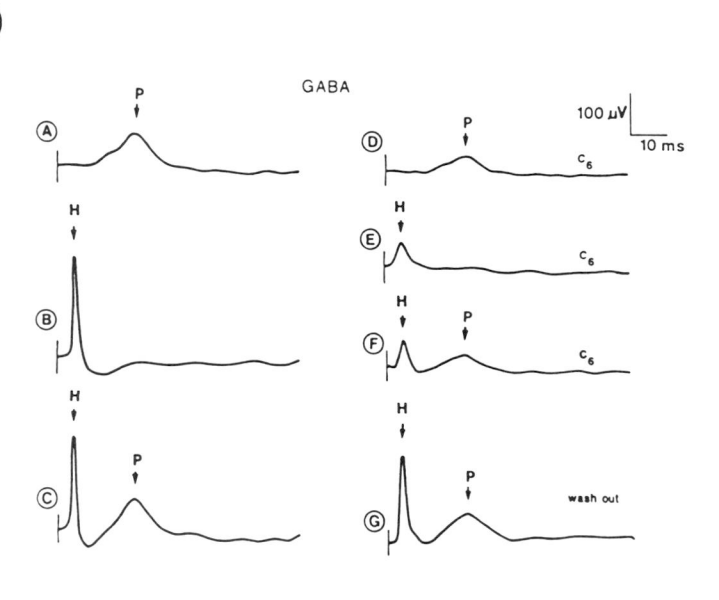

Figure 21. Action potentials, recorded in vivo from a SCG subjected to long-lasting GABA administration 3 months after implantation of the hypoglossal nerve. A : the nerve of preganglionic nerve trunk (P) stimulation. B : the effect of stimulation of the implanted hypoglossal nerve (H). C : the effect of combined P and H stimulation. D : the same experiments as A after 10 min superfusion with 1 mg/ml hexamethonium bromide (C_6). E : the same as B after C_6. F : the same as C after C_6. G : the same as F, after 15 min washing with artificial CSF. Both action potentials were reversibly sensitive to C_6, indicating new cholinergic synapses established between axons of the hypoglossal nerve and principle sympathetic neurons. Negativity upwards. (From Dames et al., 1985).

MEDIATION OF GABA EFFECTS

Second messengers

Since cyclic AMP is believed to play a role in synaptic transmission in the SCG (Libet, 1970; Greengard and Kebabian, 1974), there is much interest in understanding the control of cyclic AMP levels in this tissue. A number of neurotransmitters and hormones, including catecholamines, histamine, vasoactive intestinal peptide and prostaglandins E_1 and E_2 have been reported to raise AMP levels in the SCG of the rat (Cramer et al., 1973; Lindl and Cramer, 1974; Brown et al., 1979; Lindl, 1979; Quenzer et al., 1979; Volle and Patterson, 1982; Trevisani et al., 1982). These substances are thought to act by stimulating a receptor-linked adenylate cyclase, which has been characterized biochemically by Cahill and Perlman (1983). It was demonstrated by Ariano et al. (1982) that cGMP was localized almost exclusively in the cytoplasm of sympathetic neurons, while cAMP was confined mainly to the satellite cells. The contents of both cyclic nucleotides increased after stimulation of the preganglionic nerve trunk.

In contrast, GABA significantly increased the concentration of cAMP in a dose-dependent manner but did not influence the level of cGMP (unpublished results). SCG incubated in the presence of 10^{-4} M GABA yielded 23.0 ± 1.2 pmol cAMP/mg protein during 10 minutes, while the control value was 11.1 ± 0.4 pmol cAMP/mg protein. A GABA concentration of 10^{-6} M still activated the adenylate cyclase in the SCG and resulted in an increase of the cAMP production (20.2 ± 0.3); whereas 10^{-8} M GABA was much less effective (12.1 ± 0.9). The activation of the cAMP-generating system seems to be specific, because we did not find any detectable change in the cGMP level of SCG. Supposedly, GABA increases preferentially the cAMP production in the satellite cells (Ariano et al., 1982), and one can speculate about further consequences. Cyclic AMP derivatives have been shown to induce the synthesis of galactocerebroside, a lipid found in myelin, in Schwann cell cultures (Sobue and Pleasure, 1984). In addition, elevation of the intracellular concentrations of cAMP was shown to induce multiple process formation in rat C6 glioma cells (Edstrom et al., 1974; Oey, 1975). Thus, it is possible that the elevation by GABA of the cAMP content

in satellite cells interferes in some way with the
metabolic coupling between neuronal and glial cells and
ultimately may be involved in the induction by GABA of the
morphogenetic effects in neurons.

It remains to be determined whether the effect of GABA
on the cAMP production in the SCG is mediated through
specific GABA receptors on glia cells or neurons and, in
the latter case, even includes other transmitter systems
in the SCG. It is well-documented that exogenous GABA
induces a release of noradrenaline and probably through
this mechanism increases the level of cAMP in cerebral
cortex slices (Caciagli et al., 1984). On the other hand,
the $GABA_B$ receptor is negatively coupled to adenylate
cyclase, i.e., baclofen and GABA inhibit basal adenylate
cyclase activity in various brain areas (Wojcik and Neff,
1984). From these studies, it is conceivable that GABA
mediated by other transmitters and/or second messenger
molecules induces specific metabolic responses (e.g., the
formation of nAChR) and molecular interactions (e.g.,
protein phosphorylation) which are involved in the
regulation of synaptogenetic capacity. Further studies
are warranted along this line to elucidate the molecular
basis of metabolic and morphogenetic GABA effects.

Nerve growth factor

Nerve growth factor (NGF) is a multimeric protein that
modulates the differentiation of several neuronal cell
types in vivo and in vitro (Levi-Montalcini and Angeletti,
1968). In the rat pheochromocytoma cell line PC12, NGF
acts via a specific receptor and induces a series of
alterations that include neurite growth, modification of
cytoskeleton and changes in neurotransmitter synthesis, as
well as the induction of ornithine decarboxylase.
Interestingly, certain types of peripheral benzodiazepines
can interact with NGF to modify its action both on neurite
outgrowth and induction of ornithine decarboxylase (Morgan
et al., 1985). In addition, a specific stimulation of
c-fos messenger RNA by NGF could be increased more than
100-fold in the presence of diazepines (Curran and Morgan,
1985). These findings clearly point to a relation between
NGF and the GABA-system; an important feature that
certainly deserves further attention.

Summary

GABA seems to affect the metabolism of sympathetic neurons by interfering with secondary messenger systems and possibly with NGF. The molecular basis of this effect and its relation to morphogenetic changes seen after long term application of GABA are still unknown.

SIMULATIONS OF GABA EFFECTS BY SODIUM BROMIDE

Riker and Montoya (1978) reported that, like GABA, sodium bromide (NaBr) produces stable hyperpolarization in sympathetic ganglion cells of frogs. In a series of experiments, we studied the possibility that plastic changes, similar to that observed after GABA treatment, could be achieved by the application of NaBr.

Structural plasticity

In these experiments, the glass bulbs, used to deliver GABA or artifical CSF into the SCG (Dames et al., 1979), were filled up with NaBr (10 µl of 500 mM solution) and ethanol (0.2%) in distilled water (Joo et al., 1979). Under these conditions, free postsynaptic-like densities formed on dendrites of principle ganglion cells were frequently observed and microvesiculation was also apparent in the dendritic cytoplasm (Figs. 22-24).

Physiological plasticity

Rats were given 140 and 180 mg NaBr or NaCl (controls) in the drinking water for two weeks. Then, either the hypoglossal or the vagal nerve was implanted into the SCG, while the preganglionic nerve supply remained intact. Then, the animals received either NaBr or NaCl in the drinking water for further 1-4 months. In electrophysiological experiments, stimulation of the implanted foreign nerve was able to evoke action potentials only in animals which drank NaBr-containing water but not in controls (Fig. 25, Toldi et al., 1986).

Summary

Sodium bromide can mimic the effects of GABA on the morphology of ganglion cells and the increase in synaptogenetic capacity in the rat's SCG. These results indicate that these effects may not be specific for GABA but depend on its inhibitory effect on the ganglionic

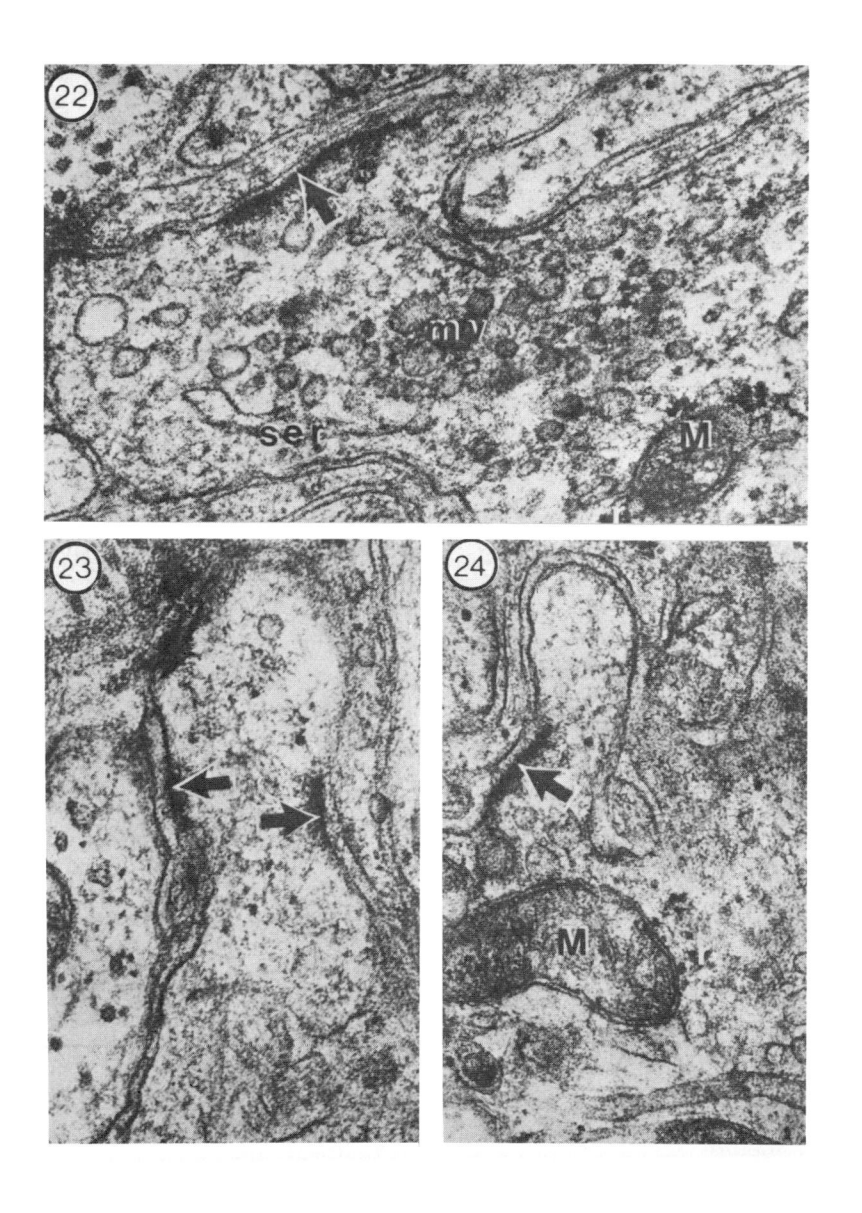

transmission which is induced by both substances.

CONCLUSIONS

I. The rat's SCG is the first case in the peripheral
    nervous system in which GABA fulfils most criteria of
    an inhibitory transmitter:

    - Endogenous GABA, synthesized probably by
      glutamate-decarboxylase, is predominantly located
      in a subset of GABAergic interneurons.
    - Release of GABA can be stimulated by depolarizing
      agents. Release sites may be vesicle-containing
      axon varicosities and glial cells.
    - $GABA_A$ and $GABA_B$ receptors, both are present on
      presynaptic and postsynaptic elements.
    - GABA inhibits the ganglionic transmission. This
      may include two effects: presynaptic inhibition of
      ACh release and postsynaptic inhibition.
    - GABA accumulation in glial cells rapidly removes
      GABA from the extracellular space and, therefore,
      may prevent receptor desensitization.

II. Long-term application of GABA induces a complex
    neuroplastic response which includes biochemical,
    metabolic and morphological changes of principle
    ganglion cells and ultimately increases their
    capacity to accept acetylcholinergic synapses.

    - GABA increases the sensitivity of ganglion cells
      for ACh (nAChR↑, AChE↓). These changes are
      similar, but not identical (e.g., mAChR not
      changed) to those induced by partial
      de-afferentation. Both conditions increase the
      number of free postsynaptic thickenings.
    - GABA increases the content of cyclic AMP (mainly
      glial) but not of cyclic GMP in the SCG. This
      suggests that GABA accumulating glial cells may be
      involved not only by preventing the desensitiza-

Figures 22-24. Non-innervated, F-POST on dendritic
surfaces of the principal ganglion cells after
implantation of glass bulbs with NaBr. M = mitochondria,
mv = microvesicles, ser = smooth endoplasmic reticulum. x
70,000.

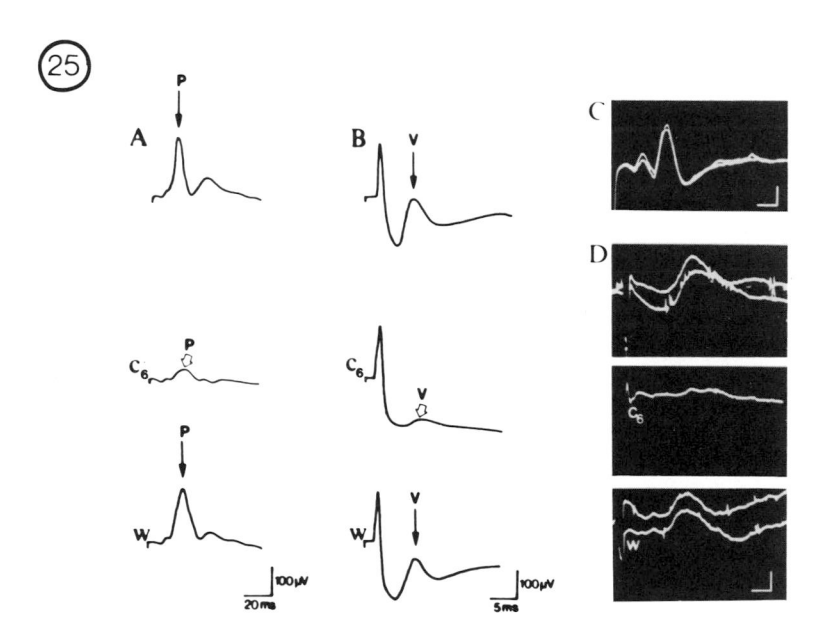

Figure 25. Action potentials recorded in vivo from the SCG of an animal which drunk NaBr-containing tap water (280 mg/ml) over a period of 3 months. A : action potentials (P) evoked by preganglionic nerve stimulation and recorded from the rostral pole of the SCG. C_6 : the effect of the same stimulus after 8-min hexamethonium infusion and after washing (W) : the same as A, with stimulation of the vagus nerve. The open arrow points to the C_6-sensitive component. C : pre-ganglionically evoked potentials photographed from the screen. Calibrations : 10 ms, 100 µV. D : the effect of stimulation of the implanted N.X. The potentials were blocked with C_6 for 8 min, and recovered after 10 min washing (W). Calibrations: 2 ms, 100 µV. Negativity upwards. (From Toldi et al., 1986).

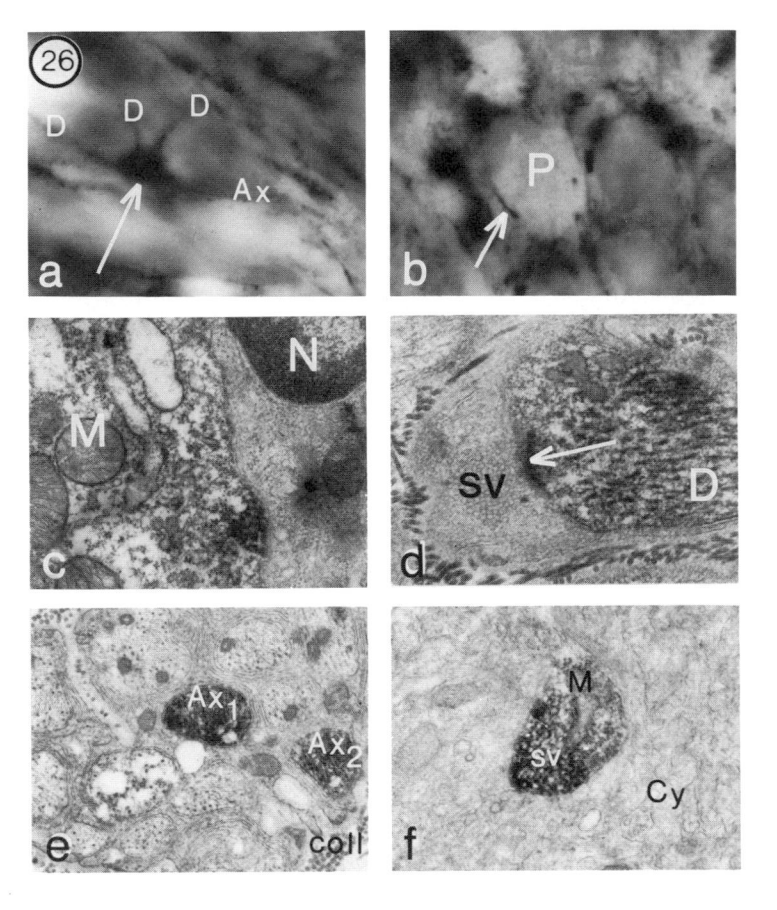

Figure 26. GABA-immunoreactivity in rat SCG. a: GABA-positive multipolar neuron (arrow) with dendrites (D) and probable axon section (Ax); x 750. b: GABA-positive structures surrounding a principle ganglion cell; x 750. c: Immunoreactive dendrite with mitochondria (M); glial nucleus (N); x 20,000. d: GABA-positive dendrite (D) making an asymmetric synapse with a non-reactive (pre-ganglionic) axon terminal containing spherical, clear vesicles (SV); x 20,000. e: Axon bundle contains reactive and non-reactive axons; collagen (coll); x 10,000. f: GABA-positive varicosity with synaptic vesicles (SV) and a mitochondrion (M). The terminal is apposed to a neuron (cy) without intervention of glial processes; x 30,000. (Modified from Wolff et al., 1986).

tion of GABA receptors.

- GABA induces several types of morphological changes in ganglionic neurons. The appearance of presynaptic-like vesicle aggregations in dendrites may indicate the induction of dendritic release of noradrenaline, i.e., the involvement of other transmitters.
- Sodium bromide mimics the neuroplastic response to GABA in the SCG. The molecular basis of this effect is unknown and, therefore, deserves further attention. Since both, GABA and NaBr, inhibit the ganglionic transmission a common effector system may be postulated.

- It is probable but has still to be proved that the endogenous GABA exerts a permanent influence on the biochemical, metabolic and morphological state of the SCG including its synaptology. If endogenous GABA would increase the "acceptance" of afferent excitatory synapses (some vacant postsynaptic densities also exist, in the normal SCG; Raisman et al., 1974; Wolff et al., 1979), then this modulator could be involved in stabilizing afferent synapses against long-term variations of afferent activity and/or in regulating the specific distribution of afferent synapses on subpopulations of sympathetic ganglion cells.

Thus, evidence is accumulating that GABA is not only a transmitter of synaptic inhibition in the central and peripheral nervous system but also serves trophic functions (see also Wolff et al., 1978). Much further work is needed to elucidate their action mechanism and the physiological role of trophic transmitter functions during ontogenesis and in the maintenance of the adult nervous system.

ACKNOWLEDGEMENTS

The authors are grateful to all co-workers, who participated in these studies. The research was carried out in the frame of an international collaboration and was supported by the Deutsche Forsungsgemeinschaft (Grants Wo 279/6-1(9) and 8-1); by the Hungarian Academy of Sciences and by the Scientific Council, Ministry of Health, Hungary

(06/4-20/457).

REFERENCES

Adams PR, Brown DA (1975). Actions of γ-Aminobutyric acid on sympathetic ganglion cells. J Physiol 250: 85-120.

Araujo DM, Collier B (1986). Evidence that endogenous catecholamines can regulate acetylcholine release in a sympathetic ganglion. Eur J Pharmac 125: 93-101.

Ariano MA, Briggs CA, McAfee DA (1982). Cellular localization of cyclic nucleotide changes in rat superior cervical ganglion. Cell Molec Neurobiol 2: 143-156.

Bertilsson L, Suria A, Costa E (1976). γ-Aminobutyric acid in rat superior cervical ganglion. Nature 260: 540-541.

Bill A, Linder J (1976). Sympathetic control of cerebral blood flow in acute arterial hypertension. Acta Physiol Scand 96: 114-121.

Birks RI, MacIntosh FC (1961). Acetylcholine metabolism of a sympathetic ganglion. Can J Biochem Physiol 39: 787-827.

Bowers CW, Zigmond RE (1979). Localization of neurons in the rat superior cervical ganglion that project into different postganglionic trunks. J Comp Neurol 185: 381-392.

Bowery NG, Brown DA (1972). γ-Aminobutyric acid uptake by sympathetic ganglia. Nature New Biol 238: 89-91.

Bowery NG, Brown DA (1974). Depolarizing actions of γ-aminobutyric acid and related compounds on rat superior cervical ganglia in vitro. Br J Pharmac 50:205-218.

Brown DA, Constantini A (1978). Interaction of pentobarbitone and γ-Aminobutyric acid on mammalian sympathetic ganglion cells. Br J Pharmacol 63:217-224.

Brown DA, Higgins AJ (1979). Presynaptic effects of γ-aminobutyric acid in isolated rat superior cervical ganglia. Br J Pharmac 66: 108P-109P.

Burt DR (1978). Muscarinic receptor binding in rat sympathetic ganglion is unaffected by denervation. Brain Res 143: 573-579.

Bulbring E (1944). The action of adrenaline on transmission in the superior cervical ganglion. J Physiol (London) 103: 55-67.

Caciagli AĪ, Lambertini L, Veratti E, Bianchi C (1984). Effect of γ-Aminobutyric acid on cyclic nucleotide content of guinea-pig cerebral cortex slice. Pharm Res Commun 16: 933-943.

Cahill AL, Perlman RL (1983). Adenylate cyclase activity in the superior cervical ganglion of rat. J Neurochem 41: 882-885.

Capuzzo A, Borasio PG, Fabri E, Ferretti ME, Trevisani A (1983). Alpha-adrenoceptor-mediated inhibition of acetylcholine release in guinea-pig superior cervical ganglion. Neurosci Lett 43: 215-219.

Chiappinelli VA, Dryer SE (1984). Nicotinic transmission in sympathetic ganglia: blockade by the snake venom neurotoxin kappa-bungarotoxin. Neurosci Lett 50:239-244.

Christ DD, Nishi S (1971a). Effect of adrenaline on nerve terminals in the superior cervical ganglion of the rabbit. Br J Pharmac 41:331-338.

Christ DD, Nishi S (1971b). Site of adrenaline blockade in the superior cervical ganglion of the rabbit. J Physiol (London) 213: 107-117.

Cramer H, Johnson DG, Hanbauer I, Silberstein ND, Kopin IJ (1973). Accumulation of adenosine-3',5'-monophosphate induced by catecholamines in the rat superior cervical ganglion in vitro. Brain Res 53: 97-104.

Curran T, Morgan JI (1985). Superinduction of c-fos by nerve growth factor in the presence of peripherally active benzodiazepines. Science 229: 1265-1268.

Dahlstrom A, Booj S, Heiwall P-O, Larsson PA (1980). The effect of chronic nicotine and withdrawal on intraneuronal dynamics of acetylcholine and related enzymes in a preganglionic neuron system of the rat. Acta Physiol Scand 110: 13-20.

Dames W, Joo F, Wolff JR (1979). A method for localized long lasting microapplication of drugs into nervous tissue of freely moving animals. Exp Brain Res 36: 259-264.

Dames W, Joo F, Feher O, Toldi J, Wolff JR (1985). γ-Aminobutyric acid enables synaptogenesis in the intact superior cervical ganglion of the adult rat. Neurosci Lett 54: 159-164.

Dawes PM, Vizi ES (1973). Acetylcholine release from the rabbit isolated superior cervical ganglion preparation. Br J Pharmacol 48: 225-232.

De Groat WC (1970). The actions of γ-Aminobutyric acid and related amino acids on mammalian autonomic ganglia. J Pharm Exp Therap 172: 384-386.

De Groat WC, Lalley PM, Block M (1971). The effect of bicuculline and GABA on the superior cervical ganglion of the cat. Brain Res 25: 665–668.

De Groat WC, Volle RL (1966). The action of the catecholamines on transmission in the superior cervical ganglion of the cat. J Pharmacol Exp Ther 154: 1–13.

Dombrowski AM, Jerkins AA, Kauffman FC (1983). Muscarinic receptor binding and oxidative enzyme activities in the adult rat superior cervical ganglion: effects of 6–hydroxydopamine and nerve growth factor. J Neurosci 3: 1963–1970.

Dun N, Karczmar AG (1977). The presynaptic site of action of norepinephrine in the superior cervical ganglion of guinea pig. J Pharm Exp Therap 200: 328–335.

Dun N, Nishi S, Karczmar AG (1976). Alteration in nicotinic and muscarinic responses of rabbit superior cervical cells after chronic preganglionic denervation. Neuropharmacol 15: 211–218.

Edstrom A, Kanje M, Walum E (1974). Effects of dibutyryl cyclic AMP and prostaglandin E1 on cultured human glioma cells. Exp Cell Res 85: 217–223.

Farkas Z, Balcar VJ, Kasa P, Joo F, Wolff JR (1984). Neuropharmacological evidence for the involvement of GABA receptors in the inhibition of ACh–release from the presynaptic axon terminals in the SCG of rat. In Vizi ES, Magyar K (eds): "Regulation of Transmitter Function: Basic and Clinical Aspect," Akademiai Kiado Budapest, p 87.

Farkas Z, Kasa P, Balcar VJ, Joo F, Wolff JR (1986). Type A and B GABA receptors mediate inhibition of acetylcholine release from cholinergic nerve terminals in the superior cervical ganglion of rat. Neurochem Int 8: 565–572.

Fonnum MF, Maehlen J, Nja A (1984). Functional, structural and chemical correlates of sprouting of intact preganglionic sympathetic axons in the guinea pig. J Physiol (London) 347: 741–749.

Fumagalli L, De Renzis G (1980). α–Bungarotoxin binding sites in the rat superior cervical ganglion are influenced by postganglionic axotomy. Neuroscience 5: 611–616.

George C, Dolivi M (1982). Regulation of acetylcholine synthesis in normal and neurotropic viral infected sympathetic ganglia. Brain Res. 242: 255–260.

Gisiger V, Vigny M, Gautron J, Rieger F (1978). Acetylcholinesterase of rat sympathetic ganglion: molecular forms, localization and effects of denervation. J Neurochem 30: 501–516.

Greengard P, Kebabian JW (1974). Role of cyclic AMP in synaptic transmission in the mammalian peripheral nervous system. Fed Proc 33: 1059-1067.

Hamori J, Somogyi J (1982). Presynaptic dendrites and perikarya in deafferented cerebellar cortex. Proc Natl Acad Sci USA 79: 5093-5096.

Hansen GH, Meier E, Schousboe A (1984). GABA influences the ultrastructure composition of cerebellar granule cells during development in culture. Int J Devl Neurosci 2: 247-257.

Hebb CJ, Waites GMH (1956). Choline acetylase on antero- and retro-grade degeneration of cholinergic nerve. J Physiol (London) 132: 667-671.

Iversen LL, Kelly JS (1975). Uptake and metabolism of γ-Aminobutyric acid by neurons and glial cells. Biochem Pharmacol 24: 933-938.

Jarvi R, Helen P, Pleto-Huikko M, Hervonen A (1986). Neuropeptide Y (NPY)-like immunoreactivity in rat sympathetic neurons and small granule-containing cells. Neurosci Lett 67: 223-227.

Joo F, Dames W, Parducz A, Wolff JR (1983). Axonal sprouts of the hypoglossal nerve implanted in the superior cervical ganglion of adult rats establish synaptic contacts under long-lasting GABA effect. An experimental degeneration study. Acta Biol Hung 34: 177-185.

Joo F, Dames W, Wolff JR (1980). Effect of prolonged sodium bromide administration on the fine structure of dendrites in the superior cervical ganglion of adult rats. In Cuenod M, Kreutzberg GW, Bloom FE (eds): "Development and Chemical Specificity of Neurons," Amsterdam: Elsevier, pp 109-115.

Joo F, Lever JD, Ivens C, Mottram DR, Presley R (1971). A fine structural and electron histochemical study of axon terminals in the rat superior cervical ganglion after acute and chronic preganglionic denervation. J Anat 110: 181-189.

Joo F, Siklos L, Dames W, Wolff JR (1987). Fine structural changes in the superior cervical ganglion of adult rats after long-term administration of GABA: A morphometric analysis. Cell Tiss Res (in press).

Kanazawa L, Iversen LL, Kelly JS (1976). Glutamate decarboxylase activity in the rat posterior pituitary, pineal gland, dorsal root ganglion and superior cervical ganglion. J Neurochem 27: 1267-1269.

Kasa P, Csernovszky E (1967). Electronmicroscopic

localization of acetylcholinesterase in the superior cervical ganglion of the rat. Acta Histochem 28: 274–285.

Kasa P, Dames W, Rakonczay Z, Gulya K, Joo F, Wolff JR (1985). Modulation of the acetylcholine system in the superior cervical ganglion of rat: Effects of GABA and hypoglossal nerve implantation after in vivo GABA treatment. J Neurochem 44: 1363–1372.

Kato E, Kuba K, Koketsu K (1978). Presynaptic inhibition of aminobutyric acid in bullfrog sympathetic ganglion cells. Brain Res 153: 398–402.

Kenny SL, Ariano MA (1986). The immunofluorescence localization of glutamate decarboxylase in the rat superior cervical ganglia. J Autonom Nerv Sys 17:211–215.

Kimura T, Imamura H, Hasimoto K (1977). Facilitatory and inhibitory effects of γ-aminobutyric acid on ganglionic transmission in the sympathetic cardiac nerves of the dog. J Pharm Exp Therap 202: 397–403.

Kobayashi H, Libet B (1970). Actions of noradrenaline and acetylcholine on sympathetic ganglion cells. J Physiol (London) 208: 353–372.

Kwok YN, Collier B (1982). Synthesis of acetylcholine from acetate in a sympathetic ganglion. J Neurochem 39: 16–26.

Levi-Montalcini R, Angeletti PU (1968): Nerve growth factor. Physiol Rev 48: 534–569.

Libet B (1970). Generation of slow inhibitor and excitatory postsynaptic potentials. Fed Proc 29: 1945–1956.

Lindl T (1979). Cyclic AMP and its relation to ganglionic transmission. A combined biochemical and electrophysiological study of the rat superior cervical ganglion in vitro. Neuropharmacol 18: 227–235.

Lindl T, Cramer H (1974). Formation, accumulation, and release of adenosine 3',5'-monophosphate induced by histamine in the superior cervical ganglion of the rat in vitro. Biochim Biophys Acta 343: 182–191.

Montoya GA, Riker W (1982). A study of the actions of bromide on frog sympathetic ganglion. Neuropharmacol 21: 581–582.

Morgan JI, Johnson MD, Wang JKT, Sonnefeld K, Spector S (1985). Peripheral-type benzodiazepines influence ornithine decarboxylase levels and neurite outgrowth in PC12 cells. Proc Natl Acad Sci USA 82: 5223–5226.

Noon JP, McAfee DA, Roth RH (1975). Norepinephrine

release from nerve terminals within the rabbit superior cervical ganglion. Naunyn-Schmiedeb Arch Pharmacol 291: 139-162.

Oey J (1975). Noradrenaline induces morphological alterations in nucleated and enucleated rat C6 glioma cells. Nature 257: 317-319.

Olschowka JA, Jacobowitz DM (1983). The coexistence and release of bovine pancreatic polypeptide-like immunore-activity from noradrenergic superior cervical ganglia neurons. Peptides 4: 231-238.

Paton WDM, Thompson JW (1953). The mechanism of action of adrenaline on the superior cervical ganglion of the cat. XIX Int Congress of Physiol Montreal, Abstract 664.

Purves D, Hadley RD (1985). Changes in the dendritic branching of adult mammalian neurones revealed by repeated imaging in situ. Nature 315: 404-406.

Quenzer L, Yahn D, Alkadhi K, Volle RL (1979). Transmission blockade and stimulation of ganglionic adenylate cyclase by catecholamines. J Pharmacol Exp Therap 208: 31-36.

Raisman G, Field PM, Ostberg AJC, Iversen LL, Zigmond RE (1974). A quantitative ultrastructural and biochemical analysis of the process of re-innervation of the superior cervical ganglion in the adult rat. Brain Res 71: 1-16.

Reinert H (1963). Role and origin of noradrenaline in the superior cervical ganglion. J Physiol (London) 167: 18-29.

Rutledge LT (1978). Effects of cortical denervation and stimulation upon axons, dendrites, and synapses. In Cotman CW (ed): "Neuronal Plasticity", New York: Raven Press, pp 273-289.

Sobue G, Pleasure D (1984). Schwann cell galactocerebro-side induced by derivatives of adenosine 3',5'-mono-phosphate. Science 224: 72-74.

Sotelo C (1977). Formation of presynaptic dendrites in the rat cerebellum following neonatal X-irradiation. Neurosci 2: 275-283.

Starke K (1977). Regulation of noradrenaline release by presynaptic receptor systems. Rev Physiol Biochem Pharmacol 77: 1-124.

Taniguchi T, Karahashi K, Fuiwara M (1983). Alterations in muscarinic cholinergic receptors after preganglionic denervation of the superior cervical ganglion in cats. J Pharmacol Exp Therap 224: 674-678.

Thoenen H, Saner A, Angeletti PU, Levi-Montalcini R

(1972). Increased activity of choline acetyltransferase in sympathetic cervical ganglia after prolonged administration of nerve growth factor. Nature 236: 26-28.

Toldi J, Joo F, Adam G, Feher O, Wolff JR (1983). Inhibition of synaptic transmission in the rat superior cervical ganglion by intracarotid infusion of bungarotoxin. Brain Res 262: 323-327.

Toldi J, Farkas Z, Feher O, Dames W, Kasa P, Gyurkovits K, Joo F, Wolff JR (1986). Promotion by sodium bromide of functional synapse formation from foreign nerves in the superior cervical ganglion of adult rat with intact preganglionic nerve supply. Neurosci Lett 69: 19-24.

Trevisani A, Biondi C, Belluzzi O, Borasio PG, Capuzzo A, Ferretti ME, Perri V (1982). Evidence for increased prostaglandin of E-type in response to orthodromic stimulation in the guinea pig superior cervical ganglion. Brain Res 236: 375-381.

Van Huizen F (1986). Significance of bioelectric activity for synaptic network formation. A quantitative electron microscopic study on rat cerebral cortex cultures. Thesis University of Amsterdam, 134 p.

Verhofstadt AAJ, Steinbusch HWM, Penke B, Varga J, Joosten HWJ (1981). Serotonin-immunoreactive cells in the superior cervical ganglion of the rat. Evidence for the existence of separate serotonic- and catecholamine containing small ganglionic cells. Brain Res. 212: 39-49.

Verdiere M, Rieger DM (1982). Multiple molecular forms of rat superior cervical ganglion acetylcholinesterase: developmental aspects in primary cell culture and during postnatal maturation in vivo. Dev Biol 89: 509-515.

Vizi ES (1979). Presynaptic modulation of neurochemical transmission. Prog Neurobiol 12: 181-290.

izi ES (1983). Release-modulating adrenoceptors: In Kunos G (ed): "Adrenoceptors and Catecholamine Action," Part B. Vol I, New York: John Wiley and Sons, p 65.

Volle RL, Patterson BA (1982). Regulation of cyclic AMP accumulation in rat sympathetic ganglion: Effects of vasoactive intestinal peptide. J Neurochem 39: 1195-1197.

Wojcik WJ, Neff NH (1984). γ-Aminobutyric acid B receptors are negatively coupled to adenylate cyclase in brain, and in the cerebellum these receptors may be associated with granule cells. Molec Pharmacol 25: 24-28.

Wolff JR, Joo F, Dames W (1978). Plasticity in dendrites shown by continuous GABA administration in superior cervical ganglion of adult rat. Nature 274: 72–74.

Wolff JR, Joo F, Dames W, Feher O (1979). Induction and maintenance of free postsynaptic membrane thickenings in the adult superior cervical ganglion. J Neurocytol 8: 549–563.

Wolff JR, Joo F, Kasa P, Storm-Mathisen J, Toldi J, Balcar VJ (1986). Presence of neurons with GABA-like immunoreactivity in the superior cervical ganglion of the rat. Neurosci Lett 71: 157–162.

Neurotrophic Activity of GABA During Development, pages 253–266
© **1987 Alan R. Liss, Inc.**

FACILITATION AND INHIBITION OF NEURITE ELONGATION BY
GABA IN CHICK TECTAL NEURONS

A. Michler-Stuke and J.R. Wolff

Department of Anatomy, Developmental
Neurobiology Unit, University of Gottingen,
3400 Gottingen, FRG

INTRODUCTION

During recent years a great number of studies has
established the role of γ-aminobutyric acid (GABA) as an
inhibitory transmitter of the central as well as of the
peripheral nervous system (Roberts et al., 1976). The
action of GABA is mediated by at least two classes of
receptors which are pharmacologically distinct. $GABA_A$
receptors are sensitive to bicuculline, whereas $GABA_B$
receptors do not recognize bicuculline but the drug (-)
baclofen (Hill and Bowery, 1981). Furthermore, they seem
to activate different ion channels. $GABA_A$ receptors are
believed to be associated with a chloride channel
mediating increase in chloride ion permeability (Dunlap,
1984) while $GABA_B$ receptors inhibit voltage-dependent
inward calcium currents (Dolphin and Scott, 1986). Both
are found on central (Bowery et al., 1980) as well as on
peripheral neurons (Dunlap, 1981; Dunlap, 1984).

In addition to its function as an inhibitory
transmitter GABA also seems to play a role in
morphogenesis of neurons. It has been shown in the
superior cervical ganglion of rat that GABA can induce the
formation of free postsynaptic membrane thickenings and
desmosome like contacts in vivo (Wolff et al., 1978; 1979;
1981; see also Wolff et al., in this volume) and in murine
neuroblastoma cells in vitro (Spoerri and Wolff, 1981).
Hansen et al. (1984) demonstrated that GABA stimulated
neurite extension in cerebellar granule cells in cell
culture. At the ultrastructural level, GABA led to an

increase of various cell organelles. The effects were accompanied by the formation of GABA$_A$ receptors being induced by the presence of GABA in the culture medium (Meier et al., 1984). Thus, long lasting GABA applications, like those applied in vivo, and those in a relatively short term range in vitro seem to have numerous and complex effects on neuronal growth and differentiation.

In the present study, the influence of GABA on the morphological development of chick tectal neurons in vitro was investigated at a time just before retinal ganglion cells had innervated the tectum (Rager, 1980). The experiments are performed in serum-supplemented as well as in serum-free, defined medium, since the latter conditions are known to facilitate neuron survival and suppress growth of non-neuronal cells (Barnes and Sato, 1980).

MATERIALS AND METHODS

Cell Culture

Tecta of 6 day embryonic chicken were dissected by carefully removing the meninges and treated with trypsin (0.25% in phosphate buffered saline) for 5 min at 37ºC. After aspiration of the trypsin solution the tissue was washed 3 times with Basal Eagle's Medium (BME) supplemented with 10 fetal calf serum (FCS) to inactivate remaining trypsin. The tissue was suspended in 1 ml fresh BME + 10 FCS and tritiated with a 1 ml Falcon plastic pipette until all tissue fragments were dissociated. Cells were plated in poly-D-lysine (0.05 mg/ml) coated plastic Petri dishes at a density of 5 x 10^5 cells/35 mm dish. Culture media were either BME + 10 FCS or serum-free, defined N2 medium (Bottenstein and Sato, 1979) consisting of BME and the following supplements: transferrin, 100 µg/ml; sodium selenite, 30 nM; putrescine, 100 µM; insulin, 5 µg/ml and progesterone 20 nM. GABA at various concentrations was added 24h after plating of cells, since its initial presence seemed to be inhibitory to plating efficiency and cell growth. In contrast, NGF, potassium or calcium ions were added immediately at the time of plating. After 3 days cultures were fixed with glutaraldehyde and analysed for neurite growth.

Cell Morphometry

The influence of various medium components on neurite growth was assayed in the following way. Fixed cell cultures were screened in an inverted Zeiss microscope equipped with phase contrast optics and the number of neurites and somata crossing defined lines in the visual field of the microscope was counted (Fig. 1). Cell clumps or processes of cell clumps were discarded. Also individual neurites crossing a line more than once were only counted as one neurite. The numbers were expressed as the quotient N/S (number of neurites N, over number of

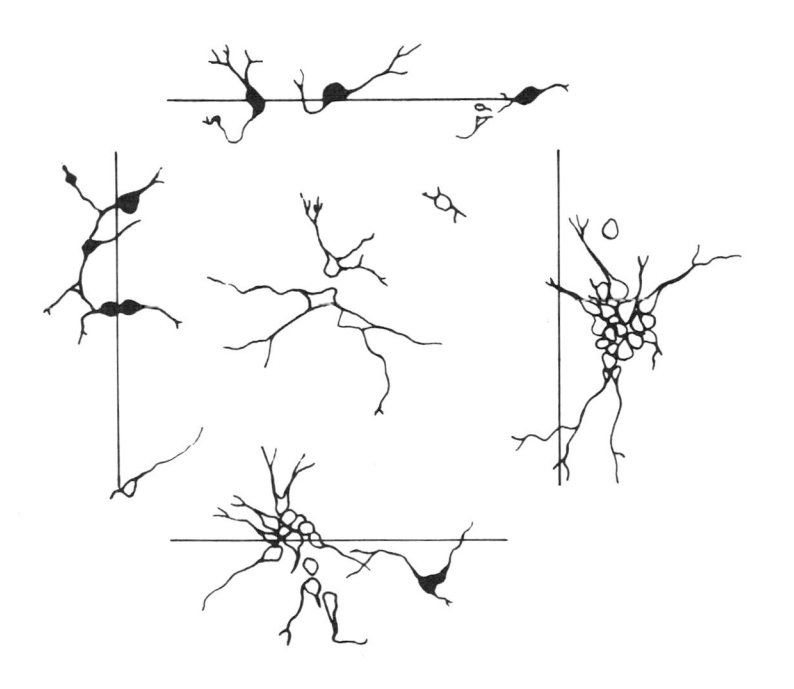

Figure 1. N/S was determined by counting the number of somata and number of neurites crossing 4 test lines in the visual field of an inverted Zeiss microscope. Cells which were counted in a situation illustrated above are marked in black. Cell clumps (white cells) and neurites of these clumps were discarded. Cell clumps consisting of 5 or less cells were regarded as single cells.

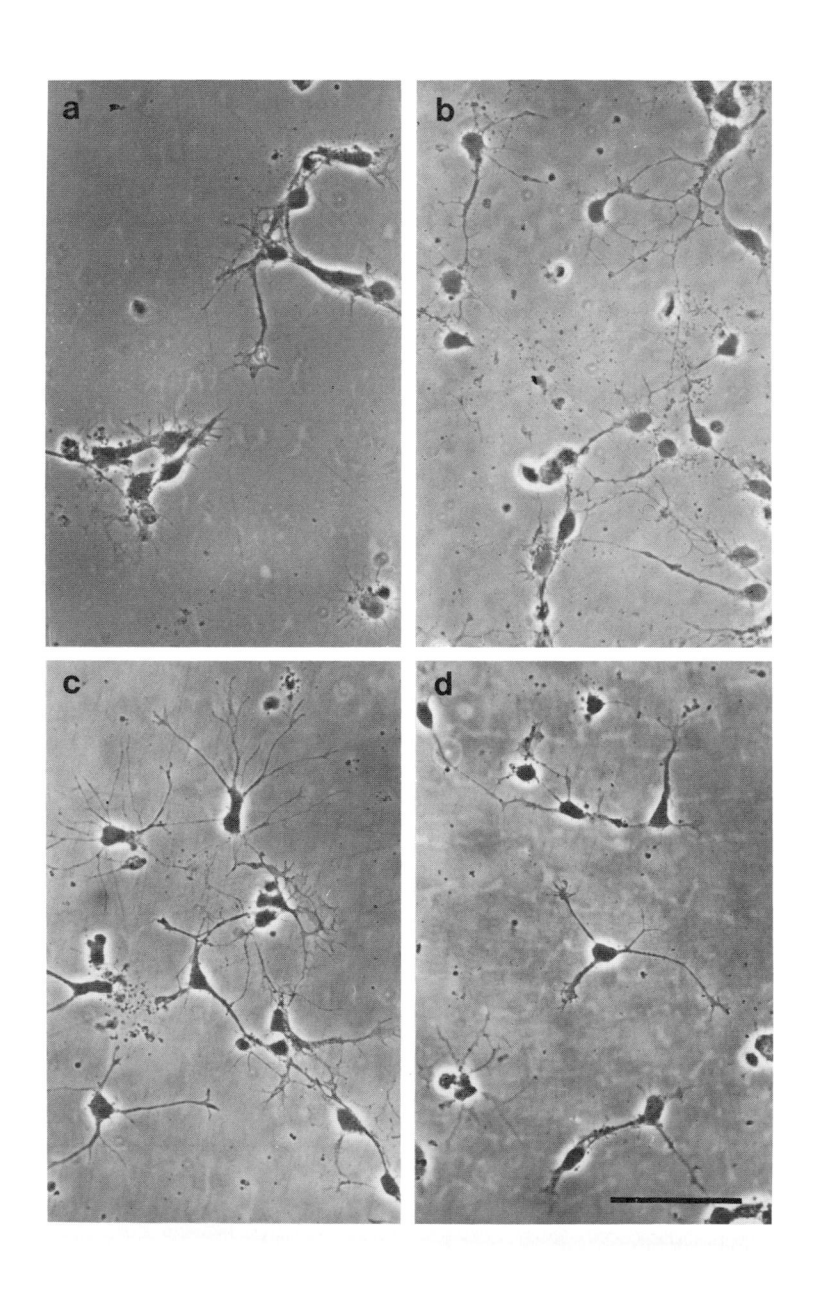

somata S), hit by the lines. In each culture dish 5 randomly chosen fields were evaluated and experiments done in triplicate were repeated twice.

RESULTS

Tectal cells, which were grown in serum-supplemented medium developed into a cell population mainly existing of phase bright neuronal cell bodies with short more or less unbranched processes (Fig. 2 a). Most of these processes reached a length not exceeding one cell diameter. In the presence of GABA, neurite outgrowth was markedly stimulated, and both neurite length and number of processes per cell were increased (Fig. 2b). Counting the number of neurites and somata crossing defined lines in the visual field of the microscope revealed that extremely high concentrations of GABA (10^{-3}M) increased N/S by a factor of about two as compared to controls which had not received a GABA treatment (Table 1). Lower concentrations of GABA (10^{-3}M, 10^{-8}M) also proved to be stimulatory on neurite outgrowth.

In serum-free N2 medium the morphology of tectal cells was quite different. As in serum-supplemented medium, a fairly uniform cell population comprised primarily of neuronal cells was present. But in contrast to the situation described above neuronal cells grew numerous, long, and branched processes (Fig. 2c). Although exact numbers were not counted it was obvious that the plating efficiency was higher in cultures grown in N2 medium. When GABA was added to those cultures a quite unexpected result was obtained. In the presence of this substance, neurite outgrowth was suppressed, resulting in a less dense network of processes (Fig. 2d). These observations were confirmed by counting the number of neurites and somata crossing the test lines. The data revealed that the quotient N/S was increased by a factor of about 4 when cells were grown in N2 medium as compared to serum-supplemented cultures. When GABA at a concentration

Figure 2. Phase contrast micrographs of tectal neurons after 3 days in vitro. Cells were grown in a) BME + 10% FCS, b) BME + 10% FCS and 10^{-3}M GABA added one day after plating, c) N2 medium or d) N2 medium and 10^{-3}M GABA added one day after plating. Bar represents 50 μm.

of 10^{-3}M was added to N2 medium, the number of neurites versus number of somata was reduced to half of that reached in N2 medium alone (Table 1). The inhibitory effect of GABA in N2 medium was dose dependent (Fig. 3) with higher (10^{-3}M) concentrations of GABA suppressing neurite growth more than lower (10^{-8}M) ones.

Effect of NGF

The reason for the opposite action of GABA in the two media was not quite clear. Since fetal calf serum contains low concentrations of NGF the obtained effects may be due to the presence of NGF in the serum-supplemented medium. Therefore, NGF was added to N2 medium at a concentration of 20 ng/ml, which is sufficient to stimulate neurite growth in sensory and sympathetic neurons. NGF alone had no significant effect on neurite growth of tectal cells. However, when GABA was present in combination with NGF the inhibitory influence of GABA was abolished (Table 2). Neurite extension was not significantly suppressed, not even at high (10^{-3}M)

Table 1

Effect of various GABA concentrations on neurite elongation in serum-supplemented and serum-free, defined medium.

concentration of GABA	culture medium	
	BME + 10% FCS	N2 medium
none (control)	0.97 + 0.2	3.74 + 0.4
10^{-3}M	1.86 + 0.3 *	2.07 + 0.6*
10^{-5}M	1.57 + 0.1 *	2.57 + 0.5
10^{-8}M	1.47 + 0.1 *	2.72 + 0.5*

Values are expressed as the quotient N/S of number of neurites versus number of somata crossing defined lines in the visual field (see Methods) + S.D. of quadruplicate cultures. Asterisks indicate statistically significant differences from control cultures ($p<0.01$, t-test).

concentrations of GABA.

Effect of elevated K$^+$ ion concentration

Raising the potassium ion concentration of the medium is known to stimulate neurite extension in neurons of the peripheral nervous system. When potassium was present in N2 medium at a concentration of 24.5 mM, the quotient N/S was also raised substantially compared to control N2

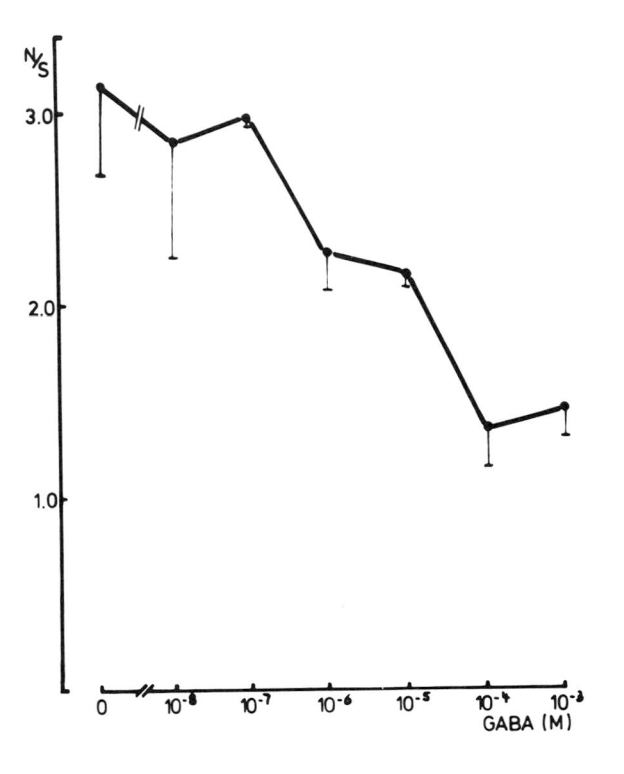

Figure 3. Dose dependent growth of neurites from chick tectal neurons in N2 medium in the presence of different GABA concentrations. For measurement of N/S values see MATERIAL AND METHODS-section.

medium (Table 2) having a standard potassium ion concentration of 5.5 mM. Addition of GABA at a concentration of 10^{-3}M to N2 medium containing high K^+ resulted in a slight decrease of N/S which was, however, not smaller than control values. With lower concentrations of GABA (10^{-5}M and 10^{-8}M) the same N/S values were obtained as with a raised potassium ion concentration alone.

Effect of elevated Ca^{++} ion concentration

The increase in N/S turned out to be even more pronounced when the calcium ion concentration was raised from 12.6 mM being standard BME concentration to 1.36 mM (Table 2). When GABA was added to high Ca^{++} medium at a concentration of 10^{-5}M, a further increase in number of neurites versus number of somata was obtained. Yet, high

Table 2
Influence of NGF, K^+ and Ca^{2+} on neurite elongation of cells grown in N2 medium.

concentration of GABA	NGF (20 ng/ml)	K^+ (24.5 mM)	Ca^{2+} (1.36 mM)
none	2.61 + 0.6	2.68 + 0.3 *	4.10 + 0.4*
10^{-3}M	2.23 + 0.2	2.20 + 0.3	−
10^{-5}M	2.27 + 0.2	2.65 + 0.3 *	4.31 + 0.5*
10^{-8}M	2.39 + 0.4	2.72 + 0.5 *	−
N2 medium without any additives	2.35 + 0.4	2.01 + 0.4	3.02 + 0.6

Values are expressed as quotient N/S of number of neurites versus number of somata crossing defined lines in the visual field + S.D. of quadruplicate cultures. Asterisks indicate statistically significant differences from cultures grown in N2 medium without any additives (p<0.01; t-test).

Ca^{++} (2 mM) in the medium proved to be deleterious. This was the only culture condition, where like in serum–supplemented medium a positive effect was induced upon addition of GABA.

DISCUSSION

The experiments described in the present report revealed that depending on the environment – serum supplemented versus serum-free, defined medium – GABA influenced neurite elongation of tectal neurons in different directions. The growth stimulating effect obtained in serum–containing medium is consistent with results reported by Hansen et al. (1984) using serum–supplemented medium in cultures of rat cerebellar granule cells. According to these authors, GABA also increased the density of rough endoplasmic reticulum and stimulated the development of Golgi–apparatus and coated vesicles in granule cells.

These structures are known to be involved in protein synthesis and incorporation of material into the outer cell membrane (Hammerschlag et al., 1982; Hammerschlag and Stone, 1983). Since GABA is also believed to play a role in the regulation of protein synthesis in brain (Snodgrass, 1973; Tapia and Sandoval, 1974), it is possible that GABA can also stimulate neurite elongation by influencing those cytological phenomena. However, the opposite effects of GABA observed in N2 medium cannot be explained by this mechanism.

Neuroblastoma cells quite frequently extend more neurites when grown in N2 medium (Bottenstein et al., 1979) as compared to their serum–supplemented counterparts. Similar observations were made in cultures of tectal neurons described in the present paper. In N2 medium the number of neurites versus number of somata was about 4 times higher than in serum–grown cultures. However, we are not aware of any studies indicating, that under these otherwise stimulating conditions, GABA suppresses protein synthesis and thereby neurite extension.

One among several hypotheses may be, that GABA in combination with supplements of the medium is affecting certain ion channels or internal ion levels which in turn stimulate or inhibit neurite growth. Such a regulative function could be mediated by a different set of GABA receptors expressed on tectal cells depending on the environment. Meier et al. (1984) showed that GABA can induce the formation of low-affinity binding sites in cultures of cerebellar granule cells, which have the pharmacological properties of GABA$_A$ receptors. These experiments were done in medium supplemented with serum. Supposing that in serum-free, defined medium GABA induces the formation of GABA$_B$ receptors on tectal cells, this might explain the contradictory results obtained in our experiments. Since the two receptor types are associated with different ion channels, neurite growth might be regulated by activation or inactivation of these channels. Neurite extension could thereby be maintained at a distinct level.

One of the substances possibly involved in such an interaction with GABA may be NGF. It is known to be present in fetal calf serum in low concentrations. A relation between NGF and peripherally active benzodiazepines has recently been described by Curran and Morgan (1985). In the presence of NGF the proto-oncogene c-fos is induced in PC 12 cells and its level is further increased by concomitant presence of certain benzodiazepines in the medium. This proto-oncogene seems to be associated with differentiated cells which have reduced proliferative capacities (Muller et al., 1985). Another kind of interaction between NGF and certain benzodiazepines involves the induction of ornithine decarboxylase and neurite outgrowth in PC 12 cells (Morgan et al., 1985).

The results obtained in tectal neurons after addition of NGF and GABA to N2 medium suggest, that some interaction may occur between these two substances, since the inhibitory effect of GABA is no longer observed in the presence of NGF. However, since no clear stimulatory effect on neurite growth was seen, other mechanisms must still be considered.

Raising the potassium ion concentration in the culture medium is known to stimulate neurite outgrowth in various types of neuronal cells (Chalazonitis and Fischbach, 1980; Nishi and Berg, 1981; Traynor, 1984). Elevated potassium levels can also induce c-fos (Morgan and Curran, 1986). When the potassium ion concentration was raised in N2 medium a stimulation of neurite growth was observed in tectal cells. Further addition of GABA resulted in a slight decrease of the N/S value which was, however, not smaller than control values. Since lower doses of GABA appeared to be less inhibitory, as it was observed in N2 medium without any other additives, an interaction of potassium ions or potassium channels with GABA seems to be equivocal. Thus, the inhibitory effect of GABA may simply be counterbalanced by the stimulatory effect of K^+ on neurite growth.

The stimulatory effect of Ca^{2+} in N2 medium may give some clues as to what the underlying mechanisms could be. There are a number of reports which state the important role of calcium with respect to neurite extension (Schubert et al., 1978; Anglister et al., 1982; Freeman et al., 1985). Evidence is provided by these authors that inward Ca^{2+} currents are involved in neurite elongation (Anglister et al., 1982; Freeman et al., 1985) and also can increase cell adhesion presumably by mobilizing intracellular Ca^{2+} pools (Schubert et al., 1978). If in N2 medium in the presence of GABA, Ca^{++} channels were affected and thus inward Ca^{++} currents were reduced the inhibitory effect of GABA could be explained.

With regard to the experiments described above a model is proposed in which the expression of $GABA_A$ and $GABA_B$ receptors on tectal cells may be differentially influenced by the environment the cells are grown in. It is likely that $GABA_B$ receptors – like $GABA_A$ receptors which are formed on granule cells in the presence of GABA – are induced on tectal cells in response to the presence or absence of certain media components. Binding of GABA to these receptors could then have changed the permeability of a Ca^{++}-channel and thereby influenced neurite extension.

Further experiments are in progress in order to define the receptor populations and to test whether or not an "imprinting mechanism" is involved and whether a critical period during development can be defined.

SUMMARY

The influence of γ-aminobutyric acid (GABA) on neurite extension was investigated in dissociated tectal neurons of embryonic chicken. Applying GABA to serum-supplemented and serum-free, defined medium rendered apparently conflicting data with regard to the effect of this substance on neurite growth in vitro. While GABA was stimulating neurite elongation in the presence of serum it was inhibitory when serum-free, defined medium was used.

A set of experiments was designed to get hints what mechanisms are responsible for this discrepancy. This involved tests attempting to define the role of NGF, potassium, and calcium in this context.

It is concluded that the effects of GABA on neuronal morphogenesis may depend on the environment the cells are growing in. A hypothetical mechanism for this phenomenon could be the involvement of a different set of GABA receptors being formed on tectal neurons depending on the circumstances under which they grow and differentiate.

Further experiments will attempt to determine whether a kind of "biochemical imprinting" is involved and whether a critical period can be affected.

ACKNOWLEDGEMENT

Ms. H. Tytko is cordially thanked for her expert technical assistance and Ms. E. Raufeisen for typing the manuscript. This work has been supported financially by grants from the German Service Foundation (DFG-grant Wo 279/6-1) to A.M-S. and J.R.W.

REFERENCES

Anglister L, Farber JC, Shadar A, Grinvald A (1982). Localization of voltage-sensitive calcium channels along developing neurites: Their possible role in regulating neurite elongation. Dev Biol 94: 351-365.
Barnes D, Sato GH (1980). Methods for growth of cultured cells in serum-free medium. Anal Biochem 102: 255-270.
Bottenstein JE, Sato GH (1979). Growth of a rat neuroblastoma cell line in serum-free, supplemented medium. Proc Natl Acad Sci (USA) 16: 514-517.
Bottenstein JE, Sato GH, Mather JP (1979): Growth of neuroepithelial-derived cell lines in serum-free, hormone-supplemented media. In Sato G, Ross R (eds): "Cold Spring Harbor Conferences on Cell Proliferation,"

Vol 6, New York: Cold Spring Harbor Laboratory, pp 531-544.

Bowery NG, Hill DR, Hudson AL, Doble A, Middlemiss DN, Shaw J, Turnball M (1980). (-) Baclofen decreases neurotransmitter release in the mammalian CNS by an action at a novel GABA receptor. Nature (Lond) 283: 92-94.

Chalazonitis A, Fischbach G (1980). Elevated potassium induces morphological differentiation of dorsal root ganglionic neurones in dissociated cell culture. Dev Biol 78: 173.

Curran T, Morgan JI (1985). Superinduction of c-fos by nerve growth factor in the presence of peripherally active benzodiazepines. Science 229: 1265-1268.

Dolphin AC, Scott RH (1986). Inhibition of calcium currents in cultured rat dorsal root ganglion neurones by (-)-baclofen. Br J Pharmacol 88: 213-220.

Dunlap K (1981). Two types of γ-aminobutyric acid receptor on embryonic sensory neurons. Br J Pharmacol 74: 579-585.

Dunlap K (1984). Functional and pharmacological differences between two types of GABA receptor on embryonic chick sensory neurons. Neurosci Lett 47: 265-270.

Freeman JA, Manis PB, Snipes GL, Mayes BN, Samson PC, Wikswo JP, Freeman DB (1985). Steady growth cone currents revealed by a novel circularly vibrating probe. A possible mechanism underlying neurite growth. J Neurosci Res 13: 257-283.

Hammerschlag R, Stone GC, Bolen FA, Lindsey JD, Elisman MH (1982). Evidence that all newly synthesized proteins destined for fast axonal transport pass through the Golgi apparatus. J Cell Biol 93: 568-575.

Hammerschlag R, Stone GC (1983). Golgi and post-Golgi events: prelude to fast axonal transport. J Neurochem 41: Suppl p 68.

Hansen GH, Meier E, Schousboe A (1984). GABA influence the ultrastructure composition of cerebellar granule cells during development in culture. Int J Dev Neurosci 2: 247-257.

Hill DR, Bowery NG (1981). ^{3}H-GABA bind to bicuculline-insensitive GABA$_B$ sites in rat brain. Nature (Lond) 290: 149-152.

Meier E, Drejer J, Schousboe A (1984). GABA induces functionally active low-affinity GABA receptors on cultured cerebellar granule cells. J Neurochem 43:

1737–1744.

Morgan JI, Johnson MD, Wang JKT, Sonnenfeld K, Spector S (1985). Peripheral-type benzodiazepines influence ornithine decarboxylase levels and neurite outgrowth in PC 12 cells. Proc Natl Acad Sci (USA) 82: 5223–5226.

Morgan JI, Curran T (1986). Role of ion flux in the control of c-fos expression. Nature (Lond.) 322: 552–555.

Muller R, Curran T, Muller D, Guilbert L (1985). Induction of c-fos during myelomonocytic differentiation and macrophage proliferation. Nature (Lond.) 314: 546–548.

Nishi R, Berg DK (1981). Effects of high K^+ concentrations on the growth and development of ciliary ganglion neurones in cell culture. Dev Biol 87: 301–307.

Rager HG (1980). Development of the retinotectal projection in the chicken. Adv Anat Embryol Cell Biol 63: 1–92.

Roberts E, Chase TN, Tower DB (1976). "GABA in nervous system function". New York: Raven Press.

Schubert D, La Corbiere M, Whitlock C, Stallcup W (1978). Alterations in the surface properties of cells responsive to nerve growth factor. Nature (Lond.) 273: 718–723.

Snodgrass SR (1973). Studies on GABA and protein synthesis. Brain Res 59: 339–348.

Spoerri PE, Wolff JR (1981). Effect of GABA-administration on murine neuroblastoma cells in the culture. Cell Tiss Res 218: 567–579.

Tapia R, Sandoval ME (1974). Possible participation of γ-aminobutyric acid in the regulation of protein synthesis in brain in vivo. Brain Res 69: 255–263.

Traynor AE (1984). The relationship between neurite extension and phospholipid metabolism in PC 12 cells. Dev Brain Res 9: 369–379.

Wolff JR, Joo F, Dames W (1978). Plasticity in dendrites shown by continuous GABA administration in superior cervical ganglion of adult rat. Nature (Lond.) 274: 72–74.

Wolff JR, Joo F, Dames W, Feher O (1979). Induction and maintenance of free postsynaptic membrane thickenings in the adult superior cervical ganglion. J Neurocytol 8: 549–563.

Wolff JR, Joo F, Dames W, Feher O (1981). Neuroplasticity in the superior cervical ganglion as a consequence of long-lasting inhibition. Adv Physiol Sci 36: 1–9.

Index